Thymus Gland Pathology
Clinical, Diagnostic, and Therapeutic Features

Corrado Lavini • Cesar A. Moran • Uliano Morandi •
Rudolf Schoenhuber (Eds)

Thymus Gland Pathology

Clinical, Diagnostic, and Therapeutic Features

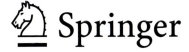

CORRADO LAVINI
Department of General Surgery
and Surgical Specialities
Division of Thoracic Surgery
University of Modena and Reggio Emilia
General Hospital
Modena, Italy

CESAR A. MORAN
Institute of Thoracic Pathology
University of Texas
Anderson Cancer Center
Houston, TX, USA

ULIANO MORANDI
Department of General Surgery
and Surgical Specialities
Division of Thoracic Surgery
University of Modena and Reggio Emilia
General Hospital
Modena, Italy

RUDOLF SCHOENHUBER
Division of Neurology
Bolzano Hospital
Bolzano, Italy

Library of Congress Control Number: 2008927451

ISBN 978-88-470-0827-4 Springer Milan Berlin Heidelberg New York   e-ISBN 978-88-470-0828-1

Springer is a part of Springer Science+Business Media
springer.com
© Springer-Verlag Italia 2008

This work is subject to copyright. All rights are reserved, whether the whole or part of the material is concerned, specifically the rights of translation, reprinting, re-use of illustrations, recitation, broadcasting, reproduction on microfilms or in other ways, and storage in data banks. Duplication of this publication or parts thereof is only permitted under the provisions of the Italian Copyright Law in its current version, and permission for use must always be obtained from Springer. Violations are liable for prosecution under the Italian Copyright Law.

The use of general descriptive names, registered names, trademarks, etc., in this publication does not imply, even in the absence of a specific statement, that such names are exempt from the relevant protective laws and regulations and therefore free for general use.

Product liability: The publisher cannot guarantee the accuracy of any information about dosage and application contained in this book. In every individual case the user must check such information by consulting the relevant literature.

Cover design: Simona Colombo, Milan, Italy
Typesetting: C & G di Cerri e Galassi, Cremona, Italy
Printer: Printer Trento Srl, Trento, Italy

Printed in Italy
Springer-Verlag Italia S.r.l.,Via Decembrio 28, I-20137 Milan

To the memory of my wonderful mother Anne Marie

C. Lavini

To my wife Susan and my daughters Kate Leticia and Elisa Jean

C.A. Moran

To the young surgeons

U. Morandi

To my patients, friends and colleagues from Modena

R. Schoenhuber

Preface

The thymus is a gland that over the last two centuries has generated great awareness not only from the anatomical perspective but also for the physiological and pathological roles it plays in many disease processes. Prior to the early studies on its anatomy and physiology in the 18th century, the thymus was believed to perform unusual and curious functions such as purification of the nervous system, providing a protective cushion for the vasculature of the superior mediastinum, fetal nourishment, or more spiritual roles such as being the seat of the soul, among others. During the 19th century important anatomical/physiological studies took place focusing on the role of the thymus in pathological conditions. However, it was not until the middle of the 19th century that a more comprehensive analysis of the role of the thymic gland and its role in pathogenesis began to emerge.

Currently, while the knowledge gained on the diverse aspects of the thymic gland has furthered our understanding of its role in a gamut of processes, more knowledge is still being sought, and by no means is a full understanding of the gland's physiology and pathology complete. Different aspects, including its purported endocrine function, its association with other autoimmune diseases like multiple sclerosis, rheumatoid arthritis, and lupus erythematosus, among others, are under evaluation and research. In addition, surgical modalities in the treatment of pathological conditions affecting the thymus gland are also under evaluation and scrutiny in order to provide the best methodology. Therefore, our daily practice regarding diseases involving the thymic gland has become a multidisciplinary approach in which experts, including radiologists, neurologists, immunologists, pathologists, oncologists, and surgeons, participate in the evaluation of patients.

Analysis of past and the present developments has afforded us the opportunity to bring you an updated version of the thymic gland – its diagnosis and treatment. This volume encompasses authors from four different continents and attempts to highlight clinical, diagnostic, and therapeutic modalities. New pathological and oncological classifications are carefully presented and discussed; the role of thymopathies with special interest on myasthenia gravis is clearly addressed; and the role of the different diagnostic imaging modalities, including PET and the different surgical techniques, is carefully reviewed. Special emphasis is given to the surgery of the thymus: the different approaches including open conventional, open video-assisted, totally endoscopic, and robotic techniques, and the types of interventions including the complex techniques in superior vena cava syndrome, and the re-interventions. As would be expected, an accurate analysis of the anesthesiological and intensive care problems is also presented. From the oncological point of view, the role of radiation, chemotherapy, and complementary treatments (steroids, octreotide) is highlighted. In the section of myasthenia gravis, the effectiveness of modern therapeutic protocols, the use of multimodal therapy, and the follow-up of patients are carefully discussed. And finally, a chapter dedicated to one of the most recent treatment modalities – thymic transplantation in the setting of some congenital thymic diseases – provides important insight to this text.

In short, we hope that the current text will provide valuable information for those involved in the diagnosis and treatment of patients with thymic pathology, and will add significantly to the understanding of this complex gland.

July 2008

Corrado Lavini
Cesar A. Moran
Uliano Morandi
Rudolf Schoenhuber

Contents

Contributors XIII

CHAPTER 1 **The Thymus from Antiquity to the Present Day: the History of a Mysterious Gland** 1
C. Lavini

CHAPTER 2 **Embriology and Anatomy of the Thymus Gland** 13
C. Palumbo

CHAPTER 3 **Physiology and Immunology of the Thymus Gland** 19
M. Nasi, M. Pinti, L. Troiano, A. Cossarizza

CHAPTER 4 **Congenital Pathology of the Thymus** 31
W. Diehl-Jones, D.F. Askin

CHAPTER 5 **Hyperplastic and Inflammatory Pathology of the Thymus** ... 39
A. Maiorana, L. Reggiani-Bonetti

CHAPTER 6 **Benign and Malignant Tumors** 55
C.A. Moran

CHAPTER 7 **Clinical Features of Thymus Pathology** 69
G. Khaleeq, H.A. Ali, A.I. Musani

CHAPTER 8 **Thymus and Myasthenia Gravis. Pathophysiological and Clinical Features** 89
L. Capone, R. Gentile, R. Schoenhuber

CHAPTER 9 **Radiologic Diagnosis : X-ray, CT and MRI** 99
M. Zanichelli, M. Gozzi, M. Bertolani

CHAPTER 10 **PET Features** 111
B. Bagni, A. Franceschetto, A. Casolo, M. Cucca

CHAPTER 11 **Minimally Invasive and Surgical Diagnosis** 121
C. Ruggiero, C. Lavini, Y. Mehd, D. Paioli, M. Patelli, M. De Santis, A. Affinita

CHAPTER 12 **Surgical Anatomy of the Thymus Gland** 133
J.B. Shrager

CHAPTER 13 **Anesthesiological Problems in Thymus Gland Surgery** 137
V.L. Indrizzi, F. Gazzotti, M.A. Fanigliulo, A. Tassi

CHAPTER 14 **Conventional Techniques: Cervicotomy** 149
P. Borasio, F. Ardissone

CHAPTER 15	**Conventional Techniques: Median Sternotomy**	157
	A. Mussi, M. Lucchi	

CHAPTER 16	**Conventional Techniques: Transthoracic Approach**	161
	U. Morandi, C. Casali	

CHAPTER 17	**Open Videoassisted Techniques: Transcervical Approach**	167
	M. De Perrot, S. Keshavjee	

CHAPTER 18	**Open Videoassisted Techniques: Subxiphoid Approach with Bilateral Thoracoscopy**	173
	C.-P. Hsu, C.-Y. Chuang	

CHAPTER 19	**Open Videoassisted Techniques: Transcervical-Subxiphoid - Videothoracoscopic Maximal Thymectomy**	181
	M. Zieliński, Ł. Hauer, J. Kużdżał, W. Sośnicki, M. Harazda, J. Pankowski, T. Nabiałek, A. Szlubowski	

CHAPTER 20	**Open Videoassisted Techniques: Thoracoscopic Extended Thymectomy with Bilateral Approach and Anterior Chest Wall Lifting**	187
	H. Shiono, M. Ohta, M. Okumura	

CHAPTER 21	**Totally Endoscopic Techniques: Left-Sided Thoracoscopic Thymectomy**	193
	K. Gellert, S. Köther	

CHAPTER 22	**Totally Endoscopic Techniques: Right-Sided Thoracoscopic Thymectomy**	201
	G.M. Wright, C. Keating	

CHAPTER 23	**Robotic Techniques**	207
	F. Rea, G. Marulli	

CHAPTER 24	**Complex Surgical Interventions in Superior Vena Cava Syndrome**	213
	Z.-D. Gu, K.-N. Chen	

CHAPTER 25	**Reinterventions for Thymoma Recurrences**	217
	P. Zannini, G. Negri, M. Casiraghi, L. Ferla, P. Ciriaco	

CHAPTER 26	**Chemotherapy in Thymic Neoplasms**	225
	P.F. Conte, F. Barbieri	

CHAPTER 27	**Radiotherapy in Thymic Neoplasms**	229
	T.Y. Eng, A.Z. Diaz, J.Y. Luh	

CHAPTER 28	**Complementary Treatments in Thymic Neoplasms: Steroids and Octreotide**	241
	L. Montella, G. Palmieri	

CHAPTER 29 **Thymus-related Myasthenia Gravis. Multimodal Therapy and Follow-up** 247
R. Gentile, L. Capone, R. Schoenhuber

CHAPTER 30 **Thymus Transplantation** 255
M.L. Markert, B.H. Devlin, E.A. McCarthy, I.K. Chinn, L.P. Hale

Subject Index 269

Contributors

ANTONIO AFFINITA
Department of Diagnostic Imaging
Division of Radiology
University of Modena and Reggio Emilia
General Hospital
Modena, Italy

HAKIM A. ALI
Department of Pulmonary Diseases and
Critical Care Medicine
Albert Einstein Medical Center
Philadelphia, PA, USA

FRANCESCO ARDISSONE
Department of Clinical & Biological Sciences
University of Turin
Thoracic Surgery Unit
San Luigi Hospital
Orbassano, TO, Italy

DEBBIE F. ASKIN
Department of Pediatrics
Faculty of Medicine
University of Manitoba
Winnipeg, MB, Canada

BRUNO BAGNI
Department of Nuclear Medicine
University of Modena and Reggio Emilia
General Hospital
Modena, Italy

FAUSTO BARBIERI
Department of Oncology and Hemathology
University of Modena and Reggio Emilia
Modena, Italy

MARIO BERTOLANI
Department of Radiology
New "S. Agostino-Estense" Hospital
Modena, Italy

PIERO BORASIO
Department of Clinical & Biological Sciences
University of Turin
Thoracic Surgery Unit
San Luigi Hospital
Orbassano, TO, Italy

LOREDANA CAPONE
Department of Neurology
Bolzano Hospital
Bolzano, Italy

CHRISTIAN CASALI
Department of General Surgery and
Surgical Specialities
Division of Thoracic Surgery
University of Modena and Reggio Emilia
General Hospital
Modena, Italy

MONICA CASIRAGHI
General Thoracic Surgery Unit
University "Vita-Salute"
Scientific Institute San Raffaele Hospital
Milan, Italy

ALESSANDRA CASOLO
Department of Nuclear Medicine
University of Modena and Reggio Emilia
General Hospital
Modena, Italy

KE-NENG CHEN
Department of Thoracic Surgery I
Peking University School of Oncology
Beijing Cancer Hospital
Beijing, China

IVAN K. CHINN
Department of Pediatrics
Duke University Medical Center
Durham, NC, USA

CHENG-YEN CHUANG
School of Medicine
National Yang-Ming University
Taipei, Taiwan, ROC

PAOLA CIRIACO
General Thoracic Surgery Unit
University "Vita-Salute"
Scientific Institute San Raffaele Hospital
Milan, Italy

PIER FRANCO CONTE
Department of Oncology and Hemathology
University of Modena and Reggio Emilia
Modena, Italy

ANDREA COSSARIZZA
Department of Biomedical Sciences
University of Modena and Reggio Emilia
Modena, Italy

MARINA CUCCA
Department of Nuclear Medicine
University of Modena and Reggio Emilia
General Hospital
Modena, Italy

MARC DE PERROT
Division of Thoracic Surgery
Toronto General Hospital
Toronto, ON, Canada

MARIO DE SANTIS
Department of Diagnostic Imaging
Division of Radiology
University of Modena and Reggio Emilia
General Hospital
Modena, Italy

BLYTHE H. DEVLIN
Department of Pediatrics
Duke University Medical Center
Durham, NC, USA

AIDNAG Z. DIAZ
Department of Radiation Oncology
Health Science Center San Antonio and
Cancer Therapy and Research Center
University of Texas
San Antonio, TX, USA

WILLIAM DIEHL-JONES
Faculty of Nursing
University of Manitoba and
Department of Biological Sciences
Faculty of Science
University of Manitoba
Winnipeg, MB, Canada

TONY Y. ENG
Department of Radiation Oncology
Health Science Center San Antonio and
Cancer Therapy and Research Center
University of Texas
San Antonio, TX, USA

MARIA A. FANIGLIULO
2nd Anesthesia and Resuscitation Service
University of Modena and Reggio Emilia
General Hospital
Modena, Italy

LUCA FERLA
General Thoracic Surgery Unit
University "Vita-Salute"
Scientific Institute San Raffaele Hospital
Milan, Italy

ANTONELLA FRANCESCHETTO
Department of Nuclear Medicine
University of Modena and Reggio Emilia
General Hospital
Modena, Italy

FABIO GAZZOTTI
2nd Anesthesia and Resuscitation Service
University of Modena and Reggio Emilia
General Hospital
Modena, Italy

KLAUS GELLERT
Department of General and Visceral Surgery
SANA Klinikum Berlin-Lichtenberg
Oskar-Ziethen-Hospital
Berlin, Germany

RICCARDA GENTILE
Department of Neurology
Bolzano Hospital
Bolzano, Italy

MANUELA GOZZI
Department of Radiology
New "S. Agostino-Estense" Hospital
Modena, Italy

ZHEN-DONG GU
Department of Thoracic Surgery I
Peking University School of Oncology
Beijing Cancer Hospital
Beijing, China

LAURA P. HALE
Department of Pathology
Duke University Medical Center
Durham, NC, USA

MARIA HARAZDA
Department of Pathology
Pulmonary Hospital
Zakopane, Poland

ŁUKASZ HAUER
Department of Thoracic Surgery
Pulmonary Hospital
Zakopane, Poland

CHUNG-PING HSU
Department of Surgery
Division of Thoracic Surgery
Taichung Veterans General Hospital
Taichung, Taiwan, ROC

VINCENZO L. INDRIZZI
2nd Anesthesia and Resuscitation Service
University of Modena and Reggio Emilia
General Hospital
Modena, Italy

CAMERON KEATING
Cardiothoracic Care Centre
St. Vincent's Hospital
Melbourne, Australia

SHAF KESHAVJEE
Division of Thoracic Surgery
Toronto General Hospital
Toronto, ON, Canada

GHULAM KHALEEQ
Department of Pulmonary Diseases
and Critical Care Medicine
Albert Einstein Medical Center
Philadelphia, PA, USA

SVEN KÖTHER
Department of General and Visceral Surgery
SANA Klinikum Berlin-Lichtenberg
Oskar-Ziethen-Hospital
Berlin, Germany

JAROSŁAW KUŻDŻAŁ
Department of Thoracic Surgery
Pulmonary Hospital
Zakopane, Poland

CORRADO LAVINI
Department of General Surgery and
Surgical Specialities
Division of Thoracic Surgery
University of Modena and Reggio Emilia
General Hospital
Modena, Italy

MARCO LUCCHI
Cardiac and Thoracic Department
Division of Thoracic Surgery
University of Pisa
Pisa, Italy

JOIN Y. LUH
Department of Radiation Oncology
Health Science Center San Antonio and
Cancer Therapy and Research Center
University of Texas
San Antonio, TX, USA

ANTONIO MAIORANA
Department of Laboratories
Pathologic Anatomy and Law Medicine
Section of Pathologic Anatomy
University of Modena and Reggio Emilia
Modena, Italy

M. LOUISE MARKERT
Department of Pediatrics and
Department of Immunology
Duke University Medical Center
Durham, NC, USA

GIUSEPPE MARULLI
Department of Cardiologic, Thoracic and
Vascular Sciences
Division of Thoracic Surgery
University of Padova
Padova, Italy

ELIZABETH A. MCCARTHY
Department of Pediatrics
Duke University Medical Center
Durham, NC, USA

YOUNES MEHD
Department of General Surgery and
Surgical Specialities
Division of Thoracic Surgery
University of Modena and Reggio Emilia
General Hospital
Modena, Italy

LILIANA MONTELLA
Medical Oncology Unit
"San Giovanni di Dio" Hospital
Naples, Italy

CESAR A. MORAN
Institute of Thoracic Pathology
University of Texas
Anderson Cancer Centre
Houston, TX, USA

ULIANO MORANDI
Department of General Surgery and
Surgical Specialities
Division of Thoracic Surgery
University of Modena and Reggio Emilia
General Hospital
Modena, Italy

ALI I. MUSANI
Pulmonary Allergy and
Critical Care Medicine
Interventional Pulmonology Program
Hospital of the University of Pennsylvania
Philadelphia, PA, USA

ALFREDO MUSSI
Cardiac and Thoracic Department
Division of Thoracic Surgery
University of Pisa
Pisa, Italy

TOMASZ NABIAŁEK
Department of Anesthesiology and
Intensive Care Medicine
Pulmonary Hospital
Zakopane, Poland

MILENA NASI
Department of Biomedical Sciences
University of Modena and Reggio Emilia
Modena, Italy

GIAMPIERO NEGRI
General Thoracic Surgery Unit
University "Vita-Salute"
Scientific Institute San Raffaele Hospital
Milan, Italy

MITSUNORI OHTA
Department of General Thoracic Surgery
Osaka University Graduate School
of Medicine
Osaka, Japan

MEINOSHIN OKUMURA
Department of General Thoracic Surgery
Osaka University Graduate School
of Medicine
Osaka, Japan

DANIELA PAIOLI
Unit of Thoracic Endoscopy and Pneumology
Maggiore-Bellaria Hospital
Bologna, Italy

GIOVANNELLA PALMIERI
Molecular and Clinical Endocrinology
and Oncology Department
University "Federico II"
Naples, Italy

CARLA PALUMBO
Department of Anatomy and Histology
Section of Human Anatomy
University of Modena and Reggio Emilia
Modena, Italy

JULIUSZ PANKOWSKI
Department of Pathology
Pulmonary Hospital
Zakopane, Poland

MARCO PATELLI
Unit of Thoracic Endoscopy and Pneumology
Maggiore-Bellaria Hospital
Bologna, Italy

MARCELLO PINTI
Department of Biomedical Sciences
University of Modena and Reggio Emilia
Modena, Italy

FEDERICO REA
Department of Cardiologic, Thoracic
and Vascular Sciences
Division of Thoracic Surgery
University of Padova
Padova, Italy

LUCA REGGIANI-BONETTI
Department of Laboratories
Pathologic Anatomy and Law Medicine
Section of Pathologic Anatomy
University of Modena and Reggio Emilia
Modena, Italy

CIRO RUGGIERO
Department of General Surgery and
Surgical Specialities
Division of Thoracic Surgery
University of Modena and Reggio Emilia
General Hospital
Modena, Italy

RUDOLF SCHOENHUBER
Department of Neurology
Bolzano Hospital
Bolzano, Italy

HIROYUKI SHIONO
Department of General Thoracic Surgery
Osaka University Graduate School
of Medicine
Osaka, Japan

JOSEPH B. SHRAGER
School of Medicine
Thoracic Surgery
University of Pennsylvania
Hospital of the University of Pennsylvania
and Pennsylvania Hospital
Philadelphia Veterans Affairs Medical Center
Philadelphia, PA, USA

WITOLD SOŚNICKI
Department of Thoracic Surgery
Pulmonary Hospital
Zakopane, Poland

ARTUR SZLUBOWSKI
Department of Anesthesiology and
Intensive Care Medicine
Pulmonary Hospital
Zakopane, Poland

ALBERTO TASSI
2nd Anesthesia and Resuscitation Service
University of Modena and Reggio Emilia
General Hospital
Modena, Italy

LEONARDA TROIANO
Department of Biomedical Sciences
University of Modena and Reggio Emilia
Modena, Italy

GAVIN M. WRIGHT
Surgical Oncology
St Vincent's Hospital
Melbourne, Australia

MATTEO ZANICHELLI
Department of Radiology
New "S. Agostino-Estense" Hospital
Modena, Italy

PIERO ZANNINI
General Thoracic Surgery Unit
University "Vita-Salute"
Scientific Institute San Raffaele Hospital
Milan, Italy

MARCIN ZIELIŃSKI
Department of Thoracic Surgery
Pulmonary Hospital
Zakopane, Poland

CHAPTER 1

The Thymus from Antiquity to the Present Day: the History of a Mysterious Gland

Corrado Lavini

The thymus is a lymphatic organ situated in the thorax, known since the 1st century AD. The officinal plant of the same name had been known for several centuries, since the time of the ancient Egyptians who, as it seems, appreciated its therapeutical properties. The name of the gland seems to come from the thyme plant, possibly due to the resemblance – fairly vague, to tell the truth – of the lobes of the gland to the plant leaves (Fig. 1.1).

According to another hypothesis, the name comes from the Greek θύμος, which means smoke, spirit and hence also soul, valor, courage: indeed, Greek physicians believed that the thymus was the seat of the soul due to the halo of mystery that surrounded it as well as due to its close proximity to the heart [1, 2].

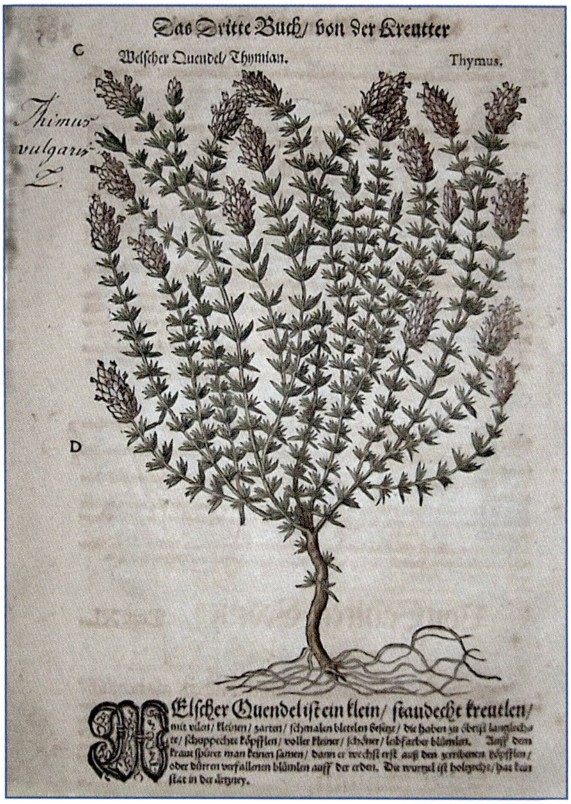

From this fanciful interpretation there comes the culinary term of Latin origin still used today for the gland in Italy, most especially if it refers to cows and horses, *animella* (i.e., small soul) equivalent to sweetbread.

The name and the first description of the thymus probably date back to **Rufus of Ephesus** (98-117 AD), a Greek physician, known to have lived in Alexandria and for some time in Rome under the Emperor Trajan [3] (Fig. 1.2).

In particular, he studied the anatomy of the inner organs and their nomenclature, writing as many as twelve treatises of which only some fragments have come down to us through Greek and Arab authors. Most especially, he devoted himself to the study of the heart, the pancreas, and the thymus. Regarding the latter, in his treatise "De corporis humani partium appellationibus," Rufus wrote "*Di ghiandole ce ne sono molte, alcune nel collo, altre sotto le ascelle, altre nel-*

Fig. 1.1 Thymus vulgaris. Etching from the German edition of "Discorsi sopra Dioscoride" by Pietro Andrea Mattioli, Prague, 1563

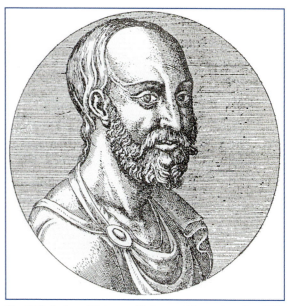

Fig. 1.2 Rufus of Ephesus. Wellcome Library, London (UK)

l'inguine, altre nel ganglio mesenterico; esse sono una sorta di carni un po' grasse e friabili. Tra queste ghiandole, c'è anche quella chiamata timo, posizionata sotto la testa del cuore, si orienta verso la settima vertebra del collo, e verso l'estremità della trachea che tocca il polmone; non la si trova in tutti gli animali" [4] ("There are many glands, some of which are in the neck, others under the axillae, others in the groins, others in the mesenteric ganglion; they are a sort of fairly fat and friable flesh. Amongst these glands there is the one called thymus, situated under the head of the heart, oriented towards the seventh vertebra of the neck and towards the end of the trachea that touches the lung; it is not to be found in all animals").

Galen of Pergamum (130-200 AD) was, together with Hippocrates, the most famous physician of antiquity. A follower of the Hippocratic theory of humours, he was the initiator of the experimental method applied to the study of anatomy and pathology and wrote over 400 texts: his propositions have dominated Western medicine for over a thousand years.

Galen only briefly dealt with the thymus in his work "De usu partium corporis humani," writing *"La vena cava si appoggia nella parete inferiore su una ghiandola assai voluminosa e molle chiamata timo"* ("The inferior wall of the vena cava rests upon a quite bulky and soft gland called thymus") [5] (Fig. 1.3).

Galen also highlighted that this organ plays an important role in the purification of the nervous system and, most importantly, that the gland *"è di dimensioni tutt'altro che trascurabili, ma anzi cospicue specialmente nei cuccioli di animali, mentre diviene progressivamente più piccola con la crescita"* ("is far from being small, instead large, most especially in young animals, and gradually dwindles with growth") [6, 7].

During the Early and Late Middle Ages, the thymus seems to have been completely forgotten by scholars: indeed, there are no descriptions of it in Western and Arab treatises until the 15th century.

It was the Italian Jacopo Barigazzi, better known as **Berengario da Carpi** (1466-1530) who rediscovered the gland, which he discussed in "Commentaria super Anatomia Mundini" (Fig. 1.4).

A most serious anatomist and surgeon – certainly the greatest one before Andrea Vesalio – Berengario became lecturer of Anatomy and Surgery at the University of Bologna.

Eustachius and Phallopius referred to him as the "refounder of Anatomy" [8].

He understood the great didactic value of anatomic plates in the teaching of medicine: as a matter of fact, his main treatises enclose detailed illustrative drawings.

Drawing inspiration from Mondino de' Liuzzi, he made several surgical dissections describing in detail the heart, the brain, the chyliferous vessels, the vermiform appendix, and the thymus.

Indeed, Berengario wrote. *"… Il mediastino è rappresentato da un pannicolo non nervoso ma legamentoso… ha la funzione di dividere il polmone ed il petto e di delimitare in tal modo eventuali danni ad un lato solo e non ad entrambi… La sua natura è fredda e secca… è situato a metà del petto e collegato posteriormente alle vertebre dorsali ed anteriormente ad una ghiandola detta mora disposta come una coperta davanti alle grandi vene ed arterie ascendenti…"* ("The mediastinum is represented by

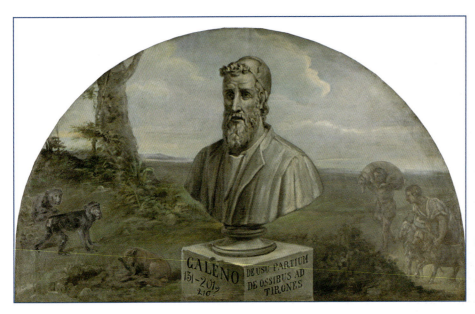

Fig. 1.3 Galen of Pergamum. Courtesy of Museum of Human Anatomy "Luigi Rolando", University of Turin (Italy)

Chapter 1 • The Thymus from Antiquity to the Present Day: the History of a Mysterious Gland

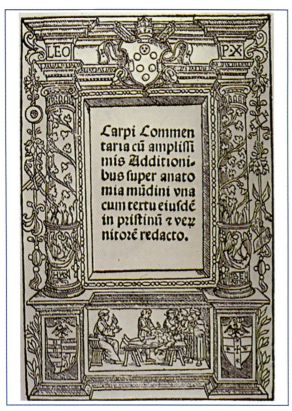

Fig. 1.4 Berengario da Carpi, "Commentaria super Anatomia Mundini", Bologna 1521. Courtesy of BEU, Modena (Italy)

a ligamentous – rather than nervous – tissue… its function is that of separating the lung from the chest thus confining any possible damage to one of the two sides only… Its nature is cold and dry… it is situated in the middle of the chest and connected posteriorly to the dorsal vertebrae and anteriorly to a gland called *mora* placed like a blanket in front of the large ascending veins and arteries") [9].

Berengario also made a curious culinary digression on the thymus in "Isagogae breves in Anatomiam humani corporis" when he wrote "…*Vicino alla vena ascendente e verso la sua parte alta, sta un organo ghiandolare che la copre a guisa di mantello. Questo organo risulta di dimensioni cospicue e viene chiamato mora o timo. Dal volgo viene denominato animella ed è tra i cibi di gusto molto saporito, soprattutto quello del vitello e dell'agnello da latte…*" ("Close to the ascending vein and towards its upper portion, there lies a glandular organ that covers it like a cloak. This organ is quite large and is called "mora" or thymus. Common people refer to it as "animella" and as food it is very tasty, most especially that from young calves and lambs") [10].

The Belgian André Vésale, better known as **Andrea Vesalio** (1514-1564), was the greatest anatomist of his time in that he laid the groundwork for modern anatomy (Fig. 1.5).

He was a lecturer of surgery in Padua and teacher in Bologna and Pisa and ended his career in Spain where he was the personal physician of Charles V and Philip II.

Vesalio discussed the thymus in his main work "De humani corporis fabrica librorum epitome" and, in particular, in Chapter III he described the protective function of the organ acting as a cushion for the vasculature of the superior mediastinum: "*La vena cava, salendo verso il giugulo, trova un organo molle e ghiandolare che i greci denominarono timo*

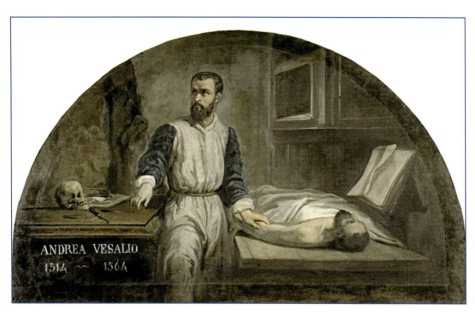

Fig. 1.5 Andrea Vesalio. Courtesy of Museum of Human Anatomy "Luigi Rolando", University of Turin (Italy)

mentre i latini lo chiamarono molto più comunemente animella. Questa stessa ghiandola viene altresì assai nobilmente collocata per proteggere da qualsivoglia danno la fitta rete di vasi che in questa sede sono sospesi..." ("The vena cava, ascending toward the jugulum, finds a soft, glandular organ that the Greeks called thymus and the Latins called, more simply, 'animella'. This same gland is also very nobly placed to protect from whatsoever damage the thick network of vessels suspended in this area..."). In Chapter VI of this work Vesalio was the first to reproduce the thymus in an anatomic table. The gland appears to be small, multilobulated in shape and lying under the sternal manubrium [11, 12] (Fig. 1.6).

The Italian **Bartolomeo Eustachio** (1500-1574) was a most distinguished anatomist, chief physician of the Pope and professor of Anatomy in Rome (Fig. 1.7). He undertook important studies on the anatomy of the inner ear, the kidney, and the teeth.

He was unable, for economic reasons, to publish his valuable "Tabulae anatomicae", which are said to have been drawn by Titian; these were published posthumously in 1714 thanks to another notable physician and anatomist, Giovanni Maria Lancisi.

Eustachio did not discuss the thymus; rather, he produced an anatomical drawing that was even more precise than that by Vesalio: the gland appears to be well defined, with an oval-shaped morphology and situated in front of the trachea (Fig. 1.8).

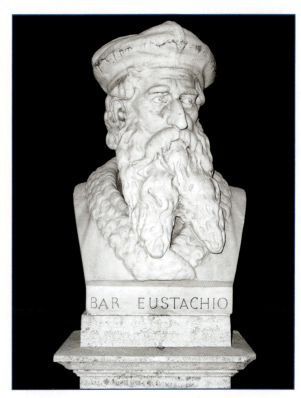

Fig. 1.7 Bartolomeo Eustachio. Courtesy of Wynn White Photographies

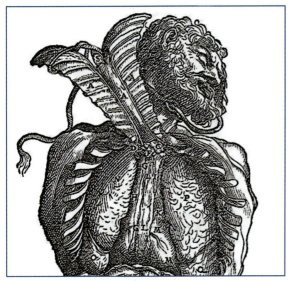

Fig. 1.6 Andrea Vesalio, De humani corporis fabrica, Representation of endothoracic organs with the thymic gland (marked by letter *F*). Courtesy of Archiginnasio Library, Bologna (Italy)

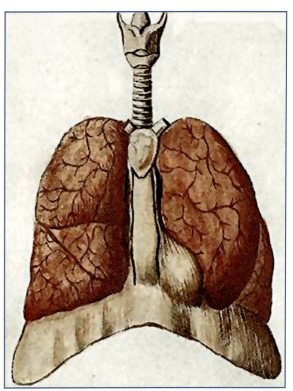

Fig. 1.8 Bartolomeo Eustachio, Tabulae anatomicae. Representation of the endothoracic organs and of the thymus (modified). Courtesy of NLM, Bethesda MD (USA)

The Frenchman **Ambroise Paré** (1510-1590) was a great surgeon and served even five kings (Fig. 1.9). He earned fame and prestige from the vast experience he had gained on battlefields as army surgeon. He devoted himself not only to surgery but also to anatomy, introducing the work of Vesalio to his contemporaries.

The title of his main treatise is "Les oeuvres d'Ambroise Paré, Conseiller et Premier Chirurgien du Roy": in book III he wrote "*La Phagoue est une glande de substance fort molle, rare et spongieuse de quantité assez notable située sur les parties supérieures du thorax, entre les divisions des veines et artères sousclavières ou iugulaires… elle servist de deffense tant'à la veine qu'à l'artère, à l'encontre de l'os du thorax… On la trouve fort notable et apparente aux bestes et ieunes gens, mais à l'homme qui est parvenu à son age, elle n'appert plus ou peu*" ("The thymus is a gland the substance of which is strong and soft, rare and spongy. It is sizable and situated in the upper part of the thorax among the subclavian and jugular arteriosus and venous branches… it protects them like a cushion from the thorax bone… The gland attains a remarkable size in the young or in animals, whereas in the elderly it is hardly visible") [13].

The Swiss anatomist and physician **Felix Plater** (1536-1614), professor in Basel, devoted himself to the study of psychiatric diseases and is considered by many to be the founder of modern psychiatry.

He was the first to discuss the thymus in a clinical context in 1614, in relation to the sudden death of a 5-month-old infant "*from suffocation from a hidden internal struma about the throat*" – bearing in mind that the term "struma" at that time referred to any type of tumor rather than solely to thyroid disease as is the case nowadays.

At autopsy, Plater reported: "*We found the gland in the region of the throat as a large protruding tumor, one ounce in weight, spongy fleshing and pendent, replete with veins, adhering by membrane to the largest vessels adjacent to the throat; these being filled with blood and flowing into the struma, dilated it to such an extent that it compressed the blood vessels in the locality; in which manner I concluded that the child was thus suffocated*" [3, 14].

Francis Glisson (1597-1677) was a famous English anatomist (Fig. 1.10). He taught at Cambridge and devoted himself to the study of the anatomy and physiology of the digestive system and of the muscles.

He wrote a fundamental treatise on the anatomy of the liver and one on children's rickets. When briefly discussing the thymus, he identified its function as that of producing a fluid for fetal nourishment and growth.

The great anatomists of the 15th, 16th, and 17th centuries had not significantly advanced the knowl-

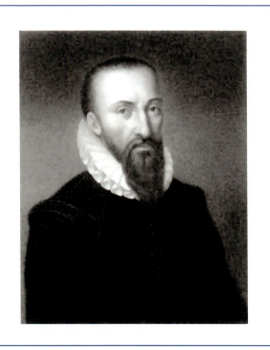

Fig. 1.9 Ambroise Paré

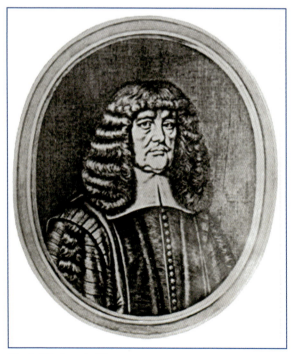

Fig. 1.10 Francis Glisson

edge of the thymus: from antiquity to the Baroque Age, the notions about thymus remained substantially unaltered.

This organ was still viewed as having a protective function, acting as a cushion for endothoracic vascular structures and it was confirmed, as Galen had said, that it could be sizable at birth and gradually dwindled with age: allegedly, this explanation was not enough to clarify its morphological and functional aspects.

More than a century away, the anatomy and physiology of this enigmatic organ started to be studied with scientific method and rigor.

For some time in the 18th century the prevalent theory was that the thymus was someway involved in regulating the fetal and neonatal pulmonary function and was defined as the "organ of vicarious respiration" [1].

Another hypothesis was that the thymus merely had the function to fill the endothoracic space that would be later on occupied by the lungs of the growing neonate [1].

Knowledge of the thymus gathered momentum with the advent of the optical microscope. It was invented by the Dutchman Antoine van Leuwenhoek (1632-1723) who was the first to study the capillary network; later on, it was used by the great Italian anatomist Marcello Malpighi (1628-1694) and enabled him to discover human cells.

The systematic use of the optical microscope soon allowed the acquisition of new important knowledge in terms of normal anatomy, physiology, and pathological anatomy.

The English surgeon, anatomist, and physiologist **William Hewson** (1739-1774) was rightfully defined as the father of hematology (Fig. 1.11).

Using the optical microscope, he gained fundamental insights into blood cells and on the physiology of coagulation. He studied the lymphatic system, the spleen, and the thymus.

In 1774 he published the first scientific treatise on the thymus, describing its change in size with aging and identifying for the first time its lymphatic nature [15]. Indeed, he noted that the gland was disseminated with "particles" similar to those found in peripheral blood and in the lymph and thought that the thymus worked in the early months of life when the organism most needed these "particles" [16]. As a matter of fact, he wrote *"The thymus gland we consider an appendage to the lymphatic glands, for the more perfectly and expeditiously forming the central particles of the blood of the foetus, and in the early part of life. We have proved that vast numbers of central particles made by the thymus and the lymphatic glands are*

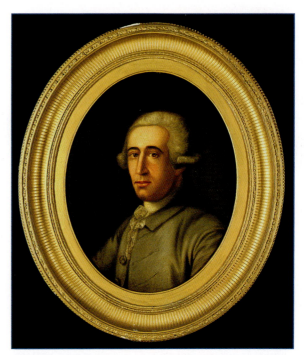

Fig. 1.11 William Hewson. Wellcome Library, London (UK)

poured into the blood vessels through the thoracic duct and if we examine the blood attentively we see them floating in it. Nature surely would not make so many particles to answer no purpose! What then becomes of these particles after they are mixed with the circulation blood?... They are, we believe, carried with the blood to the spleen... and the spleen has the power of separating them from other parts of the blood" [17].

Hewson correctly sensed that the lymphatic system was a unitary one. He pointed out that *"By the lymphatic system and its appendages we mean the lymphatic vessels, the lymphatic glands (nodes), the thymus and the spleen. At first view it may seem extraordinary that nature should have given so many and so complicated organs to form only part of the blood, when she effects other secretions by organs apparently more simple; but our surprise must cease when we reflect that upon a due formation of these particles, not only the various functions of the body but the very existence of the animal, in a great measure, depends"* [17].

Finally, he confirmed that the thymus becomes smaller with aging and assumed that some other tissue could take on its functions during mature age but he also found that the size of the organ can be rapidly reduced in the course of acute and chronic diseases [17].

The Englishman Sir **Astley Paston Cooper** (1768-1841), who was the personal physician of three kings, was the first surgeon to be appointed Baronet (Fig. 1.12).

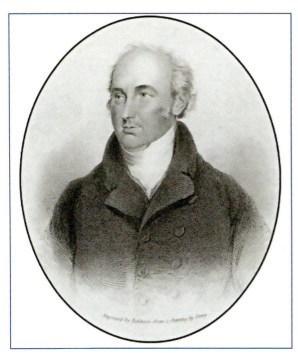

Fig. 1.12 Sir Astley Paston Cooper

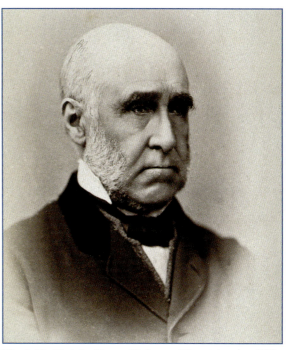

Fig. 1.13 Sir John Simon. Wellcome Library, London (UK)

He was lecturer of Anatomy in London and extensively devoted himself to the surgical practice. He wrote valuable treatises, all with elaborate illustrations, on abdominal herniations, the pathology of the breast and of the testicle, and on bone fractures.

In 1832 he published "The Anatomy of the Thymus Gland", which was a summary of its vast experience with animal dissections. The treatise comprised, besides accurate descriptions and illustrations of the thymus, also three pages focusing on the pathology of the gland, including the first description of malignant thymoma [1, 3].

Cooper confirmed the significant volumetric and structural variability of the gland over the years and disagreed with those theories that saw the thymus as an organ the mere function of which was to fill, in the fetal age, the space destined to be occupied by the lungs: *"That an important function must be performed by an organ… so large… and secreting abundantly, no one who duly considers the subject can for a moment hesitate to acknowledge…I cannot subscribe to the opinion…[that] this gland is designed merely to fill a space wich the lungs… may be destined to occupy"* [18]. Still, he did not disagree with Glisson's old theory on the role of the gland in the growth of the foetus.

Twelve years after the publication of Astley Cooper's essay, the London surgeon **Sir John Simon** (1816-1904) published a new treatise on the thymus, entitled "An Essay on the Physiology of the Thymus Gland" [19] (Fig. 1.13).

The work of John Simon represented for years a hallmark for the anatomy and physiology of the thymus, even though the author concluded, thus proving that he was still relying on outdated notions, that the thymus is *"the sinking fund in the service of respiration* [1].

Arthur Hill Hassall (1817-1894), an Englishman, was a physician and a chemist (Fig. 1.14).

He was interested in anatomy, physiology, pathological anatomy, chemistry, botany, and public hygiene.

In 1846 he published the first text in English on microscopic anatomy: "The Microscopic Anatomy of the Human Body in Health and Disease".

Hassall, using the latest and most advanced models of optical microscope, described with H. Vanarsdale the histological differences between the thymus and the other lymphatic organs [1, 20].

In 1849 he discovered, in the medullary portion, the spherical corpuscles of epithelioid cells in corneal transformation thus named [21].

On the verge of the 20th century, the anatomical and histological knowledge relating to the thymus could be said to be well established: there were no doubts on the lymphatic nature of this organ and on the fact that it was somehow of fundamental importance, most especially during fetal life and the pediatric age when it could attain a very large size.

For sure, it is peculiar that it took two millennia for the history of medicine to throw light on just two

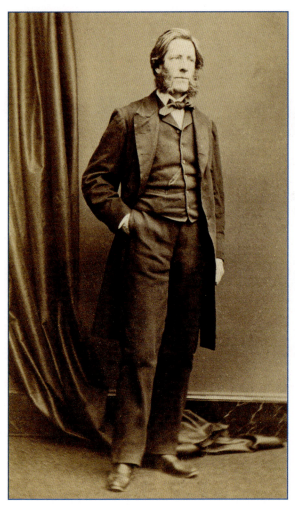

Fig. 1.14 Arthur Hill Hassall. From Science & Society Picture Library, London (UK)

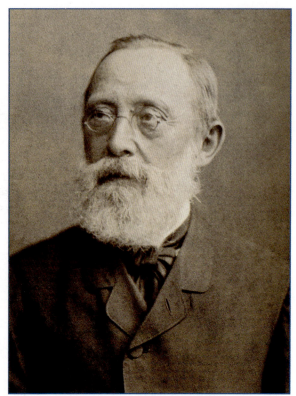

Fig. 1.15 Rudolf Virchow. Wellcome Library, London (UK)

anatomical and descriptive aspects of the gland, which had been considered as the organ of mystery for centuries.

There still lacked objective and definite data on what could be the actual role of the thymus in physiology and pathology. In particular, hypertrophic-hyperplastic and neoplastic conditions had not been clarified: for these reasons, the organ remained for years a sort of scapegoat and a victim of the scientific approximation that lingered on, and the gland was seen as the cause for a diverse range of pediatric diseases [1].

The great German pathologist **Rudolf Wirchow** (1821-1902) was interested in cellular pathology and significantly contributed to the study of leukemias and thrombosis (Fig. 1.15).

He took a minor interest in the thymus and reinstated the validity of the notion of "*thymic asthma*" (first coined by J.H. Klopp in 1830) from compression by a hypertrophic thymus of the large airways and in particular of the trachea [22].

The notion of "*thymic asthma*" was for decades associated to that of "*thymic death*": indeed, it was thought that the thymus could be involved in seemingly unexplained sudden deaths, most especially at the pediatric age. The anatomical pathologists of the early 20th century already insisted on the danger of death caused mechanically by hypertrophy and hyperplasia of the gland, either during a paroxystic fit of asphyxia or sudden syncope or during surgery. As a matter of fact, the notion of "*thymic death*" resulted from finding at autopsy a large thymus that was thought to cause compression of vital mediastinal structures like the large vessels and the trachea [23].

The Austrian medical examiner **Arnold Paltauf** (1860-1893) was the first to introduce the term "*status thymolimphaticus*" in 1889 to indicate a constitutional disorder said to entail widespread hypertrophy of the entire lymphoid tissue, including the thymus, which, thus enlarged, could cause infant sudden death [24, 25].

The notions of "*thymic asthma*", "*thymic death*" and "*status thymolymphaticus*", persisted for almost one century, leading to completely misleading conclusions in terms of diagnosis and therapy.

In 1896 the German surgeon **Ludwig Rehn** (1849-1930) did the first surgery ever done on thymus in humans on a patient suffering from respiratory distress: he did transcervical thymopexy and delivered the enlarged gland upwards fixating it to the posterior lamina of the sternal manubrium. Some time later, in light of the poor outcome of the previous thymopexy, in another, similar case, the same surgeon decided to perform a partial thymectomy [3, 26].

In the early 20th century, thymectomy in infants/children with thymic hypertrophy and respiratory distress became widely accepted [27] (Fig. 1.16).

A renowned US radiologist, **Henry K. Pancoast**, well-known for his investigations into lung cancer, at the beginning of the last century reaffirmed the notion that a large thymus could cause a range of diseases (bronchitis, bronchopneumonia, tubercular and non-tubercular adenitis, sinusitis) and suggested that prolonged preoperative fluoroscopy and significant exposure to radiation were necessary in infants/children to find enlarged thymus [28].

In 1907 the Cincinnati (USA) pediatrician **Alfred Friedländer** reported the first case of thymic hypertrophy successfully treated with irradiation of the gland. It was a 2-month-old infant with paroxystic dyspnea attacks. The author enthusiastically reported that *"the procedure is of course infinitely simpler than removal of the thymus by surgical means, and it would seem justifiable to hope that in the X-ray we have a valuable therapeutic resource for the treatment of what has heretofore been considered an almost desperate condition"* [3, 29].

Since then, thousands of children and adolescents received radiation to prevent or treat "*status thymolymphaticus*"; some pediatricians even advocated prophylactic irradiation of all neonates [3, 30-32].

Only some years later did they start to throw light on the risk for these irradiated patients to develop neoplasms, most especially of the thyroid and of the breast.

At last, in 1945, in the first edition of "Paediatric X-Ray Diagnosis," the American radiologist **John Caffey** confirmed that *"… a causal relationship between hyperplasia of the thymus and sudden unexplained death has been completely refuted… Irradiation of the thymus… is an irrational procedure at all ages"* [1, 33].

In 1899 the German neurologist **Hermann Hoppenheim** was the first to point out a possible association between myasthenia gravis and diseases of the thymus, reporting the case of a myasthenic patient with a thymoma found at autopsy [34].

The study of physiology continued in parallel with the gaining of clinical knowledge on the thymus.

The Scottish hematologist **John Beard** (1857-1924) understood, like Hewson, that the gland was part of the lymphatic system; still, he went further to say that the role of the thymus was that of parent source of all of the lymphocytes of the body. Indeed, he wrote, at the beginning of the 20th century, that *"The thymus must be regarded as the parent source of all the lymphoid structures of the body. It does not cease to exist in later life no more than would the Anglo-Saxon race disappear were the British Isles to sink beneath the waves. For just the Anglo-Saxon stock has made its way from its original home into all parts of the world, and has there set up colonies for itself and for its increase, so the original leukocytes, starting from their birth place in the thymus, have penetrated into almost every part of the body, and have there created new centres for growth, for increase, and for useful work for themselves and for the body"* [35].

It was not until the second half of the 20th century that scholars gained an insight into the central function of the organ as part of the immunocompetent system [2].

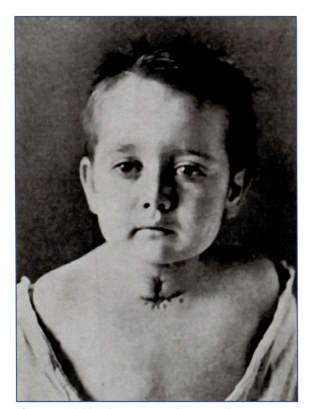

Fig. 1.16 Child with respiratory distress undergoing surgical removal of hypertrophic thymus. From a medical textbook of 1912 [27]. With kind permission of Springer Science and Business Media, Heidelberg (Germany)

Since the beginning of the last century the treatment of thymus-related diseases mainly involved surgical treatment.

The Swiss **Ernst Ferdinand Sauerbruch** (1875-1951), regarded as the father of thoracic surgery, was professor of surgery at the Universities of Zurich, Munich, and Berlin (Fig. 1.17).

He did the first cervicotomic total thymectomy in 1911 on a 19-year-old girl with myasthenia gravis and hyperthyroidism, and in 1930 he did the first thymectomy with thoracotomic approach on a patient with malignant thymoma [3].

The US surgeon **Alfred Blalock** (1899-1964) was the pioneer of heart and thoracic surgery (Fig. 1.18).

In 1936 Blalock did the first thymectomy via median sternotomy. Furthermore, he had a fortunate insight: he successfully suggested thymectomy for myasthenic patients, including those without accompanying thymoma; since then this indication was followed throughout the world [3, 36-38].

Douglas R. Gracey and co-workers, surgeons at the Mayo Clinic (Minnesota, USA), in 1982 suggested manubriotomy as a sparing procedure compared to total median sternotomy during thymectomy in patients with myasthenia gravis [39].

The advent of video-assisted thoracoscopy brought with it the first video-assisted minimally invasive surgery of the thymus: the US surgeons **Rodney J. Landreneau** and **David J. Sugarbaker** were the first to do, in 1992 and 1993 respectively, thymectomy with thoracoscopic access [40, 41].

In 2001, the Japanese **Ichiro Yoshino** did the first robotic thymectomy on a patient with a Masaoke-I thymoma [42].

The discovery of serious forms of congenital immunodeficiency from aplasia or hypoplasia of the thymus (DiGeorge's syndrome, Nezelof's syndrome) provided a stimulus, starting from the end of the 1960s, for investigations into thymus transplantation.

The US pediatricians **Charles S. August**, **William W. Cleveland** and co-workers in 1968 and **Richard Hong** in 1976 were the pioneers of this type of research.

Today, using appropriately prepared cultures of postnatal thymus to be implanted in the thigh or the omentum, very encouraging results can be obtained, especially in the DiGeorge's syndrome [43-45].

The last decades of the 1900s were devoted to further clarify the complex functions of the thymus, thus finally doing justice to a gland that had been so ill-treated in the past. Light was thrown on the neuroendocrine regulation of the gland and on its role in the maturation of immunocompetent T-cells, in the

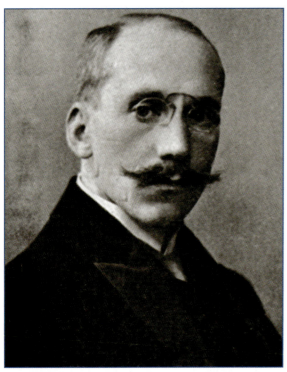

Fig. 1.17 Ernst Ferdinand Sauerbruch. Wellcome Library, London (UK)

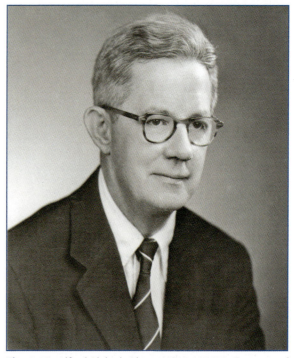

Fig. 1.18 Alfred Blalock. Photo UA24-005412. Courtesy of IUPUI University Library Special Collections and Archives, Indianapolis, IN (USA).

development of immune tolerance, in the prevention of auto-immune diseases and the supposed secretion of hormones or peptides such as *thymolin*, *thymopoietin* and *thymosin alfa-1* [46].

To conclude this brief overview of over 20 centuries, it can undoubtedly be said that the thymus has had an unusual – to say the least – history: presented as the seat of the soul by the Ancients; disrespected or forgotten altogether in the Middle Ages, the Renaissance and the Baroque Age; gradually revalued starting from the Age of Enlightenment and finally given its correct and fundamental role during the last century.

Today we know everything, or almost everything, about the thymus. Its vital function as precursor and coordinator of immunity (acting like a sort of control room of the defense systems of the organism) is widely acknowledged; likewise, we have gained well-established knowledge on the diseases of the gland and on the relationships with other autoimmune diseases, most especially myasthenia gravis.

Can we say, as a result of the foregoing, that we have come to the end of the journey that has led to knowledge of this organ?

Well, not quite, perhaps. Indeed, we believe that such a complex gland, that has remained a mystery for such a long period of time, is going to amaze us further and that in the coming years it might keep surprising us.

References

1. Jacobs MT, Frush DP, Donnelly LF (1999) The right place at the wrong time: Historical perspective of the relation of the thymus gland and pediatric radiology. Radiology 210:11-16
2. Miller JFAP (2002) The discovery of thymus function and of thymus-derived lymphocytes. Immunol Rev 185:7-14
3. Kirschner PA (2000) The history of surgery of the thymus gland. Chest Surg Clin N Am 10:153-165
4. Mazzini I (2001) Rufo di Efeso. Denominazioni delle parti del corpo. Medicina&Storia 2:81-112
5. Penso G (1985) La medicina romana. Ciba-Geigy Edizioni, Roma, p 207
6. Galen (1998) On the usefulness of the parts of the body. May MT (ed), Cornell University Press Ithaca, New York, pp 283-286
7. Singer CS (1956) Galen on anatomical procedures. Oxford University Press, London, p 250
8. De Santo NG, Bisaccia C, De Santo LS et al (1999) Berengario da Carpi. Am J Nephrol 19:199-212
9. Jacopo Berengario da Carpi (1521) Commentaria super Anatomia Mundini. Bologna
10. Jacopo Berengario da Carpi (1535) Isagogae breves perlucidae ac uberrime in anatomiam humani corporis. Venezia
11. Crotti A (1922) The thymus gland. In: Crotti A (ed) Thyroid and thymus. Lea & Febiger, Philadelphia, pp 607-693
12. Vesalius A (1950) De humani corporis fabrica. In: Sanders JB, O'Malley CD (eds) Illustrations from the works of Andrea Vesalius of Brussels, book 6. The World Publishing Co., Cleveland and New York
13. Paré Ambroise (1585) Les oeuvres d'Ambroise Paré, Conseiller et Premier Chirurgien du Roy, divisées in 28 livres avec les figures et portraicts, tant de l'anatomie que des instruments de chirurgie, et de plusieurs monsters, revues et augmenteés par l'autheur. Gabriel Buon, Paris
14. Plater F (1925) In: Ruräh J (ed) Pediatrics of the past. Paul B Hoeber Inc, New York, pp 237-239
15. Hewson W (1777) Experimental enquires III. In: Cadell T (ed) Experimental enquires into the properties of the blood. Longman, London, pp 1-223
16. Gulliver G (1846) The works of William Hewson. Sydenham Society, London
17. Doyle D (2006) William Hewson (1739-1974): The father of haematology. Br J Haematol 133:375-381
18. Cooper AP (1833) The anatomy of the thymus gland. Longmand, Rees, Orme, Green & Brown, London, pp 1-48
19. Simon J (1845) An essay on the physiology of the thymus gland. Renshaw, London
20. Hassall AH, Vanarsdale H (1846) Illustrations of the microscopic anatomy of the human body in health and disease. In: Hassall AH (ed) Microscopic anatomy of the human body in health and disease. Wood, London, pp 1-79
21. Watanabe N, Wang YH, Lee HK et al (2005) Hassall corpuscles instruct dendritic cells to induce CD4+ CD25+ regulatory T cells in human thymus. Nature 436:1181-1185
22. Kopp JK (1830) Denkwürdigkeiten in der ärztlichen praxis. Hermann, Frankfurt
23. Debré R, Lelong M (1963) Pediatria. Intermedical S.a.r.l., Roma, p 431
24. Paltauf A (1889) Über die beziehung der thymus zum plötzlichen tod. Wien Klin Wochenschr 3:877-881
25. Paltauf A (1890) Über plötzlichen tod. Wien Klin Wochenschr 3:172-175
26. Rehn L (1906) Compression from the thymus gland and resultant death. Ann Surg 44:760-768
27. Musser JH, Kelly AOJ (eds) (1912) A handbook of practical treatment. Saunders, Philadelphia, p 215
28. Gofman JW (1996) Preventing breast cancer, 2nd edn. Committee on nuclear responsibility, San Francisco
29. Friedländer A (1907) Status lymphaticus and enlargement of the thymus; with report of a case successfully treated by the X-ray. Arch Pediatr 24:490-501
30. Leonidas JC (1998) The thymus: From past misconception to present recognition. Pediatr Radiol 28:275-282
31. Moncrieff A (1937) Enlargement of the thymus in infants with special reference to clinical evidence of so-

called status thymo-lymphaticus. Proc R Soc Med 31:537-544
32. Oestreich AE, William H (1995) Crane of Cincinnati and the first irradiation of the pediatric thymus, 1905. AJR 165:1064-1065
33. Caffey J (1945) The mediastinum. In: Caffey J (ed) Pediatric X-ray diagnosis. Year Book, Chicago, pp 344-345
34. Oppenheim H (1899) Weiterer Beitrag zur Lehre von den Acuten Nicht-Eitrigen Encephalitis und der Polioencephalomyelitis. Deutsche Zeitschr Nervenheil Kande 15:1-27
35. Beard J (1900) The source of leucocytes and the true function of the thymus. Anat Anz 18:550-560
36. Hughes T (2005) The early history of myasthenia gravis. Neuromuscul Disord 15:878-886
37. Kattach H, Anastasiadis K, Cleuziou G et al (2006) Transsternal thymectomy for myasthenia gravis: Surgical outcome. Ann Thorac Surg 81:305-308
38. Kirschner PA (1987) Alfred Blalock and thymectomy for myasthenia gravis. Ann Thorac Surg 43:348-349
39. Gracey DR, Divertie MB, Howard FM Jr et al (1984) Postoperative respiratory care after transsternal thymectomy in myasthenia gravis. A 3-year experience in 53 patients. Chest 86:67-71
40. Landreneau RJ, Dowling RD, Castillo WM (1992) Thoracoscopic resection of an anterior mediastinal tumor. Ann Thorac Surg 54:142
41. Sugarbaker DJ (1993) Thoracoscopy in the management of anterior mediastinal masses. Ann Thorac Surg 56:653-656
42. Yoshino I, Hashizume M, Shimada M et al (2001) Thoracoscopic thymomectomy with the Da Vinci computer-enhanced surgical system. J Thorac Cardiovasc Surg 122:783-785
43. August CS, Rosen FS, Filler RM et al (1968) Implantation of a foetal thymus restoring immunological competence in a patient with thymic aplasia (DiGeorge's) Lancet 2:1210
44. Cleveland WW, Fogel BJ, Brown WT et al (1968) Foetal thymic transplant in a case of DiGeorge's syndrome. Lancet 2:1211
45. Hong R, Santosham M, Schulte-Wissermann H et al (1976) Reconstitution of B and T lymphocyte function in severe combined immunodeficiency disease after transplantation with thymic epithelium. Lancet 2:1270
46. Hadden JW (1998) Thymic endocrinology. Ann N Y Acad Sci 840:352-358

Embryology and Anatomy of the Thymus Gland

Carla Palumbo

Introduction

The thymus is a lymphoepithelial organ, whose function was long obscure. It is now well established that it is one of the primary central lymphoid organs, the other being the red bone marrow, from which it receives T-lymphocyte precursors. The thymus gland, while providing thymus-processed T-lymphocytes to the entire body, also produces some special humoral secretions and may thus also be regarded as an endocrine organ. Though it undergoes a drastic diminution in size with age (*vide infra*), it is now well established that it remains active even into old age. Certain diseases significantly accelerate its physiological involution.

Embryology

According to the classical view, the thymus derives from the endoderm of the 3rd pharyngeal pouch on both sides. The 3rd pharyngeal pouch gives origin ventrally to the thymus and dorsally to the 3rd parathyroid gland, whereas the 4th pharyngeal pouch gives origin to the 4th parathyroid and the ultimobranchial body. In recent years, however, most embryologists have tended to support the hypothesis that the thymic epithelium (*thymic epitheliocytes*) derives from both ectoderm and endoderm of the 3rd and often 4th pharyngeal pouches; these components are thought to interact with the associated mesenchyme, which derives from the neural crest at the stage of 10 somites (23 days) [1, 2], to trigger thymus development.

During the earlier stages of thymus descent, the related 3rd parathyroid moves down with the whole 3rd pouch thus explaining, in later stages, the normal lower position of this parathyroid as compared with the 4th parathyroid. In embryos of about 20 mm, the 3rd parathyroid separates from the corresponding pouch, thus freeing completely the ipsilateral thymic bud. Prior to this separation the thymus rudiments cannot be recognized. The two thymic buds meet ventrally to the aortic sack and are subsequently joined by connective tissue only. The connection with the 3rd pouch is then lost, but sometimes a solid cellular cord (or stalk) may persist. After the separation from the 3rd parathyroid, the cells of the thymus form a densely packed epithelial mass, endodermal in origin. Later, they are more loosely arranged to form an epithelial reticulum (*cytoreticulum*), in which lymphoid stem cells soon appear; these have migrated from the bone marrow. The vascular mesenchymal tissue, accompanied by vagal nerve fibers, invades the gland in such a way as to produce its lobulated appearance. The differentiation of thymic medulla and cortex takes place in embryos of about 40 mm in length. The medulla arises in the central portion of the thymus and the deep portions of the lobules by hypertrophy of the cytoreticulum, accompanied by degeneration or migration of thymocytes. Later Hassall's corpuscles appear as involutive clusters of the cytoreticulum. As of the 10th week, more than 95% of cells belong to T-lineage with few erythroblasts and B-lymphocytes. Cells of the macrophage lineage enter the medulla starting from the 14th week. The thymus appears to be completely differentiated by the 17th week, and thereafter the main type of thymocytes, the so-called TdT$^+$, will be produced throughout the whole life.

Gross Anatomy

The size of the thymus undergoes considerable changes with age. At birth it weighs 10-15 g; it grows until puberty when it reaches its maximum weight of 30-40 g. Thereafter, it undergoes a physiological involution and transforms into the *retrosternal adipose body*. After middle age it may weigh 10 g, but in certain cases it remains large, weighing up to 50 g [3].

The appearance of the thymus also changes with age. At birth it is pinkish; it becomes gray during infancy and yellow in adulthood. It is classically described as a single median organ with two lobes, but each lobe develops from the pharyngeal pouch of the corresponding side; thus there are, strictly speaking, a right and left thymus.

The thymus has a pyramidal shape with a lower base and two upper horns. It lies in the anterior mediastinum, extending above into the neck, where its horns may reach the lower poles of the thyroid gland; strands of connective tissue usually connect the two organs. Below it extends to the 4th-5th costal cartilages. The *anterior surface* is related to the sternum, the four upper costal cartilage and the insertions of the sternohyoid and sternothyroid muscles. In the front of the neck, the thymus is anteriorly in relation with the infrahyoid muscles ensheathed by the middle and superficial cervical fasciae. The *posterior surface* is connected to the upper pericardium, the aortic arch with its branches, the left brachiocephalic vein and the front and sides of the trachea. Laterally the thymus is related to the mediastinal pleurae, lungs and phrenic nerves, particularly the left one.

Small accessory thymic nodules may be present in the neck, as a result of their detachment from the main organ during its early descent.

Microscopic Structure

The microscopic components of the mature thymus derive from several sources: epithelial derivates from the pharyngeal wall, mesenchyme, hemolymphoid cells, and vascular tissue. These components form a network in which they interact functionally to provide the thymus with its unique immunological properties.

Thymus microarchitecture includes two distinct parts: an outer *cortex* and an inner *medulla*. Septa of loose connective tissue extend from the capsule inside the cortex, thus dividing it into lobules of various sizes, their diameter ranging between 0.5 and 2.0 μm (Fig. 2.1). Both cortex and medulla are permeated by a framework of reticular fibers and by a peculiar network of epithelial cells joined by both simple contacts and specialized junctions. As regards the lymphoid tissue, it mostly pertains to cells of T-lymphocyte lineage, known as *thymocytes*; these are numerous and closely packed in the cortex. The medulla contains few lymphoid cells and the characteristic Hassall's corpuscles (*vide infra*). The connective septa separating adjacent lobules contain blood vessels, nerves, and efferent lymphatics.

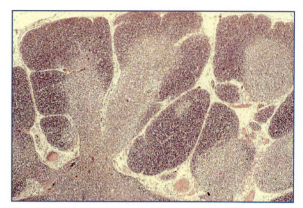

Fig. 2.1 Light micrograph of neonatal human thymus showing its lobular architecture. In each lobule a pale medullary core appears to be surrounded by a dark stained cortex. Note the higher cellular density in the cortex with respect to the medulla. Haematoxylin-Eosin stain (specimen prepared by the Department of Anatomy and Histology of University of Modena and Reggio Emilia)

Epithelial Framework

A distinct feature of the thymus with respect to other lymphoid organs, whose stroma is only composed of a reticular collagenous framework, is that it is further supported by a network of finely-branched epithelial reticular cells (*thymic epitheliocytes*) forming a three-dimensional network of meshes in which lymphoid cells are entrapped. These epitheliocytes are interconnected with each other by cell-to-cell contacts and perform a pivotal role in determining a microenvironment containing soluble factors and cytokines essential for the development of thymocytes.

Thymic epitheliocytes are present throughout the cortex and medulla; histologically, however, they are more easily identifiable in the cortex.

Six different types of thymic epitheliocytes may be distinguished (Fig. 2.2): type-1 epitheliocytes have a subcapsular and perivascular location, types 2-4 are located in the cortex and types 5-6 are present in the medulla. *Type-1 epitheliocytes* carpet the internal outline of the thymus as well as the perivascular spaces, passing through the cortico-medullary boundary. They are flat, with a well-defined basal lamina, and display a few, short cisternae of granular endoplasmic reticulum and tubular complex of unknown function. A feature of type-1 epitheliocytes is to secrete hormones [4] and factors attracting stem cells [5]; cortical epitheliocytes are often branched and separated by wide intercellular spaces. *Type-2 epitheliocytes* extend from the cortex towards the medulla; their size is larger then type-1 ep-

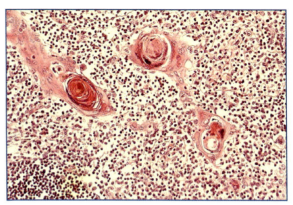

Fig. 2.3 Light micrograph of neonatal human thymus showing in the medulla three Hassall's corpuscles surrounded by many thymocytes. Haematoxylin-Eosin stain (specimen prepared by the Department of Anatomy and Histology of University of Modena and Reggio Emilia)

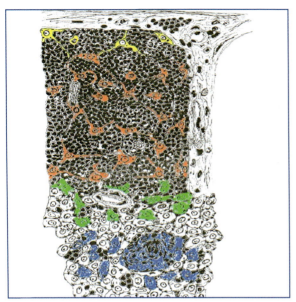

Fig. 2.2 Schematic drawing showing the location of the various types of epitheliocyte in the thymic parenchyma. Type 1 epitheliocytes in *yellow*, type 2-4 epitheliocytes in *orange*, type 5 epitheliocytes in *green*, type 6 epitheliocytes in *blue*

itheliocytes and display small Golgi apparatus and long cytoplasmic processes (up to 100 micra). *Type-3 epitheliocytes* are large and pale, while *type-4 epitheliocytes* appear dense and smaller than the former. Epitheliocytes of the medulla tend to form solid cords and often appear keratinized and stratified when forming Hassall's corpuscles. *Type-5 epitheliocytes* are very small cells without any specialized function. *Type-6 epitheliocytes* are the more common epithelial cells in medulla. They are variously shaped: the spindle ones secrete thymic hormones, while the flat ones also form Hassall's corpuscles.

Hassall's corpuscles (or thymic corpuscles), discovered by Arthur Hill Hassall in 1849, are formed by types 4 and 6 epitheliocytes. They appear as clusters of flattened cells arranged like onion skins, whose diameter ranges between 30 and 100 micra and whose center often contains cellular debris (Fig. 2.3). They start to form before birth and their number increases with age. The function of Hassall's corpuscles is currently unclear; it is known that they are a potent source of the cytokine TSLP (Thymic Stromal Lymphopoietin). In vitro, TSLP directs the maturation of dendritic cells, and increases the ability of dendritic cells to convert naïve thymocytes to a Foxp3+ regulatory T-cell lineage [6]. It is unknown whether this is the physiological function of Hassall's corpuscles in vivo.

Thymocytes

Thymic lymphocytes (thymocytes) form about 90% of total thymus weight and are located in both cortex and medulla but with a different density. They enter the thymus from the yolk sack and the liver (in their hemopoietic phase) during the life of the embryo, and from bone marrow after birth. The thymocyte precursors, which circulate in the bloodstream, are generally attracted by thymic chemotactic substances and enter the thymus parenchyma. In the cortex, thymocytes occupy both the outer and the deeper zones, where they undergo mitosis. As the differentiating T-cell clones mature, they gradually move deep into the cortex towards the medulla. It has been observed that the closer the thymocytes to the epitheliocytes, the better their conditions for proliferation and differentiation [7]; indeed, type 2 and 3 epitheliocytes are also named *thymic nurse cells* (TNC). Notwithstanding the fact that the exact nature of epitheliocyte-thymocyte interactions are still unclear, it seems likely that epitheliocytes release soluble mitogenic and differentiating factors which, in turn, are triggered by dynamic intercellular contacts with the transforming thymocytes. During the process of their maturation, thymocytes acquire in sequence the CD3+ marker and various T-cell receptors (TCR), thus switching into the different subclasses of T-cells.

The thymocytes are not immunocompetent within the cortex; as their differentiation progresses the thymocytes enter the medulla (becoming postthymic thymocytes or T-lymphocytes) and thus attain maturity. This is in line with the existence of antigen-presenting cells and plasma cells in the medulla: hence it is not surprising that T-lymphocytes can also be activated within the thymus, though few in number. Another possibility is that thymocytes achieve maturity when they reach their secondary lymphoid tissue destinations.

During the maturation process, four cell types can be recognized, each of them of different proportions corresponding to small, medium and large thymocytes. (1) *Double negative cells* (for CD4- and CD8-, besides CD3-) are located in the subcapsular cortex and are mostly large blast cells; when undergoing mitosis these cells become smaller in size, display TCR complexes and become CD3+. (2) *Double positive cells* (CD4+ and CD8+, besides CD3+) are located deep within the cortex, are mostly small cells and represent 80-90% of the thymocyte population. While acquiring their immunocompetence, most of the two types of thymocytes mentioned above will die by apoptosis due to "mistakes" in their differentiation process; they will then be removed by mononuclear macrophages (*vide infra*). Thus, a positive selection takes place, resulting in (3) *medullary single-positive cells* (positive only for one of the markers CD4 or CD8); these are exported in order to enter the peripheral lymphoid organs, where they become fully immunocompetent. (4) *Immunocompetent medullary single-positive cells* are recirculating, activated T-cells which enter the medulla secondarily [8]. Besides these T-cell types, *natural killer cell lineages* originate and are present in thymic parenchyma. *Immature B-lymphocytes* are also present in the thymus, but they come from the bloodstream; like plasmacytes they are mainly located in the medulla or around blood vessels at the cortico-medullary junction. In this connection, it is interesting to note that the contemporaneous presence of mature B-lymphocytes and recirculating activated T-cells inside the medulla supports the hypothesis that at least part of the medulla is more likely a secondary ("peripheral") rather than a primary ("central") lymphoid organ.

Thymic Macrophages

Mononuclear macrophages, which derive from the bone marrow, form an important cell population in the thymus. They are mostly located at the cortico-medullary junction, where they phagocytize a huge amount of differentiating thymocytes. Their macrophage activity is particularly devoted to remnants of apoptotic thymocytes and to those undergoing erroneous differentiation. It has been suggested that this substantial thymocyte destruction could prevent the occurrence of autoimmune diseases.

Vascularization and Microcirculation

Thymus blood supply is provided by branches from the internal thoracic artery and the inferior thyroid artery and, occasionally, from the superior thyroid artery; more rarely a posterior thymic artery derives from the aortic arch or from the brachio-cephalic or left common carotid arteries. The thymus does not have a hilum, thus the arteries enter the organ through the capsule and the interlobar septa, to reach the gland parenchyma at the cortico-medullary junction. The drainage of the gland is performed by the left brachiocephalic, internal thoracic, and inferior thyroid veins.

Thymus microcirculation differs in the cortex and medulla. In each lobe the vessels give off small capillaries to the cortex and large vessels to the medulla. The cortical capillaries run along different depths and join venous vessels at the *cortico-medullary* junction. Some of them, smaller in diameter, reach the capsule, where they join the large veins draining the blood from the thymus. The main feature of cortical capillaries is that they have a complete sheath of epithelial cells that contribute to the formation of the so-called *blood-thymic barrier* [9, 10]. *Medullary* vessels are very variable in size; they drain into larger veins that emerge medially from each thymus lobe. The medullary capillaries are not ensheathed by epithelial cells, thus the blood-thymic barrier does not exist in the medulla. At the cortico-medullary junction, some postcapillary venules are short and display a particular high endothelium similar to those observed in other lymphoid organs and tissues.

Lymphatics

Lymph vessels emerge from the cortico-medullary junction and, passing through the extravascular spaces along with blood vessels, leave the gland from the capsule. Afferent lymphatics are absent in the thymus.

Innervation

Thymus nerves are arranged in bundles and plexuses; their fibers derive from both the sympathetic chain (via the stellate ganglion) and the vagus. A further contribution to the thymus capsule innervation comes from the phrenic and *descendens cervicalis* nerves. The two lobes have separate innervations coming from their posterior, lateral, and medial sides. Sympathetic and vagal innervations reach the organ at different times: vagal branches come to the thymus before its descent into the thorax, whereas the sympathetic ones are distributed inside the gland only once it has reached its final location.

On the whole, the role of the nervous system in thymus biology is still not yet well known. Most nervous fibers are noradrenergic and associated with blood vessels, where they form intricate ramifications in their adventia; thus they clearly have a vasomotor function. The presence of cholinergic fibers among the cells, particularly in the medulla, is still a matter of speculation.

Thymic Hormones and Factors

The thymus produces a series of polypeptides which display hormone-like properties, particularly, but not exclusively, devoted to inducing immune function maturation. The main substances released by the gland are thymosins, thymulin, thymopentin and thymic humoral factor (THF). The *thymosins* are a family of biologically active peptides whose molecular weight ranges between 1,000 and 15,000 Daltons. Several of these small peptides, such as thymosin-alpha-1 and thymosin-beta-4, have been synthesized and shown to have important clinical applications. The physiological processes that these peptides affect include stimulation or suppression of immune responses, regulation of actin dynamics and cell motility, neuroplasticity, repair and remodeling of vessels of the injured tissues, angiogenesis, and stem-cell differentiation. *Thymulin* is a neuroendocrine hormone having an immunoregulatory action, originally known as "serum thymic factor" (FTS) that binds to a carrier protein and zinc to exert its biological properties; it is also essential for T-lymphocyte differentiation. Recently, thymulin has also been shown to be involved in inflammation of various etiologies. *Thymopentin*, also known as TP-5 (thymic fraction V), is a synthesized derivative of thymopoietin, a thymic hormone with immunoregulatory properties responsible for inducing T-cell precursors to differentiate and mature. *Thymic humoral factor (THF)* is a peptide hormone first isolated from calf thymus; it has been shown to increase the number of T-lymphocytes and enhance cell-mediated immunity.

Thymic factors are often said to affect also other endocrine organs and, in turn, hormones released from endocrine glands can influence thymic function and/or structure. However, the exact functional relationships between the thymus and the other endocrine glands are far from being clearly established.

Thymus in Postnatal Life

After birth, the size and weight of the thymus increase during the first year of life, achieving the mean weight of 25 g; this weight remains fairly constant up to the 6th decade of life. Thereafter, the thymus decreases in size and weight in parallel with changes in its microscopic structure (a phenomenon known as "involution"), although thymocyte production and differentiation persist throughout the whole life. The process of thymus atrophy seems to be directed by high levels of circulating sex hormones, and chemical or physical castration of an adult results in the thymus increasing in size and activity [11]. Upon atrophy, size and activity are dramatically reduced, and the organ is primarily replaced with fat, the *retrosternal adipose body* (Fig. 2.4). Four phases have been identified during thymus involvement: until the 10th year of life, the reduction on lymphatic tissue occurs at a rate of about 5% per year (*I phase*); from the 10th to the 25th year, adipocytes start to infiltrate the perivascular spaces of the medulla (*II phase*); from the 25th to the 40th year, as fatty atrophy proceeds involving the cortex, thymus involution continues at a rate of 5% per year (*III phase*); after the 40th year, however, the involution rate decreases to 0.1% per year (*IV phase*). Notwithstanding this remarkable involution, isles of functioning thymic tissue are also present in old age.

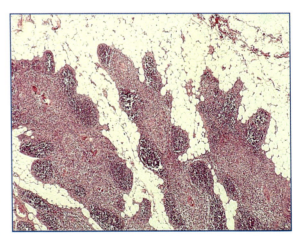

Fig. 2.4 Light micrograph of adult human thymus showing a massive adipose infiltration. Note the presence of active thymic isles. Haematoxylin-Eosin stain (specimen prepared by the Department of Anatomy and Histology of University of Modena and Reggio Emilia)

References

1. Hamilton W, Boyd JD, Mossman HW (1972) Human embryology. William and Wilkins, Baltimore
2. Stark D (1975) Embryologie, ein Lehrbuch auf Allgemein Biologischer Grundlage, 3rd edn. Thieme, Stuttgart
3. Kendall MD, Johnson HR, Singh J (1980) The weight of the human thymus gland at necropsy. J Anat 131(3):483-497
4. Dardenne M, Savino W (1990) Neuroendocrine control of the thymic epithelium modulation of thymic endocrine function, cytokine expression and cell proliferation by hormones and peptides. PNEI 3:18-25
5. Dargemont C, Dunon D, Deugnier M et al (1989) Thymatoxin, a chemotactic protein, is identical to b2-microglobulin. Science 246:803-806
6. Watanabe N, Wang Y, Lee H et al (2005) Hassall's corpuscles instruct dendritic cells to induce CD4+ CD25+ regulatory T cells in human thymus. Nature 436(7054):1181-1185
7. Janossi G, Prentice HG, Grob JP et al (1986) T lymphocyte regeneration after transplantation of R cell depleted allogeneic bone marrow. Clin Exp Immunol 63:577-586
8. Agus DB, Surh CD, Sprent J (1991) Re-entry of T cells to the adult thymus is restricted to activated T cells. J Exp Med 173:1039-1046
9. Marshall AHE, White RG (1961) The immunological reactivity of the thymus. Brit J Exp 77(8):515-524
10. Raviola E, Karnosky MJ (1972) Evidence for a blood-thymus barrier using electron opaque tracers. J Exp Med 136:466-498
11. Sutherland JS, Goldberg GL, Hammet MV et al (2005) Activation of thymic regeneration in mice and humans following androgen blockade. J Immunol 175(4):2741-2753

CHAPTER 3
Physiology and Immunology of the Thymus Gland

Milena Nasi, Marcello Pinti, Leonarda Troiano, Andrea Cossarizza

Introduction

The thymus is a gland located in the upper anterior portion of the chest cavity just behind the sternum. Under the evolutionary pressure exerted by the emergence of adaptive immunity and its inherent risk to form receptors that recognize self molecules, this gland appeared about 500 million years ago as a novel structure that had the role of instructing T-cells in order to prevent autoimmunity and orchestrate self-tolerance. The thymus has thus become a crucial lymphoid organ in which cells arriving from the bone marrow undergo a finely tuned process of selection, based on the specificity of T-cell receptors (TCRs), and differentiate into mature T-cells. The development of thymocytes involves a stringent selection in which only 1-3% of these cells succeed in survival and can leave the gland to colonize the periphery and give origin to effective immune cells [1-3]. During the maturation in the thymus, T-cells are first positively selected for "usefulness" [positive selection, driven by the affinity of the clonotypic TCR for Major Histocompatibility Complex (MHC) molecules] and then negatively selected against autoreactivity (negative selection, driven by the recognition of self peptides on self MHC by the TCR, which triggers the process of cell death). These intrathymic events are governed by sequential interactions of thymocytes with different stromal cell types during the migration through the thymus, essentially from the external to the internal part of the thymic *lobuli*. The mature T-cells, called naïve T-cells, leave the organ and contribute to the peripheral T-cell pool.

The complex process of intrathymic maturation of T-lymphocytes involves various thymic-specific factors and several other molecules. Indeed, T-cell maturation requires either direct cell-to-cell or paracrine interactions, that occur via cytokines or thymic hormones produced by the cells of the thymic microenvironment.

For a long time the functions of the thymus have remained obscure [4]. The first demonstration of its crucial role in the ontogeny and development of the immune system was provided in 1961, when it was shown that mice thymectomized immediately after birth had poorly developed lymphoid tissues, impaired immune responses and susceptibility to infections [5, 6]. Although cells present in the thymus were believed to be immunoincompetent, a few years later it was shown that they could proliferate after an antigenic challenge and produce cells unable to synthesize antibodies. Such cells were capable of enabling other lymphocytes to differentiate to antibody-forming cells. This was the first demonstration, in mammalians, of the existence of two major subsets of lymphocytes, now known as T- and B-cells. It required a re-evaluation of many immunological phenomena, such as tolerance, memory, and autoimmunity, and it was followed by a huge number of studies elucidating many of the mysteries of the immune system [4, 7, 8].

Immune Functions of the Thymus

The development of T-cells in the thymus consists of several processes that require the dynamic relocation of developing lymphocytes into, within, and out of the environments of the gland [9]. These processes include:

– Entry of lymphoid progenitor cells into the thymus;
– The generation of cells expressing both the CD4 and CD8 molecules on the plasma membrane, defined "double-positive" (DP) thymocytes, at the outer cortex of the thymus;
– The positive selection of DP thymocytes in the cortex;
– The interaction of positively selected thymocytes with medullary thymic epithelial cells (mTECs) to complete thymocyte development and ensure central tolerance (negative selection);
– The export of mature T-cells from the thymus.

Migration of Progenitors from Bone Marrow

In humans, lymphoid progenitor cells arrive into the thymus at the eightth week of gestation [10, 11], and the arrival is mediated by at least two different pathways: The vasculature-independent pathway, which probably occurs during the very early stage of embryonic development before vascularization of the thymus, and the vasculature-dependent pathway, which probably occurs in the late stage of embryogenesis and postnatally after vascularization.

It is thought that vasculature-independent colonization of the fetal thymus is regulated by the chemotactic attraction of lymphoid progenitor cells to the thymic primordium. Different chemokines are involved in fetal thymus colonization, but this process still remains unclear, and some of these chemokines (or other molecules exerting such function) are not fully characterized. In the postnatal thymus, lymphoid progenitor cells that have just entered the thymic parenchyma are found mainly in the area close to the corticomedullary junction, where the vasculature is well developed. This suggests that this area is the main port of entrance of the precursors into the organ [12].

In the adult, the seeding of the progenitors in the thymus is regulated by adhesive interaction between platelet (P)-selectin glycoprotein ligand 1 (PSGL1), which is expressed by circulating lymphoid progenitor cells, and P-selectin, which is expressed by the thymic endothelium [13]. Interestingly, the entry of lymphoid progenitor cells into the thymus is not a continuous phenomenon, but an intermittent and gated event that occurs in waves during embryogenesis and in adulthood [9, 14-16].

The Development of Conventional T-Cells Bearing an αβ-T-Cell Receptor

During thymic development, early T-cell progenitors arrive from the bloodstream and undergo a complex series of migration, proliferation, and differentiation events before returning to the circulation as mature T-cells. Each T-cell stage is characterized by the different expression of surface molecules, which contribute to the maturation. Each event that drives T-cell maturation takes place in a discrete region of the thymus, and depends upon fine interactions with specialized resident cells that are present in discrete anatomical regions. The positive selection of cells bearing as TCR a heterodimer formed by the α and the β chain (named αβ-T-cells) occurs mainly in the cortex. This selection involves a weak recognition of self-peptides bound to MHC molecules expressed on cortical thymic epithelial cells (cTECs) by the newly formed αβ-TCR expressed by on cortical thymocytes, resulting in thymocyte survival and maturation.

The central medullary region of the thymus is the main site where negative selection occurs, after a strong recognition of self peptide-MHC complexes displayed on cells such as thymic dendritic cells and mTECs. Thymocytes whose TCR recognize self antigens trigger the process of cell death/apoptosis [9, 17]. Following entry into the thymus, lymphoid progenitor cells begin their development into T-cells through the developmental pathway. Thymocytes move from the cortico-medullary junction to the subcapsular region of the thymic cortex [12]. In the first stage thymocyte progenitors are characterized by the absence of the co-receptors CD4 and CD8, and of the α chain of IL-2 receptor (CD25), and by the expression of CD44 (a glycoprotein involved in cell-cell interactions, cell adhesion, and migration). These thymocytes, called CD4–CD8–CD44+CD25-double-negative 1 (DN1) cells, are found near their site of entry, namely at the corticomedullary junction.

The slightly more mature CD4–CD8–CD44+CD25+DN2 subset (which expresses CD25) is found throughout the cortex, whereas the CD4–CD8–CD44–CD25+DN3 subset (that looses CD44) is concentrated in the outermost part of the thymus, just below the thymic capsule [12]. Several chemokine receptors, including CXCR4, CCR7, and CCR9, are likely involved in the movement of immature thymocytes [18-20]. In the thymic cortex, going to the subcapsular region, DN thymocytes begin to rearrange the locus that codifies for the TCR-β chain. Cells that succeed in generating the in-frame β rearrangement begin assembling TCR-β and pre-TCR-α (pTα) chains to form the pre-TCR complex present on the cell surface [21, 22]. The successful expression of the pre-TCR complex on the cell surface [22, 23], along with the δ-Notch interaction, initiates the signals for further development to CD4+CD8+DP thymocytes that express a TCR-αβ receptor [24]. This is the first checkpoint of T-cell development at the DN3 stage, which censors the cells that have succeeded in performing a functional TCR-β rearrangement, and allows further development of thymocytes beyond the DN3 stage. The subcapsular region of the thymus is rich in transforming growth factor-β (TGF-β), which retards the cell-cycle progression of pre-DP thymocytes and controls the generation of DP thymocytes [25], indicating that the migration of pre-DP thymocytes to the subcapsular region might have a role in regulating the rate of production of such cells.

The progression from the DN1 to DN3 stage is also regulated by an interplay of Notch1 and interleukin-7 (IL-7) receptor signaling. During these phases, rearrangements of different loci (γ, δ, and β) of the TCR occur. Successful (in-frame) TCR-β rearrangement allows DN3 thymocytes to assemble pre-TCR complexes to induce "β-selection". This process allows DN3 thymocytes to survive, proliferate, and generate a large pool of CD4+CD8+DP thymocytes that exit the cell cycle and begin the rearrangement of the TCR-α chain. However, DN2/DN3 thymocytes that make successful rearrangements of the TCR-γ and δ chain typically become DN γδ-T-cells. Along this developmental pathway, immature DN thymocytes also promote the differentiation of thymic stromal cells and trigger the formation of the cortical-epithelial environment in the thymus [26-29]. The differentiation of thymocytes from the DN1 stage to the DN3 stage regulates the differentiation of TEC precursor cells into cTECs that form the cortical environment in the thymus.

The Positive Selection of DP Thymocytes

DP thymocytes, generated in the cortex, express low levels of the αβ-TCR complex [30, 31]. These thymocytes interact through their TCR with peptide-MHC complexes, which are expressed by stromal cells, such as cTECs and dendritic cells (DC) present in the cortex [31]. Following a low avidity interaction between TCR and the MHC-peptide complex, DP thymocytes are induced to receive signals for survival and further differentiation into single positive (SP) thymocytes. This process, referred to as positive selection, enriches "useful" T-cells that are potentially reactive to foreign, but not to self, antigens presented by self-MHC molecules. By contrast, high-avidity interactions elicit signals that lead to the death of thymocytes. In order to escape a default fate of programmed cell death, DP thymocytes must express αβ-TCR complexes that can recognize self-MHC molecules presenting self-peptides on cTECs [32]. Positively selected DP thymocytes are induced to differentiate into SP (CD4+CD8− or CD4−CD8+) thymocytes and relocate to the medulla.

Cortical thymocytes move randomly before positive selection, stop and form contacts with TECs at the initiation of positive selection, and migrate rapidly to the medulla after such process. The rapid migration of positively selected thymocytes from the cortex to the medulla may help to terminate positive selection signals and to ensure that the process of screening for self-reactivity to medullary antigens begins in a timely way. The involvement of several chemokines in cell migration, as well as the expression patterns of chemokines and their receptors in the thymus underline the importance of these molecules in cell migration [33, 34]. A variety of chemokines regulate the migration of T-cell progenitors through the thymus, and in fact mutations in genes encoding chemokines or their receptors can lead to mislocalization of thymocyte populations [17].

The Negative Selection of Self-Reactive Cells

The thymic medulla provides a highly specialized microenvironment where the removal of thymocytes bearing self-reactive TCRs occurs. This microenvironment is formed by medullary thymocytes, dendritic cells, macrophages, and mTECs. The SP thymocytes spend approximately 12 days in the medulla before being exported from the thymus [2]. During this period, SP thymocytes go through a maturation process that can be identified by analyzing the expression profiles of CD62 ligand [CD62L, also known as lymphocyte (L)-selectin] and the C-type lectin receptor CD69 [35-37]. The newly generated SP thymocytes are $CD62L^{low}CD69^{hi}$ semi-mature cells that are functionally incompetent and have to undergo further maturation to become mature $CD62L^{hi}CD69^{low}$ SP functional thymocytes.

The maturation of SP thymocyte occurs in the medulla, and is accompanied by further deletion of self-reactive thymocytes. This is crucial in establishing central tolerance to tissue-specific antigens, as mTECs express tissue-specific antigens promiscuously [38]. Such expression is, at least in part, dependent on a molecule called "transcriptional factor autoimmune regulator" (AIRE) [39, 40]. Indeed, in humans, the deficiency in AIRE results in the failure in establishing central tolerance to tissue-specific antigens, and origins a syndrome defined autoimmune polyendocrinopathy-candidiasis-ectodermal-dystrophy (APECED) in humans [41, 42], and a similar autoimmune disease in mice [43-45].

The period of maturation in the medulla is essential for SP thymocytes to establish central tolerance by ensuring the deletion of autoreactive T-cells [45-47] and by producing regulatory T-cells (Treg) [48-50]. In fact, it has been shown that most forkhead box P3 (FoxP3)-expressing regulatory T-cells within the thymus are found in the medulla [48].

Interactions between medullary thymocytes and mTECs do not go in one direction only. Although mTECs can induce negative selection in medullary thymocytes, in turn thymocytes can promote the maturation of mTECs. The expression of AIRE in mTECs contributes to several functions of these cells, including the expression of tissue-restricted antigens, which are crucial to create a microenvironment where negative selection can occur efficiently.

Finally, positively and negatively selected SP thymocytes can leave the gland and form the peripheral pool of T-cells. The export of mature thymocytes from the thymic parenchyma to the circulation occurs through the perivascular space, which is channeled to postcapillary venules, arterioles, and lymphatics [51, 52]. However, it is still unclear whether T-cells in the perivascular space are subsequently released into the blood, or into the lymphatics, or both. The signals that regulate the movement of mature thymocytes back into circulation are not still clearly identified. In particular, the G protein-coupled receptor S1P1 (sphingosine 1-phosphate type 1 receptor) is key to both the exit of mature T-cells from the thymus and the exit of lymphocytes from lymph nodes [53]. Although S1P1 can function in a cell-autonomous way on lymphocytes, S1P receptors are also expressed by endothelial cells and may also act to regulate the opening of sites for exit [54, 55]. S1P is present at high concentrations in the blood and lymph but is maintained at a low concentration in the thymus and other tissues because of the action of the enzyme S1P lyase [56]. This indicates that a S1P gradient, established between the thymus and blood or lymph, could mediate the export of mature thymocytes. Other factors have been linked to the control of thymic exit. For example, a role could be played by CD69, which is normally downregulated on mature thymocytes before their exit from the thymus; its overexpression leads to the retention of these cells in the medulla [57]. A complete understanding of how thymocytes leave the thymus awaits more information about the mechanism of action of S1P, adhesion molecules, and chemokines, as well as a more detailed identification of the anatomy of thymocyte egress.

Alternative T-Lymphocyte Lineages

Although most T-cells produced in the thymus express an $\alpha\beta$-TCR and carry out MHC-restricted immune responses, the thymus also produces other alternative T-cell lineages, including regulatory T-cells (Treg cells), natural killer T (NKT) cells and $\gamma\delta$-T-cells, with distinct effector activities and specificities, and distinct developmental pathways. The production of these T-cell lineages depends on thymic microenvironments that differ from those that are required for the development of conventional $\alpha\beta$-T-cells [17].

Regulatory T-Cells

A specialized microenvironment created by crosstalk between TECs and medullary dendritic cells is crucial to the development of Treg cells. Treg cells help to maintain self-tolerance by actively suppressing immune responses [58, 59]. Many Treg cells resemble conventional CD4+ T-cells bearing an $\alpha\beta$-TCR, but can be distinguished by their expression of FoxP3 [60, 61], and by the constitutive expression of high levels of CD25 and low levels of CD127 [62]. Recent data also suggest that Treg can express other molecules such as CD39 [(nucleoside triphosphate diphosphohydrolase-1 (NTPDase 1)], an ectoenzyme that degrades ATP to AMP [63], or the chemokine receptor CCR6 [64].

Their development differs from that of conventional $\alpha\beta$-T-cells in that they appear relatively late in ontogeny and are insensitive to negatively selecting signals [65]. Hassal's corpuscles may provide a specialized microenvironment for the development of Treg cells [50]. A group of epithelial cells resident in the Hassal's corpuscles of the human thymus can regulate medullary DC function promoting the MHC-dependent conversion of CD4+CD8–CD25– thymocytes into FoxP3+CD4+CD25^{hi} Treg cells. In addition, analysis of fixed thymus sections has shown that thymocytes with a Treg cell phenotype are found in close association with Hassal's corpuscles. It is not known whether these events are relevant to the development of Treg cells in mice, in part because Hassal's corpuscle-like structures are relatively rare in mouse thymus [66]. Assuming that, in mouse, similar structures regulate Treg cell development, other cytokines may mediate the crosstalk between mTECs and DC.

Natural Killer T-Cells (NKT Cells)

Cortical DP thymocytes are crucial for the development of a subpopulation of T-cells called NKT cells. This term was used for the first time to define a subset of murine $\alpha\beta$-T-cells characterized by the expression of the NK1.1 marker and the preferential usage of Vα14 TCR [67]. In humans, a large subset of NKT cells expresses an $\alpha\beta$-TCR encoded by variable α-region 24 (Vα24) and joining α-region 18 (Jα18) gene segments, and recognizes self and foreign glycolipid antigens bound to the nonclassical MHC class I molecule CD1d [68]. Most Vα24Jα18 T-lymphocytes also express CD161 (equivalent to murine NK1.1). CD161 (NKR-P1A) is a type II disulfide-linked homodimer, expressed on most NK cells, a subset of peripheral T-cells and on invariant NKT cells. The ligand for human NKR-P1A is lectin-like transcript-1 (LLT1), and the interaction of NKR-P1A with LLT1 inhibits NK cytotoxicity [69].

NKT cells can be identified by using CD1d tetramers containing the glycolipid α-galactosylceramide, and indeed most NKT cells recognize CD1d-bound endogenous glycosphingolipids and a component of microbial cell wall, i.e., α-glycuronosylceramide [70]. This suggests that NKT cells play a key role in the protection from bacteria that are not detected by pattern recognition receptors. The development of NKT cells that bind CD1d-α-galactosylceramide is dependent on CD1d expression on hematopoietic cells [71, 72]. Notably, expression of CD1d exclusively on DP thymocytes is sufficient to promote NKT lineage expansion and NKT cell differentiation [73]. In contrast, CD1d expression on TECs is not sufficient to allow NKT cell maturation [74]. It is unclear why CD1d on cortical thymocytes but not on TECs can promote NKT cell development.

γδ-T-Cells

Conventional αβ-T-cells reside primarily in secondary lymphoid organs and play a central role in adaptive immune responses. On the contrary, most T-cells expressing a γδ-TCR reside in epithelial layers of tissues underlying internal and external surfaces of the body, such as the skin, intestinal epithelium, lung, and tongue, where they act as the first line of defense [75-78]. In these locations, the diversity of the TCR repertoire is much more limited than that observed in αβ-T-cells, or even than that of γδ-T-cells that reside in secondary lymphoid organs [77]. Furthermore, the repertoire of variable region genes differs strikingly in the various anatomical locations. The highly restricted TCR expressed by different subsets of γδ-T-cells enable them to recognize ligands that are specifically expressed in infected, diseased, or stressed cells in those anatomical sites [77, 78]. Early T-cell development in the thymus is characterized by progressive waves of differentiation of distinct γδ subsets characterized by expression of specific Vγ and Vδ genes. The underlying processes presumably evolved to produce functionally distinct sets of γδ-T-cells in an organized manner [79].

Cortical thymocytes provide signals essential to the development of adult γδ-T-cells. Several studies on the development of these lymphocytes have focused on the involvement of TCR gene rearrangements and TCR signaling, and the function of the thymic microenvironment and DP thymocytes has been emphasized [80-82]. Interactions with DP thymocytes may be one of several features that distinguish the development of γδ-T-cells in the fetus or in the adult. Although those distinctions are mostly due to the different progenitor cell populations that populate the fetal or adult thymus [83, 84], the fact that fetal γδ-T-cells develop in a thymic environment with few or no DP thymocytes may also contribute to some of their distinctive properties [85, 86].

In contrast with what happens for conventional αβ-T-lymphocytes, the absence of MHC molecules had no observable effect on the intrathymic development of γδ-T-cells [87-89]. This suggests that most γδ-T-cells are not selected by classical or non-classical MHC class I molecules that depend on $β_2$-microglobulin for expression on the cell surface. However, it cannot be excluded that MHC could play a role in selection of a subset of γδ-T-cells. In fact, since the natural ligands for γδ-T-cells are in most cases not known, it remains possible that these cells are positively selected by interactions with unidentified ligands in the thymus.

Endocrine Functions of the Thymus

The reticulo-epithelial (RE) cells play a vital role in lymphoid cell homing and development. Not only do thymic RE cells secrete numerous cytokines, including IL-1 and -6, granulocyte colony stimulating factor (G-CSF), macrophage CSF (M-CSF) and GM-CSF, which likely are important during the various stages of thymocyte activation and differentiation, but they also produce and release different hormones. As a proof of concept, several extracts that promote T-cell differentiation have been prepared from thymus tissue [90-93]. Chemical characterization of these extracts has allowed the identification of active peptides, named thymic hormones, some of which have been sequenced and synthesized. Peptides that differ in amino acid sequence and biological properties such as the thymosins, the thymopoietin, the thymulin [94], and the thymic humoral factor (THF) have been extensively investigated [95].

Thymosins

The isolation from the thymus gland of the thymosins, a family of biologically active molecules with hormone-like properties, that are biochemically and functionally distinct, was first described more than 40 years ago [96]. In the early 1970s, preclinical studies showed the immunorestorative effects of a partially purified thymosin preparation named "thymosin fraction 5" (TF5) [97]. TF5 consists of a mixture of small polypeptides. The biological activity of several isolated peptides was studied: None of the isolated peptides was really a "pure" thymic hormone, solely produced in this gland; nevertheless, they are biologically important peptides with diverse intracellular and extracellular functions. Thymosins were originally obtained from the thymus, but they are widely distributed in many tissues and cells, and studies on these functions are still in progress [98, 99]. In any case, thymosins can be divided into three main groups, namely α-, β-, and γ-thymosins.

α-thymosins (ProTα, Tα1) have nuclear localization and are involved in transcription and/or DNA replications; β-thymosins (Tβ4, Tβ10, Tβ15) have cytoplasmic localization and show high affinity to G-actin for cell mobility. Furthermore, both α- and β-thymosins play important roles in modulating immune response, vascular biology, and cancer pathogenesis. It has been suggested that thymosins might have clinical applications in cancer treatment [99]. Human serum levels of Tα1 show significant differences with age, gender, and race [100-102]. Tα1 is able to stimulate the production of lymphokines, such as migration-inhibiting factor, interferon-α, interferon-γ, interleukin-2 (IL-2), and IL-2 receptor [103-110]. In addition, Tα1 plays roles in several phenomena, including; i) the induction of T-helper cells; ii) expression of phenotypic T-cell markers; iii) modulation of lymphoproliferative responses triggered by specific antigens, alloantigens, and mitogens; iv) antibody production; v) T-cell cytotoxicity; and vi) natural killer cell activity [110-115].

Although β-thymosins have been identified as G-actin-binding proteins, their physiologic activities are largely unknown, including their role in the immune system. In general, intracellular β-thymosins may affect cell growth and migration. Tβ4 can induce expression of terminal deoxynucleotidyl transferase in T-cells [116], stimulates secretion of a luteinizing hormone (LH)-releasing factor and an LH [117, 118], inhibits the migration of macrophages in vitro [109], and induces phenotypic changes in a T-cell line [119].

Thymopoietin and Thymopentin

Thymopoietin is a polypeptide consisting of 49 amino acids. The pentapeptide thymopentin (TP-5), corresponding to amino acids 32-36 of thymopoietin (i.e., Arg-Lys-Asp-Val-Tyr), represents the active site of thymopoietin, and indeed it has all the biological activities of the native hormone. Thymopoietin has a pleiotropic action, affecting neuromuscular transmission, or early T-cell differentiation. Not only can TP-5 act as an immunomodulatory factor in cancer chemotherapy, but it also acts as a potential chemotherapeutic agent since it can inhibit the growth of human promyelocyte leukemia cells [120]. Moreover, the capability of TP-5 to associate with MHC class II molecules expressed by antigen-presenting cells has been recently shown, providing a new perspective to understand the immunomodulation mechanism induced by TP-5 [121].

The immunoregulatory actions of TP-5 on peripheral T-cells are mediated by increases in the intracellular levels of cyclic GMP, in contrast to the intracellular cyclic AMP elevations induced in precursor T-cells, which trigger their further differentiation to T-cells. Thymopoietin and thymopentin are able to normalize several immunological defects present in a number of animal models of immune dysbalance. These include the effects of thymectomy as well as the thymic involution associated with aging, or induced by other procedures in thymus-intact animals. The normalizing action of thymopentin, whether the immune dysbalance be in the direction of hyper- or hyporesponsiveness, points to its potential utility in human diseases [122].

Thymulin

Thymulin, originally named "facteur thymique sérique" or FTS, is a molecule exclusively produced by thymic epithelial cells. It consists of a nonapeptide component coupled to the ion zinc, which confers a strong biological activity to this molecule [94, 123]. After its discovery in the early 1970s, thymulin was characterized as a thymic hormone involved in several aspects of intra- and extrathymic T-cell differentiation. Subsequently, it was demonstrated that thymulin production and secretion is strongly influenced by the neuroendocrine system. Conversely, an emerging core of information points to thymulin as a hypophysotropic peptide.

Thymulin is involved in several aspects of intra- and extrathymic T-cell differentiation [124]. The control of thymulin secretion seems to be dependent on a complex network of events. Initial studies showed that the hormone itself exerts a controlling feedback effect on its own secretion both in vivo and in vitro [124, 125]. Additionally, thymulin production and secretion is influenced directly or indirectly by the neuroendocrine system. For instance, growth hormone (GH) can influence thymulin synthesis and secretion. In vitro, GH stimulates thymulin release from TEC lines [126], which are known to possess specific receptors for GH [127].

The existence of a neuroendocrine-thymic axis is well established, and strong evidence suggest that thymulin plays a physiological role as part of an ascending feedback loop in this axis [128].

Thymic Humoral Factor (THF)

Thymic humoral factor-γ2 (THF-γ2) is an immunoregulatory peptide present in thymic extracts [95, 129-131]; isolated and purified from calf thymus, it has been identified as an octapeptide [132]. It was characterized as stimulating T-cell functions such as the response to T-cell lectins [133] and mixed lymphocyte reactions [134], graft versus host reactivity [135], and cytotoxic responses both in thymus-deprived and in intact mice [136]. THF-γ2 also stimulates the production of IL-2 [137] and has been used as an immunomodulator in clinical conditions associated with immune impairment and dysregulation [138]. Addition of THF-γ2 immunotherapy to chemotherapy is more effective than chemotherapy alone in the arrest of tumor and metastatic growth [139] and THF-γ2 treatment restores the levels of T-cell subsets decreased by chemotherapy [140].

Neuroendocrine Control of Thymus Physiology

The interplay between the neuroendocrine and immune systems has been under extensive studies for several years. Hormones and neuropeptides influence the activities of this organ and its cells via endocrine and local autocrine/paracrine pathways. Receptors for a huge number of molecules are heterogeneously expressed in all subsets of thymic cells, and the communications are tuned by feedback circuitries. The immune and neuroendocrine systems use similar ligands and receptors to establish physiological intra- and intersystem communications that play an important role in homeostasis. Increasing evidence has placed hormones and neuropeptides among potent immunomodulators, participating in various aspects of immune system function, in both health and disease [141-144]. More particularly, the molecules that modulate the physiology of the thymus include steroids and polypeptidic hormones, as well as neuropeptides.

As an example, it is known that GH pleiotropically modulates thymic functions: GH upregulates proliferation of thymocytes and thymic epithelial cells [145]. GH-transgenic mice, as well as animals and humans treated with exogenous GH, exhibit an enhanced cellularity in the organ; accordingly, several studies suggest the clinical utility of GH in patients infected with HIV, who could benefit from an exogenous supplementation of this molecule to improve thymic activity, and thus better reconstitute the immune system [146-148].

GH stimulates the secretion of thymic hormones, cytokines, and chemokines by the thymic microenvironment, as well as the production of extracellular matrix proteins, leading to an increase in thymocyte migratory responses and intrathymic traffic of developing T-cells. In addition, GH stimulates the in vivo export of thymocytes from the organ, as ascertained by studies with intrathymic injection of GH in normal mice and with GH-transgenic mice. Moreover, since GH is produced by thymocytes and thymic epithelial cells, which also express GH receptors, it is likely that in addition to the classic endocrine pathway, the GH control of the thymus may include an autocrine/paracrine pathway.

This example indicates how the thymus is physiologically under neuroendocrine control. Such control is extremely complex, and, as in the aforementioned case, involves biological pathways that include the intrathymic production of a variety of hormones and neuropeptides, along with the presence, in thymic cells, of their respective receptors [149].

References

1. Scollay RG, Butcher EC, Weissman IL (1980) Thymus cell migration. Quantitative aspects of cellular traffic from the thymus to the periphery in mice. Eur J Immunol 10:210-218
2. Egerton M, Scollay R, Shortman K (1990) Kinetics of mature T-cell development in the thymus. Proc Natl Acad Sci USA 87:2579-2582
3. Goldrath AW, Bevan MJ (1999) Selecting and maintaining a diverse T-cell repertoire. Nature 402:255-262
4. Miller JF (2002) The discovery of thymus function and of thymus-derived lymphocytes. Immunol Rev 185:7-14
5. Miller JF (1961) Analysis of the thymus influence in leukaemogenesis. Nature 191:248-249
6. Miller JF (1961) Immunological function of the thymus. Lancet 2:748-749

7. Miller JF (1965) The role of the thymus in immune processes. Int Arch Allergy Appl Immunol 28:61-70
8. Miller JF (1967) The thymus. Yesterday, today, and tomorrow. Lancet 2:1299-1302
9. Takahama Y (2006) Journey through the thymus: Stromal guides for T-cell development and selection. Nat Rev Immunol 6:127-135
10. Owen JJ, Ritter MA (1969) Tissue interaction in the development of thymus lymphocytes. J Exp Med 129:431-442
11. Haynes BF, Heinly CS (1995) Early human T cell development: Analysis of the human thymus at the time of initial entry of hematopoietic stem cells into the fetal thymic microenvironment. J Exp Med 181:1445-1458
12. Lind EF, Prockop SE, Porritt HE, Petrie HT (2001) Mapping precursor movement through the postnatal thymus reveals specific microenvironments supporting defined stages of early lymphoid development. J Exp Med 194:127-134
13. Rossi FM, Corbel SY, Merzaban JS et al (2005) Recruitment of adult thymic progenitors is regulated by P-selectin and its ligand PSGL-1. Nat Immunol 6:626-634
14. Le Douarin NM, Jotereau FV (1975) Tracing of cells of the avian thymus through embryonic life in interspecific chimeras. J Exp Med 142:17-40
15. Havran WL, Allison JP (1988) Developmentally ordered appearance of thymocytes expressing different T-cell antigen receptors. Nature 335:443-445
16. Foss DL, Donskoy E, Goldschneider I (2001) The importation of hematogenous precursors by the thymus is a gated phenomenon in normal adult mice. J Exp Med 193:365-374
17. Ladi E, Yin X, Chtanova T, Robey EA (2006) Thymic microenvironments for T cell differentiation and selection. Nat Immunol 7:338-343
18. Plotkin J, Prockop SE, Lepique A, Petrie HT (2003) Critical role for CXCR4 signaling in progenitor localization and T cell differentiation in the postnatal thymus. J Immunol 171:4521-4527
19. Misslitz A, Pabst O, Mintzen J et al (2004) Thymic T cell development and progenitor localization depend on CCR7. J Exp Med 200:481-491
20. Benz C, Heinzel K, Bleul CC (2004) Homing of immature thymocytes to the subcapsular microenvironment within the thymus is not an absolute requirement for T cell development. Eur J Immunol 34:3652-3663
21. Raulet DH, Garman RD, Saito H, Tonegawa S (1985) Developmental regulation of T-cell receptor gene expression. Nature 314:103-107
22. von Boehmer H, Fehling HJ (1997) Structure and function of the pre-T cell receptor. Annu Rev Immunol 15:433-452
23. Irving BA, Alt FW, Killeen N (1998) Thymocyte development in the absence of pre-T cell receptor extracellular immunoglobulin domains. Science 280:905-908
24. Ciofani M, Zuniga-Pflucker JC (2005) Notch promotes survival of pre-T cells at the beta-selection checkpoint by regulating cellular metabolism. Nat Immunol 6:881-888
25. Takahama Y, Letterio JJ, Suzuki H et al (1994) Early progression of thymocytes along the CD4/CD8 developmental pathway is regulated by a subset of thymic epithelial cells expressing transforming growth factor beta. J Exp Med 179:1495-1506
26. Hollander GA et al (1995) Developmental control point in induction of thymic cortex regulated by a subpopulation of prothymocytes. Nature 373:350-353
27. van Ewijk W, Hollander G, Terhorst C, Wang B (2000) Stepwise development of thymic microenvironments in vivo is regulated by thymocyte subsets. Development 127:1583-1591
28. Klug DB, Carter C, Crouch E et al (1998) Interdependence of cortical thymic epithelial cell differentiation and T-lineage commitment. Proc Natl Acad Sci USA 95:11822-11827
29. Klug DB, Carter C, Gimenez-Conti IB, Richie ER (2002) Cutting edge: Thymocyte-independent and thymocyte-dependent phases of epithelial patterning in the fetal thymus. J Immunol 169:2842-2845
30. Witt CM, Raychaudhuri S, Schaefer B et al (2005) Directed migration of positively selected thymocytes visualized in real time. PLoS Biol 3:e160
31. Bousso P, Bhakta NR, Lewis RS, Robey E (2002) Dynamics of thymocyte-stromal cell interactions visualized by two-photon microscopy. Science 296:1876-1880
32. Guidos C (2006) Thymus and T-lymphocyte development: What is new in the 21st century? Immunol Rev 209:5-9
33. Bleul CC, Boehm T (2000) Chemokines define distinct microenvironments in the developing thymus. Eur J Immunol 30:3371-3379
34. Campbell JJ, Butcher EC (2000) Chemokines in tissue-specific and microenvironment-specific lymphocyte homing. Curr Opin Immunol 12:336-341
35. Reichert RA, Weissman IL, Butcher EC (1986) Phenotypic analysis of thymocytes that express homing receptors for peripheral lymph nodes. J Immunol 136:3521-3528
36. Bendelac A, Matzinger P, Seder RA et al (1992) Activation events during thymic selection. J Exp Med 175:731-742
37. Ramsdell F, Jenkins M, Dinh Q, Fowlkes BJ (1991) The majority of CD4+8- thymocytes are functionally immature. J Immunol 147:1779-1785
38. Kyewski B, Derbinski J (2004) Self-representation in the thymus: An extended view. Nat Rev Immunol 4:688-698
39. Derbinski J et al (2005) Promiscuous gene expression in thymic epithelial cells is regulated at multiple levels. J Exp Med 202:33-45
40. Zuklys S, Balciunaite G, Agarwal A et al (2000) Normal thymic architecture and negative selection are associated with Aire expression, the gene defective in the autoimmune-polyendocrinopathy-candidiasis-ectodermal dystrophy (APECED). J Immunol 165:1976-1983
41. Aaltonen J et al (1997) High-resolution physical and transcriptional mapping of the autoimmune polyen-

docrinopathy-candidiasis-ectodermal dystrophy locus on chromosome 21q22.3 by FISH. Genome Res 7:820-829
42. Nagamine K, Peterson P, Scott HS et al (1997) Positional cloning of the APECED gene. Nat Genet 17:393-398
43. Anderson MS, Venanzi S, Klein L et al (2002) Projection of an immunological self shadow within the thymus by the aire protein. Science 298:1395-1401
44. Kuroda N, Mitani T, Takeda N et al (2005) Development of autoimmunity against transcriptionally unrepressed target antigen in the thymus of Aire-deficient mice. J Immunol 174:1862-1870
45. Liston A, Lesage S, Wilson J et al (2003) Aire regulates negative selection of organ-specific T cells. Nat Immunol 4:350-354
46. Anderson MS, Venanzi ES, Chen Z et al (2005) The cellular mechanism of Aire control of T cell tolerance. Immunity 23:227-239
47. Gallegos AM, Bevan MJ (2004) Central tolerance to tissue-specific antigens mediated by direct and indirect antigen presentation. J Exp Med 200:1039-1049
48. Fontenot JD, Rasmussen JP, Williams LM et al (2005) Regulatory T cell lineage specification by the forkhead transcription factor Foxp3. Immunity 22:329-341
49. Sakaguchi S (2004) Naturally arising CD4+ regulatory T cells for immunologic self-tolerance and negative control of immune responses. Annu Rev Immunol 22:531-562
50. Watanabe N et al (2005) Hassall's corpuscles instruct dendritic cells to induce CD4+CD25+ regulatory T cells in human thymus. Nature 436:1181-1185
51. Kato S (1997) Thymic microvascular system. Microsc Res Tech 38:287-299
52. Muller KM, Luedecker CJ, Udey MC, Farr AG (1997) Involvement of E-cadherin in thymus organogenesis and thymocyte maturation. Immunity 6:257-264
53. Cyster JG (2005) Chemokines, sphingosine-1-phosphate, and cell migration in secondary lymphoid organs. Annu Rev Immunol 23:127-159
54. Mandala S, Hajdu R, Bergstrom J et al (2002) Alteration of lymphocyte trafficking by sphingosine-1-phosphate receptor agonists. Science 296:346-349
55. Wei SH, Rosen H, Matheu MP et al (2005) Sphingosine 1-phosphate type 1 receptor agonism inhibits trans-endothelial migration of medullary T cells to lymphatic sinuses. Nat Immunol 6:1228-1235
56. Schwab SR, Pereira JP, Matloubian M et al (2005) Lymphocyte sequestration through S1P lyase inhibition and disruption of S1P gradients. Science 309:1735-1739
57. Feng C, Woodside KJ, Vance BA et al (2002) A potential role for CD69 in thymocyte emigration. Int Immunol 14:535-544
58. Paust S, Cantor H (2005) Regulatory T cells and autoimmune disease. Immunol Rev 204:195-207
59. Sakaguchi S (2005) Naturally arising Foxp3-expressing CD25+CD4+ regulatory T cells in immunological tolerance to self and non-self. Nat Immunol 6:345-352
60. Fontenot JD, Gavin MA, Rudensky AY (2003) Foxp3 programs the development and function of CD4+CD25+ regulatory T cells. Nat Immunol 4:330-336
61. Khattri R, Cox T, Yasayko SA, Ramsdell F (2003) An essential role for Scurfin in CD4+CD25+ T regulatory cells. Nat Immunol 4:337-342
62. Banham AH (2006) Cell-surface IL-7 receptor expression facilitates the purification of Foxp3(+) regulatory T cells. Trends Immunol 27:541-544
63. Borsellino G et al (2007) Expression of ectonucleotidase CD39 by Foxp3+ Treg cells: Hydrolysis of extracellular ATP and immune suppression. Blood 110:1225-1232
64. Kleinewietfeld M, Puentes F, Borsellino G et al (2005) CCR6 expression defines regulatory effector/memory-like cells within the CD25(+)CD4+ T-cell subset. Blood 105:2877-2886
65. Fontenot JD, Rudensky AY (2005) A well adapted regulatory contrivance: Regulatory T cell development and the forkhead family transcription factor Foxp3. Nat Immunol 6:331-337
66. Farr AG, Dooley JL, Erickson M (2002) Organization of thymic medullary epithelial heterogeneity: Implications for mechanisms of epithelial differentiation. Immunol Rev 189:20-27
67. Makino Y, Kanno R, Ito T et al (1995) Predominant expression of invariant V alpha 14+ TCR alpha chain in NK1.1+ T cell populations. Int Immunol 7:1157-1161
68. Kronenberg M (2005) Toward an understanding of NKT cell biology: Progress and paradoxes. Annu Rev Immunol 23:877-900
69. Rosen DB et al (2005) Cutting edge: Lectin-like transcript-1 is a ligand for the inhibitory human NKR-P1A receptor. J Immunol 175:7796-7799
70. Zhou D, Mattner J, Cantu C IIIrd et al (2004) Lysosomal glycosphingolipid recognition by NKT cells. Science 306:1786-1789
71. Bendelac A (1995) Positive selection of mouse NK1+ T cells by CD1-expressing cortical thymocytes. J Exp Med 182:2091-2096
72. Coles MC, Raulet DH (2000) NK1.1+ T cells in the liver arise in the thymus and are selected by interactions with class I molecules on CD4+CD8+ cells. J Immunol 164:2412-2418
73. Wei DG, Lee H, Park SH et al (2005) Expansion and long-range differentiation of the NKT cell lineage in mice expressing CD1d exclusively on cortical thymocytes. J Exp Med 202:239-248
74. Forestier C, Park SH, Wei D et al (2003) T cell development in mice expressing CD1d directed by a classical MHC class II promoter. J Immunol 171:4096-4104
75. Raulet DH (1989) The structure, function, and molecular genetics of the gamma/delta T cell receptor. Annu Rev Immunol 7:175-207
76. Haas W, Pereira P, Tonegawa S (1993) Gamma/delta cells. Annu Rev Immunol 11:637-685
77. Allison JP, Havran WL (1991) The immunobiology of T cells with invariant gamma delta antigen receptors. Annu Rev Immunol 9:679-705
78. Hayday AC (2000) Gamma delta cells: A right time and a right place for a conserved third way of protection. Annu Rev Immunol 18:975-1026

79. Xiong N, Raulet DH (2007) Development and selection of gammadelta T cells. Immunol Rev 215:15-31
80. Haks MC, Lefebvre JM, Lauritsen JP et al (2005) Attenuation of gammadeltaTCR signaling efficiently diverts thymocytes to the alphabeta lineage. Immunity 22:595-606
81. Hayes SM, Li L, Love PE (2005) TCR signal strength influences alphabeta/gammadelta lineage fate. Immunity 22:583-593
82. Robey E (2005) The alphabeta versus gammadelta T cell fate decision: When less is more. Immunity 22:533-534
83. Havran WL, Carbone A, Allison JP (1991) Murine T cells with invariant gamma delta antigen receptors: Origin, repertoire, and specificity. Semin Immunol 3:89-97
84. Ikuta K, Kina T, MacNeil I et al (1990) A developmental switch in thymic lymphocyte maturation potential occurs at the level of hematopoietic stem cells. Cell 62:863-874
85. Pennington DJ, Silva-Santos B, Shires J et al (2003) The inter-relatedness and interdependence of mouse T cell receptor gammadelta+ and alphabeta+ cells. Nat Immunol 4:991-998
86. Silva-Santos B, Pennington DJ, Hayday AC (2005) Lymphotoxin-mediated regulation of gammadelta cell differentiation by alphabeta T cell progenitors. Science 307:925-928
87. Grusby MJ, Auchincloss H Jr, Lee R et al (1993) Mice lacking major histocompatibility complex class I and class II molecules. Proc Natl Acad Sci USA 90:3913-3917
88. Correa I, Bix M, Liao NS et al (1992) Most gamma delta T cells develop normally in beta 2-microglobulin-deficient mice. Proc Natl Acad Sci USA 89:653-657
89. Bigby M, Markowitz JS, Bleicher PA et al (1993) Most gamma delta T cells develop normally in the absence of MHC class II molecules. J Immunol 151:4465-4475
90. Dardenne M, Pleau JM, Blouquit JY, Bach JF (1980) Characterization of facteur thymique serique (FTS) in the thymus. II. Direct demonstration of the presence of FTS in thymosin fraction V. Clin Exp Immunol 42:477-482
91. Goldstein G (1975) The isolation of thymopoietin (thymin). Ann N Y Acad Sci 249:177-185
92. Hooper JA, McDaniel MC, Thurman JB et al (1975) Purification and properties of bovine thymosin. Ann N Y Acad Sci 249:125-144
93. Kook AI, Yakir Y, Trainin N (1975) Isolation and partial chemical characterization of THF, a thymus hormone involved in immune maturation of lymphoid cells. Cell Immunol 19:151-157
94. Dardenne M, Pléau JM, Nabarra B et al (1982) Contribution of zinc and other metals to the biological activity of the serum thymic factor. Proc Natl Acad Sci USA 79:5370-5373
95. Goso C, Frasca D, Doria G (1992) Effect of synthetic thymic humoral factor (THF-gamma 2) on T cell activities in immunodeficient ageing mice. Clin Exp Immunol 87:346-351
96. Goldstein AL (2007) History of the discovery of the thymosins. Ann N Y Acad Sci 1112:1-13
97. Goldstein AL, Badamchian M (2004) Thymosins: Chemistry and biological properties in health and disease. Expert Opin Biol Ther 4:559-573
98. Hannappel E, Huff T (2003) The thymosins. Prothymosin alpha, parathymosin, and beta-thymosins: Structure and function. Vitam Horm 66:257-296
99. Chen C, Li M, Yang H et al (2005) Roles of thymosins in cancers and other organ systems. World J Surg 29:264-270
100. Hirokawa K, McClure JE, Goldstein AL (1982) Age-related changes in localization of thymosin in the human thymus. Thymus 4:19-29
101. Naylor PH, Friedman-Kien A, Hersh E et al (1986) Thymosin alpha 1 and thymosin beta 4 in serum: Comparison of normal, cord, homosexual and AIDS serum. Int J Immunopharmacol 8:667-676
102. Weller FE, Shah U, Cummings GD et al (1992) Serum levels of immunoreactive thymosin alpha 1 and thymosin beta 4 in large cohorts of healthy adults. Thymus 19:45-52
103. Hsia J, Sarin N, Oliver JH, Goldstein AL (1989) Aspirin and thymosin increase interleukin-2 and interferon-gamma production by human peripheral blood lymphocytes. Immunopharmacology 17:167-173
104. Huang KY, Kind PD, Jagoda EM, Goldstein AL (1981) Thymosin treatment modulates production of interferon. J Interferon Res 1:411-420
105. Leichtling KD, Serrate SA, Sztein MB (1990) Thymosin alpha 1 modulates the expression of high affinity interleukin-2 receptors on normal human lymphocytes. Int J Immunopharmacol 12:19-29
106. Serrate SA, Schulof RS, Leondaridis L et al (1987) Modulation of human natural killer cell cytotoxic activity, lymphokine production, and interleukin 2 receptor expression by thymic hormones. J Immunol 139:2338-2343
107. Svedersky LP, Hui A, May L et al (1982) Induction and augmentation of mitogen-induced immune interferon production in human peripheral blood lymphocytes by N alpha-desacetylthymosin alpha 1. Eur J Immunol 12:244-247
108. Sztein MB, Serrate SA (1989) Characterization of the immunoregulatory properties of thymosin alpha 1 on interleukin-2 production and interleukin-2 receptor expression in normal human lymphocytes. Int J Immunopharmacol 11:789-800
109. Thurman GB, Seals C, Low TL, Goldstein AL (1984) Restorative effects of thymosin polypeptides on purified protein derivative – Dependent migration inhibition factor production by the peripheral blood lymphocytes of adult thymectomized guinea pigs. J Biol Response Mod 3:160-173
110. Zatz MM, McClure JE, Goldstein AL et al (1984) Thymosin increases production of T-cell growth factor by normal human peripheral blood lymphocytes. Proc Natl Acad Sci USA 81:2882-2885

111. Ahmed A, Wong DM, Thurman GB et al (1979) T-lymphocyte maturation: Cell surface markers and immune function induced by T-lymphocyte cell-free products and thymosin polypeptides. Ann N Y Acad Sci 332:81-94
112. Baxevanis CN, Reclos GJ, Perez S et al (1987) Immunoregulatory effects of fraction 5 thymus peptides. I. Thymosin alpha 1 enhances while thymosin beta 4 suppresses the human autologous and allogeneic mixed lymphocyte reaction. Immunopharmacology 13:133-141
113. Frasca D, Adorini L, Doria G (1987) Enhanced frequency of mitogen-responsive T cell precursors in old mice injected with thymosin alpha 1. Eur J Immunol 17:727-730
114. Schulof RS, Naylor PH, Sztein MB, Goldstein AL (1987) Thymic physiology and biochemistry. Adv Clin Chem 26:203-292
115. Sztein MB, Goldstein AL (1986) Thymic hormones – A clinical update. Springer Semin Immunopathol 9:1-18
116. Low TL, Hu SK, Goldstein AL (1981) Complete amino acid sequence of bovine thymosin beta 4: a thymic hormone that induces terminal deoxynucleotidyl transferase activity in thymocyte populations. Proc Natl Acad Sci USA 78:1162-1166
117. Hall NR, McGillis JP, Spangelo BL, Goldstein AL (1985) Evidence that thymosins and other biologic response modifiers can function as neuroactive immunotransmitters. J Immunol 135:806s-811s
118. Rebar RW, Miyake A, Low TL, Goldstein AL (1981) Thymosin stimulates secretion of luteinizing hormone-releasing factor. Science 214:669-671
119. Kokkinopoulos D, Perez S, Papamichail M (1985) Thymosin beta 4 induced phenotypic changes in Molt-4 leukemic cell line. Blut 50:341-348
120. Fan YZ, Chang H, Yu Y et al (2006) Thymopentin (TP5), an immunomodulatory peptide, suppresses proliferation and induces differentiation in HL-60 cells. Biochim Biophys Acta 1763:1059-1066
121. Liu Z, Zheng X, Wang J, Wang E (2007) Molecular Analysis of Thymopentin Binding to HLA-DR Molecules. PLoS ONE 2: e1348
122. Goldstein G, Audhya TK (1985) Thymopoietin to thymopentin: Experimental studies. Surv Immunol Res 4 Suppl 1:1-10
123. Gastinel LN, Dardenne M, Pleau JM, Bach JF (1984) Studies on the zinc binding site to the serum thymic factor. Biochim Biophys Acta 797:147-155
124. Savino W, Dardenne M, Bach JF (1983) Thymic hormone containing cells. III. Evidence for a feed-back regulation of the secretion of the serum thymic factor (FTS) by thymic epithelial cells. Clin Exp Immunol 52:7-12
125. Cohen S, Berrih S, Dardenne M, Bach JF (1986) Feedback regulation of the secretion of a thymic hormone (thymulin) by human thymic epithelial cells in culture. Thymus 8:109-119
126. Timsit J, Savino W, Safieh B et al (1992) Growth hormone and insulin-like growth factor-I stimulate hormonal function and proliferation of thymic epithelial cells. J Clin Endocrinol Metab 75:183-188
127. Ban E, Gagnerault MC, Jammes H et al (1991) Specific binding sites for growth hormone in cultured mouse thymic epithelial cells. Life Sci 48:2141-2148
128. Goya RG, Brown OA, Pleau JM, Dardenne M (2004) Thymulin and the neuroendocrine system. Peptides 25:139-142
129. Kook AI, Trainin N (1974) Hormone-like activity of a thymus humoral factor on the induction of immune competence in lymphoid cells. J Exp Med 139:193-207
130. Small M, Trainin N (1967) Increase in antibody-forming cells of neonatally thymectomized mice receiving calf thymus extract. Nature 216:377-379
131. Bramucci M, Miano A, Quassinti L et al (2003) Degradation of thymic humoral factor gamma2 by human plasma: Involvement of angiotensin converting enzyme. Regul Pept 111:199-205
132. Burstein Y, Buchner V, Pecht M, Trainin N (1988) Thymic humoral factor gamma 2: purification and amino acid sequence of an immunoregulatory peptide from calf thymus. Biochemistry 27:4066-4071
133. Rotter V, Trainin N (1975) Increased mitogenic reactivity of normal spleen cells to T lectins induced by thymus humoral factor (THF). Cell Immunol 16:413-421
134. Umiel T, Trainin N (1975) Increased reactivity of responding cells in the mixed lymphocyte reaction by a thymic humoral factor. Eur J Immunol 5:85-88
135. Trainin N, Small M (1970) Studies on some physicochemical properties of a thymus humoral factor conferring immunocompetence on lymphoid cells. J Exp Med 132:885-897
136. Umiel T, Altman A, Trainin N (1976) Augmentation of cell mediated lysis (CML) by THF. Adv Exp Med Biol 66:639-643
137. Umiel T, Pecht M, Trainin N (1984) THF, a thymic hormone, promotes interleukin-2 production in intact and thymus-deprived mice. J Biol Response Mod 3:423-434
138. Handzel ZT, Burstein Y, Buchner V et al (1990) Immunomodulation of T cell deficiency in humans by thymic humoral factor: From crude extract to synthetic thymic humoral factor-gamma 2. J Biol Response Mod 9:269-278
139. Rashid G, Ophir R, Pecht M et al (1996) Inhibition of murine Lewis lung carcinoma metastases by combined chemotherapy and intranasal THF-gamma 2 immunotherapy. J Immunother Emphasis Tumor Immunol 19:324-333
140. Ophir R, Pecht M, Keisari Y et al (1996) Thymic humoral factor-gamma 2 (THF-gamma 2) immunotherapy reduces the metastatic load and restores immunocompetence in 3LL tumor-bearing mice receiving anticancer chemotherapy. Immunopharmacol Immunotoxicol 18:209-236
141. Besedovsky HO, del Rey A (1996) Immune-neuro-endocrine interactions: Facts and hypotheses. Endocr Rev 17:64-102

142. Blalock JE (1994) The syntax of immune-neuroendocrine communication. Immunol Today 15:504-511
143. Madden KS, Felten DL (1995) Experimental basis for neural-immune interactions. Physiol Rev 75:77-106
144. Savino W, Dardenne M (1995) Immune-neuroendocrine interactions. Immunol Today 16:318-322
145. Min H, Montecino-Rodriguez E, Dorshkind K (2006) Reassessing the role of growth hormone and sex steroids in thymic involution. Clin Immunol 118:117-123
146. Viganò A, Saresella M, Trabattoni D et al (2004) Growth hormone in T-lymphocyte thymic and postthymic development: A study in HIV-infected children. J Pediatr 145:542-548
147. Koutkia P, Eaton K, You SM et al (2006) Growth hormone secretion among HIV infected patients: Effects of gender, race and fat distribution. Aids 20:855-862
148. Goldberg GL, Zakrzewski JL, Perales MA, van den Brink MR (2007) Clinical strategies to enhance T cell reconstitution. Semin Immunol 19:289-296
149. Savino W, Dardenne M (2000) Neuroendocrine control of thymus physiology. Endocr Rev 21:412-443

CHAPTER 4

Congenital Pathology of the Thymus

William Diehl-Jones, Debbie F. Askin

Introduction

Given its central role in the production and maturation of thymocytes, congenital anomalies of the thymus invariably result in some degree of impairment in immune function. The thymus is the largest lymphoid organ relative to body size during fetal life, and is chiefly concerned with the production of immunocompetent T-cells, with their repertoire of helper, cytotoxic, suppressor, and inducer functions in the immune system. In this context, congenital anomalies of the thymus may have a profound impact on neonatal health.

This paper focuses on two of the more common congenital anomalies associated with primary immune deficiencies (PID): DiGeorge anomaly (DGA, formerly, DiGeorge Syndrome) and Nezelof syndrome. The former is, in general, more thoroughly characterized and attributed to concrete developmental defects, while the embryonic origins of the latter are more difficult to ascribe. In contrast to these syndromes, which frequently manifest as thymic aplasia or hypoplasia, rare cases of thymic hypertrophy have been described, and will also be discussed herein. Finally, one of the more common thymic anomalies, ectopic thymus, will be described. For each of these congenital abnormalities, a summary of what is currently known about the incidence, etiology, pathophysiology, and treatment will be presented.

Overview of Thymus Development

Before discussing congenital malformations and disorders of the thymus, it is useful to review the basic origins of this lymphoid organ. The thymus has its beginnings in the pharyngeal pouches, structures which are associated with the early pharynx. By 5 weeks postconception, all five pharyngeal pouches are recognizable, and it is the third and fourth pharyngeal pouches which ultimately will give rise to either a portion of the parathyroid gland or the thymus. During the 6th and 7th weeks of embryonic development, epithelial cells which will comprise the thymus segregate into bilateral cords, which elongate and resolve into multiple side branches, thus forming the future lobes of the thymus. Small groups of cells cluster around a central locus, forming "thymic corpuscles" or "Hassall Corpuscles". Mesenchymal tissue forms divisions between these cords and it is in these septa that lymphocytes take up residence. Each of these lobes will be separately innervated, and will receive its own blood supply and lymphatic drainage. The future thymus extends inferiorly into the mediastinum, where it will remain throughout life.

Congenital Malformations of the Thymus

When the complex developmental programming that underpins these events goes awry, congenital anomalies in thymus structure and/or function are the result. DGA is an example of a failure of neural crest cell migration. These cells, which give rise to the mesenchyme and epithelial components of the thymus, constitute a critical element in the histogenesis of the thymus. In a subsequent section, we discuss specific elements of the genome which are strongly implicated in this particular disorder.

DiGeorge Anomaly

DiGeorge Anomaly (DGA) is a disorder encompassing both thymic and parathyroid dysfunction, as well as abnormalities in cardiac outflow. This is not surprising, in view of the commonality in embryonic origin of these structures: all of these defects can be attributed to perturbed migration of neural crest cells into the pharyngeal arches and associated structures [1]. Chief among the clinical signs of DGA in the neonatal period are hypocalcemic seizures and compromised immunity. In 1965, Angelo DiGeorge first recognized the connection between the absence of the parathyroid gland and the immunological deficiencies which are also commonly seen in this condition [2]. Since that time, advances in molecular biology have provided insights into the genetic basis for this anomaly.

Genetics

In 35-90% of patients with DGA, there is a microdeletion in the proximal long arm of chromosome 22, called a 22q11.2 deletion after the specific region of the affected chromosome [3]. This region is particularly susceptible to microdeletions due to the presence of low-copy repeat DNA sequences, which results in unequal crossing over with sister chromatids during meiosis [4]. There are approximately 30-40 genes which map to this region of chromosome 22, and patients with this type of deletion are left with only one copy (rather than two) of these genes, a condition referred to as a hemizygous deletion. This results in a decrease in the concentration of specific gene products which are required for normal neural crest cell migration.

It is important to note that, while most cases of DGA are associated with the 22q11.2 deletion, there is some confusion in the literature over the nomenclature of this anomaly. DGA is only one of several syndromes associated with a 22q11.2 deletion, others include, velocardiofacial syndrome (VCFS) and CHARGE syndrome. VCFS includes pharyngeal dysfunction, cardiac anomaly and dysmorphic facies, while CHARGE syndrome includes coloboma (a pupillary malformation), heart defects, atresia of coronary vessels, growth retardation, genitourinary defects and ear abnormalities [5]. In short, 22q11.2 defect and DGA are not interchangeable terms, although there is a great degree of commonality in the manifestations of the two. Some authors have coined the term 22q11.2 deletion syndromes, which can encompass DGA, CHARGE, and VCFS [6]. In fact, DGA likely presents as several overlapping phenotypes, including VCFS and CHARGE, which complicates the diagnosis of DGA.

With respect to DGA, it is not currently known whether a decrease in one or in multiple genes are associated with the DGA phenotype, although recent studies point to the TBX1 gene, which codes for a T-box transcription factor, as having a key role in the disorder [7, 8]. The T-box 1 protein appears to be necessary for the normal development of muscles and bones of the face and neck, large arteries, structures in the ear, and both the thymus and parathyroid. As with other congenital anomalies associated with DGA and 22q11.2 microdeletions, however, further work is needed to fully characterize gene products involved in these disorders [1].

Frequency of DGA

Consistent estimates of the frequency of DGA are difficult to obtain. The frequency of patients diagnosed with DGA ranges from 1:20,000 people to 1:66,000 people [9]. However, with the development of newer diagnostic techniques such as fluorescent in situ hybridization (FISH), it is possible to accurately detect 22q11.2 microdeletions in as many as 1:3,000 patients [9]. However, this figure does not represent DGA alone, and in fact a variety of symptoms not necessarily ascribed to the syndromes previously mentioned are associated with 22q11.2 anomalies.

Clinical Features of DGA

Characteristic features of DGA include hypocalcemia, abnormal facies, conotruncal heart defects, and immune deficiencies secondary to thymic hypoplasia. Additionally, cognitive, behavioral, and psychiatric abnormalities and recurrent infections have been noted in cases of DGA. In subsequent sections below, we elaborate on each of these traits.

Oro-facial Defects Associated with DGA

Facial dysmorphias may include the following: auricular abnormalities such as abnormal helices and preauricular tags, small mouth, micrognathia, prominent nose root, short forehead and midfacial flattening [2]. These features in and of themselves may be difficult to detect in the neonate, becoming apparent only in toddlers or school-age children (Fig. 4.1). Furthermore, other congenital abnormalities involving the pharyngeal arches or pouches may present with similar features, and alone are not diagnostic of DGA.

The hard and soft palates are also derived from the pharyngeal arches. Defects in these structures are also common in DGA, and afflict approximately 80% of patients diagnosed with a 22q11.2 deletion [2]. Clefts in the hard and/or soft palates are common, and frequently associated with a cleft uvula. Furthermore, defects in the velopharyngeal valve are very common, and are manifested by hypernasal speech and articulation disorders, Not surprisingly, feeding disorders are also frequently concomitant with DGA

usually near-normal, IgA fractions may be diminished and IgE lower than normal [11].

As a consequence of thymic insufficiency, patients often present with chronic or repeated viral and bacterial respiratory tract infections. Depending on the degree of expression of DGA, systemic infections resembling (but not as pronounced as) the severe combined immunodeficiency (SCID) phenotype have been noted. Although there is no specific pattern of autoimmune diseases associated with 22q11.2 deletions, the incidence of juvenile rheumatoid arthritis, idiopathic thrombocytopenic purpura, and autoimmune hemolytic anemia tends to be higher in this population [9].

Cardiac Anomalies Associated with DGA

The most common cardiac defects associated with DGA include conotruncal defects such as Tetralogy of Fallot, truncus arteriosus and interrupted aortic arch, and ventricular septal defects [12]. Other authors have noted that anomalies of the subclavian arteries were also common [10], as are hypoplastic left heart, valvular pulmonary stenosis, and bicuspid aortic valve [2].

Neurological Deficits Associated with DGA

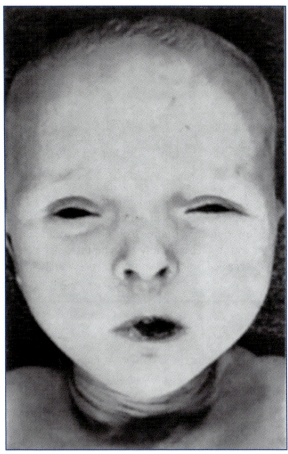

Fig. 4.1 Facial features in DiGeorge Anomaly [10]

Most patients with DGA have average to below-average IQ scores, ranging from 31% borderline IQ scores, 23% low-average and 13% average IQ scores [2]. Increased frequency of behavioral and psychiatric disorders are also commonly observed in DGA and other 22q11.2 syndrome patients, including autism spectrum disorders, attention deficit and hyperactivity, anxiety disorders, depression, and schizophrenia. These appear to be associated with the 22q11.2 deletion rather than being secondary to other anomalies, highlighting the functional and developmental significance of this chromosomal region.

and with other 22q11.2, deletion syndromes, and include nasopharyngeal reflux, gastroesophageal reflux, and disorders of motility which may or may not require feeding by nasogastric or orogastric tubes [2].

Immunological Implications of DGA

As has already been described in other chapters, the thymus gland plays an essential function in the development of immunologic function early in life. Antigen-reactive T-cells released by the thymus, as well as thymic secretions, are vital for immune function. In DGA, the gland itself typically has Hassall's corpuscles and a normal density of thymocytes, and lymphoid follicles usually appear normal, but paracortical regions of lymph nodes and thymus-dependent regions of the spleen are depleted to varying degrees [11]. Most patients born with 22q11.2 deletions have significant decreases in T-cell function, although B-cell function is usually preserved, albeit with some alterations in immunoglobulin titers. While serum concentrations of immunoglobulins are

Endocrine Disorders Associated with DGA

The primary endocrine-related symptom found with this disorder is hypoparathyroidism, which usually manifests as hypocalcemia. Other endocrine abnormalities reported in this population include growth hormone deficiency and thyroid disorders. Whether the latter are a direct consequence of the 22q11.2 deletion or are secondary to hypoparathyroidism are unknown [11].

Diagnosis

Owing to the variation in severity of DGA, and its overlap with other phenotypes, the age at diagnosis is also variable. Serious cardiac defects, hypocalcemia, and immune defects may be diagnosed during the neonatal period. Infants with facial anomalies and cardiac outflow defects or a history of recurrent infections should be investigated for DGA. Frequently, the first indications of morbidity arise when a neonate presents with hypocalcemic tetany [13] although the hypocalcemia accompanying DGA may be intermittent and resolve in infancy [14]. Laboratory investigations will usually reveal a low T-cell count, normal B-cell levels, and normal IgM titers, with serum levels of other immunoglobulins generally low. Typical T-cell mitogens such as concanavalin A and phytohemagglutinin usually fail to stimulate peripheral lymphocytes, and T-cell areas in lymph nodes are frequently lacking. In more profound cases, the thymic shadow can be absent in X-ray.

Recurrent infections generally present in patients older than 3-6 months. Persistent, refractory mucocutaneous candidiasis and recurrent viral infections are often associated with DGA. However, in cases of only mild cardiac defects, minimal anomalies, and normal immune function, a diagnosis may only be made in late childhood or even adulthood [9]. In addition to lab and imaging studies, the FISH technique is a powerful tool which has a high accuracy in detecting 22q11.2 deletions.

Treatment

The initial management of the infant with DGA is directed toward stabilization of the cardiac status. In cases of critical cardiac defects immediate surgery may be required. Calcium supplements may be required to manage hypocalcemia. 1,25-cholecalciferol or parathyroid hormone supplements may be needed to achieve normal serum calcium levels [15]. Infants with DGA should be protected from exposure to communicable diseases and should not receive live vaccines. Steroid therapy should also be avoided. When blood transfusions are required irradiated blood should be used to avoid the risk of graft-versus-host disease [14].

Continuous prophylactic antibiotic therapy in addition to regular immunoglobulin therapy may be helpful in avoiding infections. Lymphocyte infusions using donor lymphocytes that are matched to the neonate's lymphocyte antigens (HLA) are also helpful in T-cell disorders [16]. Periodic (about every 3-6 months) injections of thymic hormones have been effective in ameliorating viral and/or fungal infections. Fetal thymic tissue transplantation has also been used with some success [17], and will be discussed in another chapter.

Nezelof Syndrome

On the continuum of thymic anomalies, yet distinct from DGA, is Nezelof syndrome. Also known variously as thymic dysplasia, Nezelof syndrome is essentially a disorder of thymic function. While the thymus is essentially intact, Hassal's corpuscles are often absent, which is a manifestation of a lack of differentiation of the thymic epithelium [18].

Similar to DGA, peripheral T-cell populations (in particular CD1+ cells) are low while B-cells tend to be normal. T-cell mitogens also usually fail to elicit a lymphocyte response. Immunoglobulin titers have been reported as being normal or elevated [11, 13]. In contrast to DGA, T-cells tend to be somewhat more mature. What further distinguishes Nezelof syndrome from DGA is a lack of parathyroid gland involvement. Less is known about the specific developmental defects responsible for Nezelof syndrome, although it is generally assumed that specific secreted thymic factors are missing or absent. One of the early pioneers in thymic dysfunction is Dr. Ch. Nezelof, who first noted that children who succumbed to certain fungal infections often had some degree of thymic dysplasia and altered T-cell counts [18].

While Nezelof syndrome can be distinguished from DGA through the absence of cardiac abnormalities, parathyroid involvement, and 22Q11.2 deletions, it is not a clearly delineated disease with discrete markers. In fact, the degree of expression of Nezelof syndrome can vary from relatively minor immune dysfunction to states which are similar to that seen with severe combined immunodeficiency (SCID) [19]. What does distinguish Nezelof syndrome from SCID is that it rarely presents with the same degree of immune dysfunction, and does not per se involve B-cell anomalies. This latter finding remains an enigma, with no clear explanation as to why B-cell function can remain intact with such profound T-cell dysfunction [13]. In fact, lymphopenia in the presence of normal gamma globulins is another diagnostic factor.

Etiology

Although the etiology is unclear, some forms of Nezelof syndrome are associated with nucleoside phosphorylase (NP) deficiency. NP is involved in protein catabolism, specifically in purine-salvage pathways, and one of the diagnostic indicators of Nezelof syndrome can be low serum and urine uric acid levels [13]. Unlike DGA, there is a heritable element to Nezelof syndrome. Both autosomal recessive and X-linked patterns of inheritance have been described in cases of Nezelof syndrome [11, 20, 21].

Diagnosis

The presentation of Nezelof syndrome is one of chronic or recurrent infections in infancy including oral or cutaneous candidiasis, chronic diarrhea, pulmonary and skin infections, urinary tract infections and failure to thrive [11]. Because of the presentation of recurrent infections, Nezelof syndrome may be confused with acquired immunodeficiency syndrome. However, the distinguishing features of Nezelof syndrome include atrophy of the thymus gland and depressed cell-mediated immunity, with normal concentrations of gamma globulins [18].

Treatment

Early attempts at restoring thymic function have been unsuccessful [13]. Enzyme replacement therapies are generally not successful. Thymus transplants and bone marrow transplants are more promising therapeutic approaches.

Frequency

The true frequency of Nezelof syndrome is difficult to determine. The National Institute of Health estimates that it affects less than 200,000 individuals in the USA [22].

Congenital Hyperplasia of the Thymus

At birth, the thymus weighs 10-15 g, which is its largest size relative to total body mass. By puberty, it is approximately 35 g, but regresses through the remainder of life to become gradually replaced by fat [23]. Thymic enlargement is a fairly common radiologic finding in healthy newborns, and is usually not associated with any clinical symptoms [24]. However, thymic hyperplasia is the most common finding for enlargement of the anterior mediastinum.

Three variants of newborn thymic enlargement have been described: hyperplastic lymph follicles independent of gland size; true thymic hyperplasia (beyond normal limits for age) with normal histology; and hyperplasia representing more than 2% of body mass, also with normal histology. In the latter, the thymus is several times the normal weight, and appears on chest X-ray to be larger than the heart shadow [24].

Etiology

The etiology of thymic hyperplasia is varied, but "true" thymic hyperplasia should be distinguished from "reactive" hyperplasia in that the latter generally results from a pre-existing disease, such as hemorrhagic disease of the newborn, myasthenia gravis or hyperthyroidism; or it may arise after chemotherapy. True thymic hyperplasia essentially implies an enlarged gland that has histologically normal cortical and medullary components [25].

Clinical Presentation

Thymic hyperplasia is most commonly diagnosed in children or young adults; however, the presentation is variable. In a review, Linegar and colleagues reported that in 38% of cases, infants were asymptomatic; in 35% they had pulmonary infections; and in 29% there was evidence of respiratory distress. To this end, coughing, lymphocytosis, dysphagia, splenomegaly, and chest discomfort are associated symptoms [26]. Interestingly, B-cell counts are usually normal.

Treatment

Treatment of thymic hyperplasia is controversial. Intravenous or oral steroids have been used in an attempt to shrink the thymus, although with little effect [27]. Currently, the strategy is to closely follow symptomatic children for up to 18 months during a trial of corticosteroids. If there is poor response, and the thymus continues to enlarge and/or elicit severe symptoms, a thyrectomy may be attempted, although this should be avoided in the neonate since it can have the effect of reducing peripheral T-cell numbers [24].

Ectopic Thymus

A few cases of ectopic thymus tissue have been reported in the literature. Normally the thymus forms from the third and fourth pharyngeal pouches and descends to the mediastinum along a pathway from the mandible [28, 29]. An ectopic thymus occurs when the thymus fails to descend appropriately. In general, such lesions are either cystic or solid. The vast majority are cystic and can occur at variable locations along the embryologic path of descent, which spans the angle of the mandible to the mediastinum. Approximately half of these will connect with normal thymic tissue in the mediastinum. There are, however, reports of ectopic tissue that occur elsewhere in the body, away from the path of embryologic descent [29].

Incidence and Associated Anomalies

Cervical thymic anomalies are relatively uncommon; there are only about 100 cases reported in children who presented with a primary neck mass; however, it is felt that, because they are usually asymptomatic, this is likely much more common lesion than is reported [30].

In a study of 3,236 children at autopsy, ectopic thymic tissue was noted in 34 children (1%) and was most commonly found near the thyroid gland. Of the 34 cases found in this study, 71% of the children had features of DGA and only 5 of the 10 remaining children had a normal thymus present in the mediastinum [31].

Zarbo [32] proposed seven categories of thymic ectopy, based on anatomic location, structure (cystic or solid) and whether or not a thymopharyngeal duct is present. The least common form is the purely ectopic thymus, which is solid thymic tissue in abnormal locations off the normal embryologic path of descent. Locations where this type of anomaly has been described include the base of the skull, and within the pharynx or the trachea [33].

Diagnosis and Management

Aberrant thymic tissue seldom causes clinical symptoms but cases of airway obstruction and respiratory distress have been reported [28, 34, 35]. MRI evaluation may help to delineate the location of the exogenous tissue. Unless the extra glandular mass is symptomatic, surgical removal of ectopic thymus is not recommended, due to the possible impact on peripheral T-cells, and the risk of removing excessive glandular tissue [29]. Generally, most cases of ectopic thymus are also benign [36, 37], although there are case reports of malignant transformation in thymic cysts [38].

When an ectopic thymus does become symptomatic, in the neonate it can present as an airway obstruction causing respiratory distress [39] or as severe bleeding [26]. In the former, the actual site of the airway obstruction is variable; there have been reports of subglottal, tracheal [40], and retropharyngeal cysts [28]. With respect to thymic cysts which induce bleeding, the cause is not always clear, although it may include vitamin K deficiency, or invasion of a vascular tissue. Still other clinical symptoms associated with thymic cysts can include tachydyspnea, anemia, and even shock [26]. In most cases of thymic cysts, total surgical excision is often the most efficacious approach, although it is important to reinforce the need for caution, given the possibility of inducing a hypothymic state.

Summary

This article presents an overview of the most common thymic disorders in the neonate. In some of these, such as DGA, there are reasonably well-characterized genetic alterations which interrupt the migration of neural crest cells in the embryonic period, concomitant with changes in parathyroid structure/function. The particular genetic locus of this alteration is mapped to 22q11.2, an area associated with a number of syndromes. Nezelof syndrome, on the other hand, is not nearly as well characterized as DGA, although its heritable link has been demonstrated. Finally, although thymic hyperplasia and ectopic thymus have a relatively low incidence, an awareness of their possible patterns is essential for the practitioner.

References

1. Gruber PJ (2005) Cardiac development: New concepts. Clin Perinatol 32:845-855
2. Goldmuntz E (2005) DiGeorge syndrome: New insights. Clin Perinatol 32:963-978
3. Scrambler PJ, Carey AH, Wyse RK et al (1991) Microdeletions within 22q11.2 associated with sporadic and familial DiGeorge syndrome. Genomics 10(1):201-206
4. Bawle EV, Fratarelli DAC (2006) DiGeorge syndrome. Emedicine (retrieved on July 20, 2007 from http://www.emedicine.com/ped/topic589.htm)
5. Kobrynski LJ, Sullivan KE (2007) Velocardial syndrome, DiGeorge syndrome: The chromosome 22q11.2 deletion syndromes. Lancet 370:1443-1452
6. Hay BN (2007) Deletion 22q11: Spectrum of associated disorders. Semin Pediatr Neurol 14:136-139
7. Zhang Z, Cerrato F, Xu H et al (2005) Tbx1 expression in pharyngeal epithelia is necessary for pharyngeal arch artery development. Development 132(23):5307-5315

8. Zhang Z, Huynh T, Baldini A (2006) Mesodermal expression of Tbx1 is necessary and sufficient for pharyngeal arch and cardiac outflow tract development. Development 133(18):3587-3595
9. Hussain I, Win PH (2006) DiGeorge syndrome (retrieved on July 20, 2007 from http://emedicine.com/med/topic567.htm)
10. Moerman R, Goddeeris P, Lauwerijns J, Van Der Hauwaert LG (1980) Cardiovascular malformations in DiGeorge syndrome (congenital absence or hypoplasia of the thymus). Br Heart J 44:452-459
11. Buckley RH (1987) Immunodeficiency diseases. JAMA 258(20):2841-2850
12. Plageman TF Jr, Ytuzey KE (2005) T-box genes and heart development: Putting the "T" in heart. Dev Dyn 232:11-20
13. Cooper MD, Buckley RH (1982) Developmental immunology and immunodeficiency diseases. JAMA 248(20):2658-2669
14. Online Mendelian Inheritance in Man (OMIM) http://www.ncbi.nlm.nih.gov/entrez/dispomim.cgi?id=188400 Revised 10/25/2007, Accessed January 4, 2008
15. Ammann AJ (1977) T Cell and T-B Cell Immunodeficiency Disorders. Pediatr Clin North Am 24(2):293-311
16. Askin DF, Young S (2002) The thymus. Neonatal Netw 20(8):7-13
17. Markert ML, Devlin BH, Alexieff MJ et al (2007) Review of 54 patients with DiGeorge anomaly enrolled in protocols for thymus transplantation: outcome of 44 consecutive transplants. Blood 109(10):4539-4547
18. Nezelof C (1992) Thymic pathology in primary and secondary immunodeficiencies. Histopathology 21:499-511
19. Haynes BF, Warren RW, Buckley RH et al (1983) Demonstration of abnormalities in expression of thymic epithelial surface antigens in severe cellular immunodeficiency diseases. J Immunol 130(3):1182-1188
20. World Health Organization (1986) Primary Immunodeficiency diseases: Report of a World Health Organization scientific group. Clin Immunol Immunopathol 40:166-196
21. Rosen FS, Cooper MD, Wedgwood RJ (1984) The primary immunodeficiencies. N Eng J Med 311:235-242
22. National Institutes of Health Office of Rare Disease (http://rarediseases.info.nih.gov/asp/diseases/diseaseinfo.asp; retrieved January 22, 2008)
23. Williams H (2006) The normal thymus and how to recognize it. Arch Dis Child Ed Pract 91:25-28
24. Eifinger F, Ernestus K, Benz-Nohm G et al (2007) True thymic hyperplasia associated with severe thymic cyst bleeding in a newborn: Case report and review of the literature. Ann Diagn Pathol 11:358-362
25. Rice HE, Flake AW, Hori T et al (1994) Massive thymic hyperplasia: Characterization of a rare mediastinal mass. J Pediatr Surg 29(12):1561-1564
26. Linegar AG, Odell AJ, Fennell WM et al (1993) Massive thymic hyperplasia. Ann Thorac Surg 55(5):1197-1201
27. Gow KW, Kobrynski L, Abramowsky C, Lloyd D (2003) Massive benign thymic hyperplasia in a six-month-old girl: case report. Am Surgeon 69:717-719
28. Shah SS, Lai SY, Ruchelli E et al (2001) Retropharyngeal aberrant thymus. Pediatrics 108(5):e94-e97
29. He Y, Zhang Z-Y, Zhu H-G et al (2008) Infant ectopic cervical thymus in submandibular region. Int J Oral Maxillofac Surg 1263:1-4
30. Wagner CW, Vinocur CD, Weintraub WH, Golladay ES (1988) Respiratory complications in cervical thymic cysts. J Pediatr Surg 23:657-660
31. Bale PM, Sotelo-Avila C (1993) Maldescent of the thymus: 34 necropsy and 10 surgical cases, including 7 thymuses medial to the mandible. Pediatr Pathol 13:181-190
32. Zarbo RJ, McClatchey KD, Areen RG, Baker SB (1983) Thymopharyngeal duct cyst: A form of cervical thymus. Ann Otol Rhinol Laryngol 92:284-289
33. Millman B, Pransky S, Castillo J III et al (1999) Cervical thymic anomalies. Int J Pediatr Otorhinolaryngol 47:29-39
34. Raines JM, Rowe LD (1981) Progressive neonatal airway obstruction secondary to cervical thymic cyst. Otolaryngol Head Neck Surg 89:723-725
35. McLeod DM, Karandy EJ (1981) Aberrant cervical thymus. A rare cause of acute respiratory distress. Arch Otolaryngol 107:179-180
36. Park JJ, Kim JW, Kim JP et al (2005) Two cases of ectopic cervical thymus: Case reports and a review of the literature. Auris Nasus Laryns 33:101-105
37. Loney DA, Bauman NM (1998) Ectopic cervical thymic masses in infants: A case report and review of the literature. Int J Pediatr Otorhinolaryngol 43:77-84
38. Leong AS, Brown JH (1984) Malignant transformation in a thymic cyst. Am J Surg Pathol 8:471-475
39. Rosevear WH, Singer MI (1981) Symptomatic cervical thymic cyst in a neonate Otolaryngol Head Neck Surg 89:738-741
40. Sahhar HS, Marra S, Boyd C, Akhter J (2003) Ectopic subglottic thymic cyst: A rare cause of congenital stridor. Ear Nose Throat J 82(11):873-874

CHAPTER 5
Hyperplastic and Inflammatory Pathology of the Thymus

Antonio Maiorana, Luca Reggiani-Bonetti

Introduction

Thymic hyperplasia describes a nonneoplastic condition of the thymus, characterized by an increased number of the constituent cells of the organ. This concept was initially introduced by Castleman in the late 1940s to define the thymic changes seen in association with myasthenia gravis [1]. Years later, Rosai and Levine [2] in the A.F.I.P. fascicle on "Tumors of the thymus" identified two distinct types of thymic hyperplasia on the basis of histopathologic criteria: true thymic hyperplasia, defined by an increase in the size and weight of the organ that retains a normal microscopic morphology, and lymphoid (or follicular) hyperplasia, characterized by the presence of lymphoid follicles with active germinal centers in the thymic medulla. In the last case, the size and weight of the thymus can be increased, but in most instances they are within normal limits. The term thymitis (or autoimmune thymitis), originally coined by Goldstein in 1966 [3], has been used interchangeably by some authors to denote the lymphoid hyperplasia of the thymus, since its morphological features, both at the light and electron microscopic levels, are markedly similar to those observed in any chronic inflammatory process of other organs [4, 5], being characterized by the presence of peripheral B lymphocytes, lymphoid follicles, and diffuse plasmacytosis.

True Thymic Hyperplasia

True thymic hyperplasia (TTH) is defined as an increase in the weight and volume of the thymus beyond the upper limits of normality. In order to establish the correct diagnosis, reference must be made for comparison to standard tables of thymic weight in relation to age [6, 7]. The most recent evaluation of the thymus weights and volumes was done by Steinman, who examined, at necropsy, the thymuses of 136 apparently healthy persons who had died suddenly [7]. Since thymic weights can vary widely at any age in comparison to those expected from the standard tables [8], Judd and Welch [9] suggested to use a cut-off value of 2 standard deviations above the average weight for age as the upper limit of normality.

Weights in TTH are extremely variable, ranging from 40 to more than 1,000 g [10]. When thymus weight exceeds 100 g, TTH has been termed "massive" [11]. Maximum dimensions vary from 10 mm [12] to 18 cm and more [13, 14].

The gross aspect is that of a well-circumscribed, encapsulated mass that can reflect the normal thymic shape with two distinct enlarged lobes. More frequently, the thymus appears oval or discoid and the typical bilobate shape of the organ is no longer recognizable [13] (Fig. 5.1). Isolated cases with only one lobe enlargement [12] or a multiple nodular aspect [15] have also been described. An unusual case

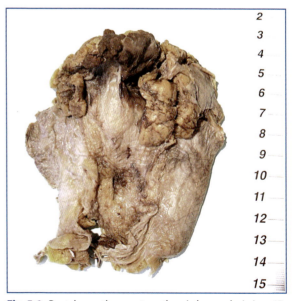

Fig. 5.1 Postchemotherapy true thymic hyperplasia in a 42-year-old man who died from rupture of cerebral artery aneurysm. Eleven months before death, the patient had been treated with chemotherapy for Hodgkin's lymphoma. At autopsy, the thymus measured 11×7×3 cm and weighed 94 g

of focal TTH featured an oval mass pendulous from the right thymic lobe [16].

The cut surface color varies from gray-yellow to reddish-brown and shows different degrees of lobulation, at times prominent at the periphery but absent in the center of the organ [13, 17, 18]. The consistency is parenchymatous or slightly increased.

The microscopic aspect of TTH is similar to that of the normal thymic tissue [19] (Fig. 5.2). The lobular architecture is well maintained, as is the distinction between cortical and medullary areas. At times, prevalence of the medullary areas is noted and Hassall's bodies can be present even within the cortex [13]. Cellular components of the thymus are conserved, but show hyperplastic changes. Lymphoid follicles with activated germinal centers are not present.

The lymphoid cell population is represented by small and medium-sized CD3+ T-lymphocytes intermingled with scattered CD20+ B-elements. Cortical lymphocytes show the expression of CD4 and CD8 antigens in the same cell. By contrast, in medullary areas, lymphocytes express either CD4 or CD8 antigens. Cortical areas exhibit an intense nuclear staining for Ki67 and contain numerous tingible-body macrophages with a starry-sky appearance [20]. Staining for cytokeratins shows a normal network of epithelial thymic cells throughout the mass.

Approximately 55% of patients present with an asymptomatic anterior mediastinal mass [21], whereas in remaining cases dyspnoea, chest pain [22, 23], respiratory distress and/or other signs of compression of the nearby tracheo-bronchial tree can be observed [13]. Bronchial compression with subsequent atelectasis [24, 13] or irreversible changes in the lung tissue [24] have also been described. Concomitant leukocytosis with absolute lymphocytosis [13], sometimes associated with bone marrow lymphocytosis [17] that disappears after thymectomy [25], have also been reported. No severe defects of cellular immunity are usually found. In the peripheral blood, there is no specific constellation of lymphocytic markers which could point to the diagnosis of TTH [26].

At radiologic examination, TTH can mimic other pathologic conditions arising in the anterior mediastinal area, such as Castleman's disease, lymphomas, germ cell tumors, thymomas, and thymic carcinomas. The differential diagnosis has usually required surgical exploration with either thymectomy or surgical biopsy for histopathologic examination [12, 27, 28]. In the majority of patients, careful clinical and radiological follow-up is sufficient and no specific treatment is needed, since TTH undergoes spontaneous regression within a few months. Longstanding cases have been reported [29, 30]. When the risk of malignancy in the mediastinum is low, some authors [31, 32] have suggested a conservative approach with an initial oral steroid treatment followed by serial radiological examinations. Shrinkage or disappearance of the anterior mediastinal mass indicates that it was a benign thymus enlargement. Steroid challenge, however, is not helpful in cases in which the initial diagnosis was steroid-sensitive leukemia or lymphoma [31].

Fine needle aspiration biopsy (FNAB) was claimed to represent an easy-to-perform and inexpensive procedure for the diagnosis of TTH. Moreover, it has the advantage of being able to obtain diagnostic material without requiring general anesthesia. Riazmontazer and Bedayat [33] used FNAB to evaluate an anterior mediastinal mass in a 12-year-old girl. The smears showed two different cell populations, consisting of lymphocytes and epithelial cells. Although the cytologic criteria to differentiate TTH from thymoma can overlap, the authors pointed out that the finding of different shapes and sizes in the epithelial cell nuclei and the presence of lymphocytes encircling individual epithelial cells are uncommon features in smears of thymomas and might help differentiate between the two entities. Another case of TTH in a 5-month-old child was diagnosed using combined radiologic imaging and FNAB [34]. Bangerter et al. [35] reported a series of eight cases of TTH diagnosed through FNAB. In all patients, the cytologic smears showed mixed populations of lymphoid cells and the cytologic diagnoses of TTH were confirmed by follow-up studies. According to the authors, FNAB is a useful front-line procedure in diagnosing TTH.

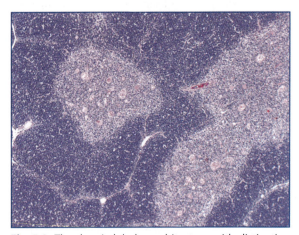

Fig. 5.2 The thymic lobular architecture, with distinction between cortical and medullary areas, is maintained in true thymic hyperplasia. Hematoxylin and eosin, ×4 (original magnification)

Although rare, the occurrence of spontaneous hemorrhage in TTH has been reported in the literature. A case of TTH with massive intrathymic bleeding and hemothorax was described in a 41-year-old man who was on peritoneal dialysis after kidney transplant removal [36]. The patient had experienced acute left chest pain and dyspnoea that simulated pericardial or myocardial disease. The authors explained TTH as a rebound phenomenon after termination of immunosuppression following transplant removal. TTH with hemorrhage simulating recurrent Hodgkin disease was reported by Langer [37] after chemotherapy-induced complete remission, whereas Eifinger et al. [38] described severe thymic cyst bleeding in a 5-week-old male infant who had recurrent respiratory distress since birth and congenital TTH. The enlarged thymus, removed via median sternotomy, weighed 29.4 g (normal controls, <20 g) and, at histopathological examination, showed normal architecture with extensive interstitial hemorrhages and small cysts. The etiology of the thymic bleeding in the infant remained enigmatic, since the coagulation status was normal.

Of interest, a case of solitary fibrous tumor arising from the hyperplastic thymus was described in a 37-year-old female [39]. The tumor was located on a pedicle that arose from the postero-inferior thymus surface.

TTH was reported in association with several clinical conditions, such as recovery from thermal burns [40], cardiovascular surgery [41], and infections. Isolated reports described the occurrence of TTH in an infant with Beckwith-Wiedemann syndrome [42], a neonate with Perlman syndrome [43], and in two infants with Pena-Shokeir syndrome type I [44, 45]. Idiopathic cases were reported in children [13]. The most common associations are with malignancies, endocrine diseases and autoimmune disorders.

TTH and Malignancies

The development of TTH in patients with malignant tumors has been described in two different clinical situations, either after chemotherapy treatment (so-called postchemotherapy TTH) or in newly-diagnosed cancers before the initiation of systemic therapy.

Postchemotherapy TTH

TTH has been described in children and young adults who received cytotoxic chemotherapy for treatment of different malignancies, particularly leukemias [46], Hodgkin's and non-Hodgkin's lymphomas [47-50], testicular germ cell tumors [51-54], Wilm's tumor [55], and different bone or soft tissue sarcomas [56, 57]. Less frequently, it can also occur in adult patients treated with chemotherapy for malignant tumors, including breast cancer, both in early and advanced stages [58, 59], prostatic carcinoma [15], testicular germ cell tumors [60-62], leukemias [63, 64], Hodgkin's and non-Hodgkin's lymphomas [64-70], ovarian tumors [70], and pulmonary metastases of sarcoma [71].

The development of TTH after chemotherapy appears to be more common in younger people because the residual thymic tissue is greater in such patients. TTH is usually responsible for the appearance of a significant mediastinal mass on CT scans that sometimes can mimic metastatic disease. All authors point out that awareness of this side effect in patients treated with chemotherapy may prevent surgical procedures and other unnecessary investigation. A "rebound phenomenon" appears to be a plausible explanation for postchemotherapy TTH. The hyperplasia would be caused by excessive regrowth of the thymus after the initial atrophy determined by cytotoxic therapy and immunosuppression. The factor(s) responsible for thymic overgrowth are uncertain. Another explanation postulates that in patients treated with chemotherapy TTH is caused by a chemotherapy-induced gonadal atrophy, which results in increase of luteinizing hormone secretion [12, 58, 72]. The increase in thymic volume is variable as are the rate of growth and the period over which enlargement occurs.

Different studies showed the changes in thymic volume to be related to the timing of chemotherapy. The greatest increase in thymic volume occurs in the last postchemotherapy period, whereas reduction of thymic volume is observed in the immediate postchemotherapy phase. Rebound thymic hyperplasia usually occurs within the first, or rarely second, year following chemotherapy.

Thymic volumes were determined by CT scan in 22 consecutive oncologic patients (2-35 years old) treated with cycles of chemotherapy [64]. Primary tumors included different types of lymphomas, sarcomas, or testicular neoplasias, excluding cases in which the mediastinum was directly involved by the tumor. In 20 of 22 patients, the thymic volume was found to decrease by an average of 43% during the first course of chemotherapy, but regrowth was observed between the first and second course. In patients who received a second course of chemotherapy, a further 36% decrease was detected. Rebound thymic enlargement, defined as a greater than 50% increase in volume over baseline, was observed in five patients, occurring an average of 4.2 months (range 3 to 8 months) after the end of the treatment. Similar data were reported by Kissin et al. [73], who reviewed serial CT scans of 200 patients with malignant testicular teratoma. Thymic enlargement was found 3-14 months after the commencement of the treatment in 14 of 120 cases (11.6%) treated with chemotherapy for metastatic disease, but only in one of 80 untreated patients with no evidence of metastases. The greatest increase in thymic volume occurred in the late postchemotherapy period. The enlarged thymus was excised in a patient and the histologic study showed TTH of the cortex and medulla. In the series of Ruether et al. [26], thymic enlargement was observed 3-20 months after initiation of treatment in 15 of 124 patients with malignant testicular tumors. An isolated case of rebound TTH was detected 5 years after cessation of chemotherapy for Wilm's tumor [55].

The development of TTH after treatment of malignancy has been claimed [73] to represent a good prognostic sign. In a group of 120 patients with metastatic testicular tumors who were treated with chemotherapy, 93% of those showing thymic enlargement were well and disease free after a mean follow-up of 45 months, whereas the frequency of disease-free survival dropped to 78% in patients with no thymic enlargement. The difference was statistically significant ($p<0.02$). According to Kissin [73], TTH in these patients may indicate the presence of an active T-cell-mediated immune response against neoplastic cells and serve as a favorable prognostic marker. Different results, however, were reported by Hara et al. [59] in a group of 102 breast cancer patients treated with high-dose chemotherapy followed by autologous stem cell transplantation. TTH was observed in 11 patients (11%), being minimal in eight of them, and it was not associated with improved survival, since no significant difference in survival probability was found in women with and women without TTH revealed by CT scans ($p=0.769$).

TTH in Patients with Untreated Tumors

TTH has been reported in patients with newly diagnosed cancer before the initiation of systemic therapy [53]. TTH was discovered in four of 221 patients (1.8%) with low-stage testicular germ cell tumors, among whom three of 100 (3.0%) were affected by seminoma and one of 121 (0.8%) by non-seminomatous neoplasias. TTH was detected at staging evaluation approximately 18-37 days after orchiectomy, but before the administration of other oncologic treatments. In these cases, the development of TTH was explained as an early rebound response to the stress either of the neoplasm or of the recent orchiectomy, although other possibilities, such as cytokine responses to the tumor, were also postulated.

An unusual case of TTH, developed in a 25-year-old man approximately 22 months after orchiectomy for malignant mesothelioma of the tunica vaginalis, was described by Wenger et al. [12]. Since the anterior mediastinal mass was confused with metastatic disease, the patient underwent right mediastinotomy, but a wedge biopsy of the thymus evidenced only hyperplasia. TTH was explained as a rebound phenomenon but no obvious cause for it was found since the patient had had no chemotherapy or infection.

TTH and Endocrine Diseases

The great majority of TTH cases in patients with endocrine diseases has been reported in association with thyroid diseases, especially Graves' disease. Only rare reports point to the association with hypercortisolism and acromegaly.

TTH and Thyroid Diseases

TTH has been recognized as a complication of hyperthyroidism, especially in young women. In most cases, the increase in thymic size is minimal, but massive enlargements have also been reported [74-76]. Murakami et al. [77] studied thymic size and density by means of computed tomography in 23 untreated patients with Graves' disease and 38 control subjects. Thymic size in mm^2 ranged from 630.4 to 977.9 in different age-matched groups of Graves' disease patients, whereas in control subjects it ranged from 142.8 to 219.9 mm ($p<0.01$). Thymic size and density significantly dropped after treatment with antithyroid drugs administered for a period of 5-24 months.

Several mechanisms can be involved in the pathogenesis of TTH in Graves' disease. Thyroid-stimulating hormone (TSH) receptors were demonstrated to be expressed in human thymic tissues by PCR amplification and Northern and Western blot analysis [77]. Their nucleotide sequence was found to be identical to that of the human TSH receptor found in thyroid cells. Immunohistochemistry of thymic tissue using anti-TSH receptor monoclonal antibodies evidenced immunostaining of epithelial cells. Thymic TSH receptors were postulated to play a role in the development of TTH in patients with Graves' disease [77]. Moreover, Wortsman et al. [78] showed that immunoglobulins from a patient with Graves' disease were able to stimulate thymocyte mitogenesis in vitro, suggesting an autoimmune mechanism in the development of TTH.

TTH may also be caused by the direct action of thyroid hormones on the thymus. Hyperplasia of the thymus was induced in mice treated with triiodothyronine (T3) during the first month of life [79]. After T3 administration, the number of thymic epithelial cells almost doubled in both cortex and medulla, whereas lymphocytes mainly increased in the cortex. Moreover, nuclear receptors for T3 can be detected in primary cultures of both mouse and human thymic epithelial cells [80, 81]. The direct action of T3 on thymic cells might explain the occasional development of TTH in children during therapy for primary hypothyroidism [82]. In such cases, the thymic enlargement arises during the transition from hypo- to euthyroidism.

An enlarged thymus can be frequently observed on CT scans of thyroid cancer patients and may raise the suspicion of metastatic disease. In the study of Niendorf et al. [83], the thymus was identified in 24 of 57 patients who had had a previous diagnosis of differentiated thyroid cancer and imaging criteria for TTH were met in 19 (33%) of them. Evidence of thyroid metastatic disease was observed in 17 patients, two of whom also showed TTH, whereas of the 40 patients without metastatic disease 22 had TTH. In the majority of cases, the enlarged thymus showed a pyramidal configuration on CT, which permitted an easy distinction of this entity from metastatic cancer. Of interest, anterior mediastinal uptake of iodine-131 has also been observed in some patients with thyroid cancer [84, 85]. The mediastinal uptake disappeared after surgical removal of the thymus and, at histopathological examination, the thymuses showed hyperplasia with no evidence of metastatic foci of thyroid carcinoma or thyroid tissue.

The mechanism for TTH associated with thyroid cancer appears to be different from the classic rebound TTH observed in other malignancies in which hyperplasia usually develops after chemotherapeutic treatment. TTH in patients with thyroid cancer does not appear to be related to the presence of stimulation of intrathymic TSH receptors, because the routine treatment of such patients with supraphysiologic doses of thyroid hormones results in low TSH levels via a negative feedback mechanism. Niendorf et al. [83] postulated that TTH in patients with thyroid cancer can rather be directly induced by the excess thyroid hormone usually administered for suppressive therapy.

TTH and Growth Hormone

Longstanding overproduction of growth hormone (GH) can induce TTH. Bazzoni et al. [86] reported the case of a 23-year-old female acromegalic patient with a mediastinal mass, that after surgical removal was diagnosed as TTH. Polgreen et al. [87] described a 7-year-old patient with TTH diagnosed after initiation of recombinant human GH therapy for the treatment of GH deficiency. The girl had a history of embryonal rhabdomyosarcoma of the rhinopharynx diagnosed at the age of 3 years and treated with radiotherapy and chemotherapy. After 3 months of GH therapy, a chest CT scan evidenced 89% increase in the thymic volume that turned out to be hyperplasia at thoracoscopic biopsy. According to the authors, the close temporal relationship between initiation of GH treatment and development of TTH suggests an etiologic effect of GH, making the probability of postchemotherapy rebound TTH unlikely. Accordingly, experimental in vitro studies have shown that the thymus is a target organ for GH [88]. Both T-lymphocytes and thymic epithelial cells express GH receptors [88, 89], whereas other studies have shown that GH modulates thymocyte development in vivo [90] and induces proliferation of thymic epithelial cells [91]. Of interest, administration of exogenous GH in a GH-sufficient adult man was shown to cause partial thymic regeneration with reversal of the normal age-related involution [92].

TTH and Cushing's Syndrome

TTH has been described in patients with Cushing's syndrome when cortisol levels drop after surgical resection of an ACTH-secreting pituitary adenoma or cortisol-producing tumor. The mechanism involved is that of a classic "rebound" hyperplasia that follows thymic depletion resulting from elevated plasma glucorticoid concentrations. Oral administration of corticosteroids in infants induces rapid atrophy of the thymus, which is followed by fast regrowth after cessation of steroid treatment [93]. Three cases of TTH after remission of Cushing's syndrome were reported by Doppman et al. [94]. The authors pointed out that, when hypercortisolism results from ectopic ACTH production by a tumor of the lung or mediastinum, the appearance of a mediastinal mass after surgery may be confused with tumor recurrence and lead to diagnostic thoracotomy. Tabarin et al. [95] described five cases of pseudo-tumors of the thymus after correction of hypercortisolism in patients with ectopic ACTH syndrome. In patients that underwent exploratory thoracotomy, histological examination showed TTH with negative immunostaining for ACTH. The time course of TTH after treatment of Cushing's syndrome cannot be predicted. TTH has been observed as early as 3-4 weeks after decline of cortisol levels and has persisted for several months [94]. In Tabarin's cases, it developed 6-14 months after remission of hypercortisolism. In a patient who did not undergo thoracotomy [95], it spontaneously disappeared 11 months after its demonstration in CT scans and magnetic resonance imaging of the thorax. The case reported by Ohta et al. [96] is unusual, since TTH was shown to be the source of ectopic ACTH production. A thymic mass was evidenced in a 26-year-old man, who had undergone both trans-sphenoidal exploration of the pituitary with no evidence of microadenoma and bilateral adrenalectomy because of progressive hypercortisolism. Skin pigmentation had gradually developed with marked elevation of plasma ACTH levels. After thoracotomy, the mediastinal mass was found to be an ACTH-producing TTH. Northern blot analysis and in situ hybridization evidenced the expression of proopiomelanocortin transcripts in the thymic lymphocytes. No increase of the thymic weight was observed in a study of 37 necropsies of patients with Addison's disease [97].

TTH and Autoimmune Diseases

The presence of TTH in autoimmune diseases has been observed in some anecdotal reports, but rarely investigated in large series of patients. Ferri et al. [98] studied thymus alterations in 34 consecutive patients with systemic sclerosis by means of unenhanced multidetector computed tomography. Major thymus alterations (abnormally enlarged or nodular thymus) were detected in a statistically significant percentage of cases compared with controls (7/34, i.e., 21%, vs. 0/34; p=0.011). They were observed in patients with shorter disease duration and were usually associated with serum anti-Scl70 antibodies. Thymectomy was carried out in two patients and histopathological examination revealed TTH, whereas an additional patient developed myasthenia gravis. Overlap with follicular hyperplasia of the thymus cannot be excluded in this last case.

Histologically confirmed TTH was also associated with sarcoidosis in a 34-year-old woman [99] who was found to have a mediastinal mass at chest radiographs.

Massive Thymic Hyperplasia

Massive thymic hyperplasia (MTH), also known as "thymic hyperplasia with massive enlargement" or "massive thymic enlargement", is an extremely rare variant of TTH characterized by a "massive" increase in the size and weight of the thymus. There are no generally accepted criteria for the definition of this entity. According to Arliss et al. [11], TTH is called massive when the thymus weight exceeds 100 g. Linegar et al. [10] applied the following criteria for its diagnosis: (1) the thymus should be larger than the heart shadow on chest radiographs; (2) the thymus weight should exceed several times the expected weight for the patient's age; (3) the thymus mass should represent more than 2% of the body mass.

MTH has been described in infants and adolescents. The great majority of cases are idiopathic, occurring in the absence of any known provocative systemic stress [10], although isolated reports describe its development in connection with systemic diseases, such as non-Hodgkin's lymphoma [100] and lymphocytosis with hypogammaglobulinemia. Virus infections or reduced level of circulating corticotropins were postulated as possible explaining mechanisms [101]. Thymus weights range from 125 g to 1260 g [10, 13] (Fig. 5.3). The majority of patients are

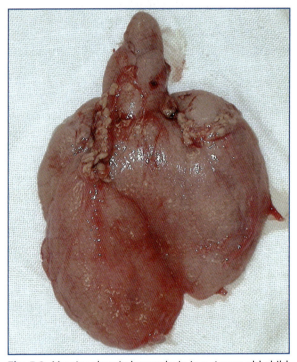

Fig. 5.3 Massive thymic hyperplasia in a 4-year-old child, who underwent thymectomy because of mild dyspnoea. CT scans evidenced an ovoid mass in the antero-superior mediastinum. The thymus weighed 210 g

asymptomatic, but chest pain and mild dyspnoea with reduction of pulmonary vital capacity and lobar atelectasis have been reported [13]. Dysphagia due to esophageal compression can also occur [102]. An interesting case of recurrent MTH was reported by Pompeo et al. [18] in a 20-year-old man who had been treated with steroid therapy at age 4 because of massive enlargement of the thymus. No apparent cause that could explain the recurrence was found.

Histological analysis typically reveals normal thymic tissue with preservation of the cortical and medullary architecture. Immunohistological features are similar to those of TTH. Nezelof and Normand [103], using cytoenzymatic methods to identify mature T-lymphocytes, evidenced a quantitative reduction in mature T-cells and postulated that MTH is caused by an abnormal intrathymic accumulation of immature T-lymphocytes. The presence of myoid cells in MTH has been documented with ultrastructural and immunohistochemical methods [102].

Follicular Thymic Hyperplasia (So-called Thymitis)

Follicular hyperplasia (also known as lymphoid or lympho-follicular hyperplasia) (FH) is characterized by the occurrence of an increased number of B-lymphocytes and lymphoid follicles with active germinal centers in the thymus. In contrast to TTH, the weight and size of the organ can be within the normal range (Fig. 5.4). Besides lymphoid follicles, plasma cell infiltration and an increased amount of reticulin fibers are also present.

Although B-lymphocytes were initially thought not to occur in the normal thymus, subsequent studies were able to disclose the presence of B-cell antigen-expressing cells in the thymic medulla of control thymuses of different ages (Fig. 5.5). According to Hofmann et al. [104], such cells can be subdivided into small lymphocytes and larger asteroidally shaped cells. In 1943, Sloan [4] showed that lymphoid follicles can be detected in approximately 10% of normal thymuses. Similar data were observed by Henry [105], whereas a higher incidence was reported by Middleton [106] in an autopsy study. Follicular structures were found in the thymus of 50% of people with no evidence of autoimmune diseases who had died from road traffic accidents, but the percentage rose to 70% in the 6-39 years age group [106]. In normal thymuses, however, lymphoid follicles are small, inactive and widely scattered, averaging less than 1 per low-power field. In FH, the density and size of lymphoid follicles are obviously increased (Fig. 5.6), although their

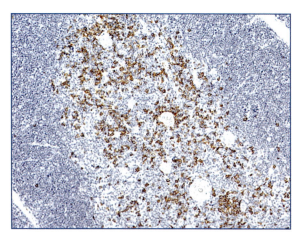

Fig. 5.5 Collection of B-lymphocytes in the medulla of normal thymus. Immunohistochemistry (streptavidin-biotin-peroxidase method) with anti-CD20 antibody. Original magnification: ×6

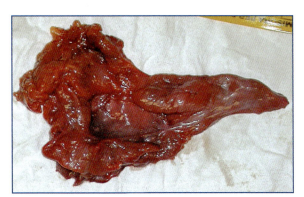

Fig. 5.4 Follicular hyperplasia of the thymus in a 32-year-old woman with myasthenia gravis. The thymus featured a triangular shape and weighed 32 g

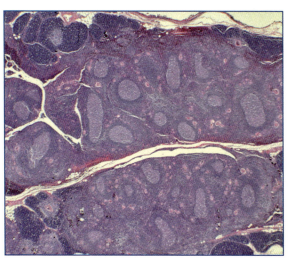

Fig. 5.6 Macrosection of the thymus with follicular hyperplasia. Numerous lymphoid follicles are present in the medulla. Hematoxylin and eosin, ×1.4 (original magnification)

number can vary from patient to patient and even in different areas of the same person. Objective criteria for the diagnosis of FH are lacking. Judd and Bueso-Ramos [107] reported an average of 3-4 lymphoid follicles per low-power field in two cases of FH of the thymus in Graves' disease. In a morphometric analysis of 26 cases of thymic FH in patients with myasthenia gravis, Moran et al. [108] found that the number of germinal centers can range from 2 to 19 per case. In this study, germinal centers showed an average diameter of 0.02-0.43 mm, a perimeter of 0.38-1.35 mm, and a cross-sectional area of 0.01-0.14 mm^2.

Lymphoid follicles are structurally identical to those found in peripheral lymphoid tissues, being composed of germinal centers surrounded by mantle zones (Fig. 5.7). The typical cellular composition of centroblasts, centrocytes, follicular dendritic cells, and tingible-body macrophages is observed in germinal centers. Their immunophenotype is similar to that detected in peripheral lymphoid tissues (Fig. 5.8). Of interest, CD23 was found to be strongly expressed in germinal center cells of hyperplastic thymuses from patients with myasthenia gravis [109], being absent in tonsillar germinal centers from nonmyasthenia gravis patients. An increased number of B-lymphocytes, polyclonal plasma cells, and mature peripheral type T-lymphocytes have also been reported [110].

Although initially thought to infiltrate the thymic medulla, lymphoid follicles and B-lymphocytes were demonstrated to be located in the perivascular space, adjacent to but outside of the epithelial network [111]. The basal lamina that separates the perivascular space from the thymic epithelial space appears to be frequently disrupted in FH of the thymus [112], allowing mixing of cells from the two compartments. The cortex of the thymus in these cases shows a normal age-dependent morphology.

FH of the thymus is usually associated with myasthenia gravis and other autoimmune diseases. Less frequent associations have been described with endocrine diseases.

Myasthenia gravis (MG) is an autoimmune disorder affecting the neuromuscular junction, characterized by the presence of either autoantibodies against the nicotinic acetylcholine receptor in the postsynaptic muscle endplate (seropositive disease) or autoantibodies against unknown targets (seronegative disease). The disease typically develops in the second to fourth decades being more frequent in women, although recent epidemiologic studies have shown an increased number of elderly-onset cases [113, 114].

The thymus plays a crucial role in the pathogenesis of MG (see Chap. 8). Approximately 10-20% of patients with MG harbor a thymoma, whereas thymic FH with expansion of thymic perivascular space by B-lymphocytes and lymphoid follicles is observed in more than 60% of them [115, 116]. Myoid cells in thymic FH from MG patients express acetylcholine receptors (AChR) but do not appear to be increased, as compared to normal thymuses [117], whereas mature dendritic cells are more numerous in nonmedullary areas, such as the outer cortex and around germinal centers [118]. Interleukin production by thymic epithelial cells and perifollicular macrophages has been postulated to play a role in the development of FH in MG patients [119]. Recurrence of thymic FH after thymectomy, probably due to incomplete surgery, has been reported [120]. Diffuse B-cell proliferation lacking germinal centers can also be observed in some MG patients, particularly after aza-

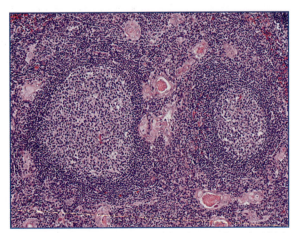

Fig. 5.7 Follicular hyperplasia of the thymus: lymphoid follicles show germinal centers surrounded by mantle zones. Hematoxylin and eosin, ×10 (original magnification)

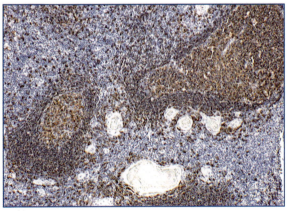

Fig. 5.8 Expression of CD20 in lymphoid follicles in thymic follicular hyperplasia. Immunohistochemistry (streptavidin-biotin-peroxidase method), with anti-CD20 antibody. Original magnification: ×10

thioprine treatment [121]. Since clusters of follicular dendritic cells can be evidenced with immunohistochemistry, these cases have been interpreted as early stages of thymic FH [122]. Quite different is the histologic aspect of the thymus in seronegative MG patients, since it shows an increase in mature T lymphocytes with normal number of B-cells in the expanded perivascular space. Thymic atrophy is detected in 10-20% of patients of MG [121], especially in elderly-onset cases [123].

FH of the thymus has also been associated with other autoimmune diseases, such as systemic lupus erythematosus [124, 125], progressive systemic sclerosis [126], rheumatoid arthritis [127], and Behçet's syndrome [128]. FH was described in two patients with Sjogren's syndrome showing elevated serum antinuclear antibody levels [129]. In these cases, the thymus contained also several cystic spaces separated by thick walls and lined by flattened cuboidal epithelium. The actual percentage of FH of the thymus in patients with autoimmune diseases (other than MG) is not available in the literature. Radiological and/or histopathological studies have not been performed in large series of patients. Aarli et al. [130] studied three groups of thymectomized patients with MG, observing FH of the thymus in 32 cases and thymoma in 16 of them. Among the 32 patients with FH, systemic lupus erythematosus was associated in two cases, whereas rheumatoid arthritis and juvenile diabetes mellitus were detected in two patients and one patient, respectively. Polymyositis was observed in two patients with thymoma. A retrospective analysis of 79 patients with juvenile-onset MG was carried-out by Lindner et al. [131], the mean age of onset being 13.7 years. Histopathological analysis was available in 65 thymectomized patients. FH was detected in 89% of the thymectomized patients and the most frequently associated immune-mediated diseases were hyperthyroidism (six cases), diabetes mellitus (two cases) and rheumatoid arthritis (two cases) [131].

Unusual associations, such as thymic FH with histiocytosis X (eosinophilic granuloma) and MG [132] or FH with pure red cell aplasia and secondary erythropoietin resistance [133], have also been reported.

The occurrence of thymic hyperplasia in Graves' disease has been known for long time. Histopathologic anomalies of the thymus characterized by the presence of lymphoid follicles in the medulla were stated to occur in approximately one third of patients with thyrotoxicosis [134]. However, the exact nature of the thymic changes in Graves' disease has been obscured by the frequent lack of histopathologic descriptions. The occurrence of lymphoid follicles is specifically mentioned in a few reports of thymectomy specimens [74, 135-138], but the majority of reported cases were based on radiologic studies only, with no thymic tissue available for histopathologic analysis [107]. The approximate quantification of the involvement of true hyperplasia versus lymphoid hyperplasia in the thymus of patients with thyrotoxicosis is, therefore, difficult. The confusion in the literature on this topic is properly underlined by Judd and Bueso-Ramos [107]. The authors described two patients with Graves' disease who underwent thymectomy because of an anterior mediastinal mass. Combined TTH and FH was diagnosed, since histopathologic studies evidenced an increase in thymic weight with expansion of cortical and medullary regions, consistent with TTH, together with prominent lymphoid follicles in the medulla with active germinal centers, typical of FH.

Isolated reports described the occurrence of thymic FH in patients with liver cirrhosis [139] or ulcerative colitis [140]. Thymectomy has been suggested by some Japanese authors in patients with ulcerative colitis who are resistant to conventional therapy. In 78 patients with ulcerative colitis treated by thymectomy, histological examination disclosed hyperplasia of the thymic epithelial cells and presence of lymphoid follicles [141].

Thymic Changes in Infectious Diseases

Little is known about the morphological changes that occur in the thymus in infectious diseases. The most documented alterations were described in patients with HIV infection and only sporadic reports deal with those occurring in other diseases.

HIV Infection

Thymus tissues removed from adult patients who died from acquired immunodeficiency syndrome (AIDS) show pronounced involution and loss of normal thymic architecture. The cortex and medulla are effaced and the normal cortico-medullary demarcation is lost [142, 143]. Both thymocytes and epithelial elements are markedly depleted. Epithelial cells are spindle-shaped and consist mainly of thin cords and small nests, exhibiting at times pyknotic nuclei [143, 144]. Striking paucity of Hassall's bodies was noted in all reported cases. In 14 thymuses removed from people who died from AIDS, Grody et al. [144] evidenced absence of Hassall's bodies in four cases and marked calcification in the remaining ten cases. Changes in Hassall's bodies were not observed in control cases (patients with chronic or debilitating illnesses other than AIDS) [144]. Additional reported alterations were the presence of variable degrees of plasma cell infiltration and patchy fibrosis [142], accompanied by vascular changes, such as hyalinization and onion-skin patterns [144]. At immunohistochemistry, cells positive for HIV-1 *gag* and *env* proteins were detected in low numbers, both inside the thymic epithelial space and in the perivascular space [145]. Increased numbers of CD8+ T-lymphocytes, especially in perivascular areas, were described [146, 147].

The histopathologic findings of the thymus in pediatric HIV infection are similar to those detected in adults. Precocious involution, often mimicking dysplasia, and lymphomononuclear or plasmacytic infiltrates with medullary lymphoid follicles were observed in thymic biopsies of 11 children with AIDS [148]. In 29 pediatric autopsies of AIDS patients (mean age: 1.77 years), Quijano et al. [149] evidenced severe lymphoid depletion of the thymus with plasmacytic infiltrates and Warthin-Finkeldey multinucleated giant cells. Hassall's bodies were absent in three cases and calcified in three patients, whereas they showed microcystic transformation in four cases.

The early phases of thymic changes were studied in juvenile rhesus monkeys (*Macaca mulatta*) experimentally infected with simian immunodeficiency virus [150]. The first changes were observed 12-24 weeks after infection and consisted of narrowing of the thymic cortex, characterized by widespread loss of cortical epithelial cells and reduction of the immature CD4+/CD8+ double-positive T-cells. No increase of pyknotic T-cells, but rather a decrease in their proliferation rate was detected [151]. A few reports describe the histological features of the thymus in the initial stages of HIV infection in human adults. In a 28-year-old man with thymus enlargement and early AIDS, thymic biopsy revealed persistence of many Hassall's bodies and lymphoid follicular hyperplasia, almost identical to that seen in myasthenia gravis. HIV RNA and *p24* HIV protein were evidenced in the germinal centers, both in lymphoid cells and in follicular dendritic cells [152]. Similar findings were observed by Burke et al. [153] in the thymic tissue collected from 11 HIV-1 seropositive drug users who had died suddenly from drug intoxication or trauma, but had never shown AIDS symptoms. Lymphoid follicles were present in all thymuses, sometimes accompanied by Warthin-Finkeldey multinucleated giant cells. In situ hybridization demonstrated viral RNA in hyperplastic follicles and in scattered medullary lymphocytes [153]. The authors concluded that lymphoid follicular hyperplasia, similar to that observed in lymph nodes and spleen, characterizes the early stages of HIV infection in the thymus, thus preceding the marked involution usually detected in all AIDS fatal cases.

Histopathologic changes similar to those described in late AIDS patients have been observed in primary immunodeficient states, and in patients with graft-versus-host disease or after cyclosporine therapy. In malnourished people, the thymus appears atrophic, but shows a normal number of cystically dilated Hassall's bodies [146].

An unusual form of thymic lesion associated with HIV infection in children is the multilocular thymic cyst. The architecture of the thymus is distorted by the presence of multiple cystic cavities, usually lined by squamous epithelium, associated with follicular hyperplasia with prominent germinal centers and diffuse plasmacytosis. Islands of residual thymic tissue can be seen within the cyst walls, together with cholesterol granulomas and fibrovascular proliferation [154-156]. Eight cases of multilocular thymic cysts in HIV-infected pediatric patients (age range: 2.1 to 12.1 years) were reported by Kontny et al. [154]. The anterior mediastinal mass had been incidentally discovered in all cases and its multiloculated appearance was well depicted at computed tomography. At follow-up, the mass resolved completely or decreased in size in five patients. In another series of four cases of multilocular thymic cysts in HIV-infected children, described by Avila [156], the mass decreased in volume in two patients, did not change in one, and increased in size in the remaining one. It was postulated that aberrant immunoregulation in HIV-infected children can lead to follicular hyperplasia and cystic transformation of Hassall's bodies and thymic epithelial cells [154].

Multilocular thymic cysts were also described in HIV-negative patients in association with Sjogren's syndrome [157], mediastinal yolk sac tumors [158], mediastinal seminomas [159], thymoma [160], or follicular hyperplasia of the thymus [129].

Other Infectious Diseases

Thymic alterations were studied in 35 patients who died from infectious mononucleosis [161]. The largest group of patients was affected by the X-linked lymphoproliferative syndrome, but 14 of them were not. The most important changes were described in Hassall's bodies, which were either moderately reduced in number or markedly depleted. In seven cases, no Hassall's bodies were identified. The destruction of Hassall's bodies was similar in appearance to that evidenced in other immune deficiency disorders. Effacement of the thymic architecture by massive lymphoproliferation was detected in six cases. Epstein-Barr virus was visualized in B-cells surrounded by cytotoxic T-cells in one patient only [161].

Miliary tuberculosis and brucellosis have been sporadically reported to affect the thymus, causing the same histopathologic changes usually observed in other lymphoid organs [162]. Of interest, after aerogenic or intravenous infection in mice, the thymus has been found to be consistently colonized by mycobacteria, such as M. tuberculosis, M. avium and M. bovis [163]. Granulomatous lesions, although present in lungs, were not identified in thymic tissues. The authors postulated that direct infection of the thymus might alter the host's immune response to mycobacteria.

References

1. Castleman B (1955) Atlas of tumor pathology. Tumors of the thymus gland, fascicle 19. Armed Forces Institute of Pathology, Washington, DC
2. Rosai J, Levine GD (1976) Atlas of tumor pathology. Tumors of the thymus, Second series, fascicle 13. Armed Forces Institute of Pathology, Washington, DC
3. Goldstein G (1966) Thymitis and myasthenia gravis. Lancet 2:1164-1167
4. Sloan HE (1943) The thymus in myasthenia gravis with observations in normal anatomy and histology of the thymus. Surgery 13:154-174
5. Simpson JA (1958) An evaluation of thymectomy in myasthenia gravis. Brain 81:112-144
6. Young M, Turnbull HM (1931) An analysis of the data collected by the status lymphaticus investigation committee. J Pathol Bacteriol 34:213-258
7. Steinmann GG, Müller-Hermelink HK (1984) Lymphocyte differentiation and its microenvironment in the human thymus during aging. Monogr Dev Biol 17:142-155
8. Kendall MD, Johnson HR, Singh J (1980) The weight of the human thymus gland at necroscopy. J Anat 131:483-497
9. Judd RL, Welch SL (1988) Myoid cell differentiation in true thymic hyperplasia and lymphoid hyperplasia. Arch Pathol Lab Med 112:1140-1144
10. Linegar AG, Odell JA, Fennell WM et al (1993) Massive thymic hyperplasia. Ann Thorac Surg 55:1197-1201
11. Arliss J, Scholes J, Dickson PR et al (1988) Massive thymic hyperplasia in an adolescent. Ann Thorac Surg 45:220-222
12. Wenger MC, Cohen AJ, Greensite F (1994) Thymic rebound in a patient with scrotal mesothelioma. J Thorac Imaging 9:145-147
13. Ricci C, Pescarmona E, Rendina EA et al (1989) True thymic hyperplasia: A clinicopathological study. Ann Thorac Surg 47:741-745
14. Lamesch AJ (1983) Massive thymic hyperplasia in infants. Z Kinderchir 38:16-18
15. Tatebe S, Oka K, Uehara A et al (2006) Unusual remnant thymic tissue in an adult mimicking malignant neoplasm: Escape from age-related involution. Thorac Cardiovasc Surg 54:138-140
16. Yoshitake T, Itoyama S, Masunaga A et al (1994) Focal thymic hyperplasia in an adult: Report of a case. Surg Today 24:72-74
17. Katz SM, Chatten J, Bishop HC et al (1977) Report of a case of gross thymic hyperplasia in a child. Am J Clin Pathol 68:786-790
18. Pompeo E, Cristino B, Mauriello A et al (1999) Recurrent massive hyperplasia of the thymus. Scand Cardiovasc J 33:306-308
19. Ruco LP, Rosati S, Palmieri B et al (1989) True thymic hyperplasia: A histological and immunohistochemical study. Histopathology 15:640-643
20. Miniero R, Busca A, Leonardo E et al (1993) Rebound thymic hyperplasia following high dose chemotherapy and allogeneic BMT. Bone Marrow Transplant 11:67-70
21. Marchevsky AM, Kaneko M (1992) Surgical pathology of the mediastinum, 2 edn. Raven Press, New York
22. Sauter ER, Arensman RM, Falterman KW (1991) Thymic enlargement in children. Am Surg 57:21-23
23. Filler RM, Simpson JS, Ein SH (1979) Mediastinal masses in infants and children. Pediatr Clin North Am 26:677-690
24. Pedroza Meléndez A, Larenas-Linnemann D (1997) Thymus hyperplasia, differential diagnosis in the wheezing infant. Allergol Immunopathol (Madr) 25:59-62
25. O'Shea PA, Pansatiankul B, Farnes F (1978) Giant thymic hyperplasia in infants: Immunologic, histologic, and ultrastructural observations. Lab Invest 38:391
26. Rüther U, Müller HA, Nunnensiek C et al (1990) Thymus hyperplasia in patients with malignant testicular tumors. Med Klin (Münich) 85:72-77
27. Pagliai F, Rigacci L, Briganti V et al (2003) PET scan evaluation of thymic mass after autologous peripheral blood stem-cell transplantation in an adult with non-Hodgkin's lymphoma. Leuk Lymphoma 44:2015-2018
28. Hessissen L, Nachef MN, Kili A et al (2006) Thymic hyperplasia following treatment for nephroblastoma. Arch Pediatr 13:358-360
29. Peylan-Ramu N, Haddy TB, Jones E et al (1989) High frequency of benign mediastinal uptake of gallium-67 after completion of chemotherapy in children with high-grade non-Hodgkin's lymphoma. J Clin Oncol 7:1800-1806
30. Hermann R, Greminger P, Dommann-Scherrer C et al (1994) Diffuse thymus hyperplasia following chemotherapy for nodular sclerosing Hodgkin lymphoma. Schweiz Med Wochenschr 124:1666-1671
31. Ford EG, Lockhart SK, Sullivan MP et al (1987) Mediastinal mass following chemotherapeutic treatment of Hodgkin's disease: Recurrent tumor or thymic hyperplasia? J Pediatr Surg 22:1155-1159

32. Caffey J, de Liberti C (1959) Acute atrophy of the thymus induced by adrenocorticosteroids. AJR Am J Roentgenol 82:530-540
33. Riazmontazer N, Bedayat G (1993) Aspiration cytology of an enlarged thymus presenting as a mediastinal mass. A case report. Acta Cytol 37:427-430
34. Hoerl HD, Wojtowycz M, Gallagher HA et al (2000) Cytologic diagnosis of true thymic hyperplasia by combined radiologic imaging and aspiration cytology: A case report including flow cytometric analysis. Diagn Cytopathol 23:417-421
35. Bangerter M, Behnisch W, Griesshammer M (2000) Mediastinal masses diagnosed as thymus hyperplasia by fine needle aspiration cytology. Acta Cytol 44:743-747
36. Gerhardt S, Gehling G, Schuster P (2004) Rebound hyperplasia of the thymus with secondary intrathymic bleeding. Rare differential diagnosis of acute chest pain. Dtsch Med Wochenschr 129:1916-1918
37. Langer CJ, Keller SM, Erner SM (1992) Thymic hyperplasia with hemorrhage simulating recurrent Hodgkin disease after chemotherapy-induced complete remission. Cancer 70:2082-2086
38. Eifinger F, Ernestus K, Benz-Bohm G et al (2007) True thymic hyperplasia associated with severe thymic cyst bleeding in a newborn: Case report and review of the literature. Ann Diagn Pathol 11:358-362
39. Tangthangtham A, Chonmaitri I, Subhannachart P et al (1998) Solitary fibrous tumor arising from hyperplastic thymus. J Med Assoc Thai 81:708-711
40. Gelfand DW, Goldman AS, Law EJ et al (1972) Thymic hyperplasia in children recovering from thermal burns. J Trauma 12:813-817
41. Rizk G, Cueto L, Amplatz K et al (1972) Rebound enlargement of the thymus after successful corrective surgery for transposition of the great vessels. Am J Roentgenol Radium Ther Nucl Med 116:528-530
42. Balcom RJ, Hakanson DO, Werner A et al (1985) Massive thymic hyperplasia in an infant with Beckwith-Wiedemann syndrome. Arch Pathol Lab Med 109:153-155
43. Schilke K, Schaefer F, Waldherr R et al (2000) A case of Perlman syndrome: Fetal gigantism, renal dysplasia, and severe neurological deficits. Am J Med Genet 91:29-33
44. Itoh H, Chuganji Y, Kodama Y et al (2000) Pena-shokeir type I syndrome with thymic and systemic lymphoid hyperplasia: Report of an autopsy case. Hum Pathol 31:1321-1324
45. Elias S, Boelen L, Simpson JL (1978) Syndromes of camptodactyly, multiple ankylosis, facial anomalies, and pulmonary hypoplasia. Birth Defects Orig Artic Ser 14:243-251
46. Cohen M, Hill CA, Cangir A et al (1980) Thymic rebound after treatment of childhood tumors. AJR Am J Roentgenol 135:151-156
47. Young GA, Grace J, Williams BG et al (1991) An unusual cutaneous lymphoma with B and T cell characteristics showing gallium-67 positive benign thymic hyperplasia following intensive chemotherapy. Aust N Z J Med 21:447-450
48. Scheinpflug K, Schmitt J, Jentsch-Ullrich K et al (2003) Thymic hyperplasia following successful treatment for nodular-sclerosing Hodgkin's disease. Leuk Lymphoma 44:1615-1617
49. Akaki S, Shinya T, Sato S et al (2006) Positive gallium-67 and thallium-201 scans in thymic rebound after chemotherapy for lymphoma. Ann Nucl Med 20:161-163
50. Leibundgut K, Willi U, Plüss HJ (1992) Thymic rebound following successful chemotherapy of B-lymphoma in an adolescent boy. Eur J Pediatr 151:95-97
51. Düe W, Dieckmann KP, Stein H (1989) Thymic hyperplasia following chemotherapy of a testicular germ cell tumor. Immunohistological evidence for a simple rebound phenomenon. Cancer 63:446-449
52. Dieckmann KP, Düe W, Bauknecht KJ et al (1988) Reactive benign thymus hyperplasia following cytostatic chemotherapy. Dtsch Med Wochenschr 113:598-601
53. Moul JW, Fernandez EB, Bryan MG et al (1994) Thymic hyperplasia in newly diagnosed testicular germ cell tumors. J Urol 152:1480-1483
54. Hansen LJ, Madsen EL, Moller MN (1993) Benign enlargement of the thymus after chemotherapy of metastasizing testicular cancer. Ugeskr Laeger 155:1141-1142
55. Chertoff J, Barth RA, Dickerman JD et al (1991) Rebound thymic hyperplasia five years after chemotherapy for Wilms' tumor. Pediatr Radiol 21:596-597
56. Bell BA, Esseltine DW, Azouz EM (1984) Rebound thymic hyperplasia in a child with cancer. Med Pediatric Oncol 12:144-147
57. Panadero MA, Cruz JJ, Gomez A et al (1996) Mediastinal mass following chemotherapy in patient with Ewing sarcoma and osteosarcoma. J Intern Med 239:457-460
58. Sehbai AS, Tallaksen RJ, Bennett J et al (2006) Thymic hyperplasia after adjuvant chemotherapy in breast cancer. J Thorac Imaging 21:43-46
59. Hara M, McAdams HP, Vredenburgh JJ et al (1999) Thymic hyperplasia after high-dose chemotherapy and autologous stem cell transplantation: Incidence and significance in patients with breast cancer. AJR Am J Roentgenol 173:1341-1344
60. Simmonds P, Silberstein M, McKendrick J (1993) Thymic hyperplasia in adults following chemotherapy for malignancy. Aust N Z J Med 23:264-267
61. Suzuki K, Kurokawa K, Suzuki T et al (1997) Anterior mediastinal metastasis of testicular germ cell tumor: Relation to benign thymic hyperplasia. Eur Urol 32:371-374
62. Tobisu K, Kakizoe T, Takai K et al (1987) Thymic enlargement following treatment for a metastatic germ cell tumor: A case report. J Urol 137:520-521
63. Rossi D, Franceschetti S, Capello D et al (2007) Simultaneous diagnosis of CD3+ T-cell large granular lymphocyte leukaemia and true thymic hyperplasia. Leuk Res 31:1019-1021
64. Choyke PL, Zeman RK, Gootemberg JE et al (1987) Thymic atrophy and regrowth in response to chemotherapy: CT Evaluation. AJR Am J Roentgenol 149:269-272

65. Shin MS, Ho KJ (1983) Diffuse thymic hyperplasia following chemotherapy for nodular sclerosing Hodgkin's disease. An immunologic rebound phenomenon? Cancer 51:30-33
66. Anchisi S, Abele R, Guetty-Alberto M et al (1998) Management of an isolated thymic mass after primary therapy for lymphoma. Ann Oncol 9:95-100
67. Michel F, Gilbeau JP, Six C et al (1995) Progressive mediastinal widening after therapy for Hodgkin's disease. Acta Clin Belg 50:282-287
68. Pendlebury SC, Boyages S, Koutts J et al (1992) Thymic hyperplasia associated with Hodgkin disease and thyrotoxicosis. Cancer 70:1985-1987
69. Edington H, Salwitz J, Longo DL et al (1986) Thymic hyperplasia masquerading as recurrent Hodgkin's disease: Case report and review of the literature. J Surg Oncol 33:120-123
70. Carmosino L, DiBenedetto A, Feffer S (1985) Thymic hyperplasia following successful chemotherapy. A report of two cases and review of the literature. Cancer 56:1526-1528
71. Hendriks JM, Van Schil PE, Schrijvers D et al (1999) Rebound thymic hyperplasia after chemotherapy in a patient treated for pulmonary metastases. Acta Chir Belg 99:312-314
72. Sperandio P, Tomio P, Oliver RT et al (1996) Gonadal atrophy as a cause of thymic hyperplasia after chemotherapy. Br J Cancer 74:991-992
73. Kissin CM, Husband JE, Nicholas D et al (1987) Benign thymic enlargement in adults after chemotherapy: CT demonstration. Radiology 163:67-70
74. White SR, Hall JB, Little A (1986) An approach to mediastinal masses associated with hyperthyroidism. Chest 90:691-693
75. Nakamura T, Murakami M, Horiguchi H et al (2004) A case of thymic enlargement in hyperthyroidism in a young woman. Thyroid 14:307-310
76. Budavari AI, Whitaker MD, Helmers RA (2002) Thymic hyperplasia presenting as anterior mediastinal mass in two patients with Graves diseases. Mayo Clin Proc 77:495-499
77. Murakami M, Hosoi Y, Negisci T et al (1996) Thymic hyperplasia in patient with Graves' disease. Identification of thyrotropin receptors in human thymus. J Clin Invest 98:2228-2234
78. Wortsman J, McConnachie P, Baker JR Jr et al (1988) Immunoglobulins that cause thymocyte proliferation from a patient with Graves' disease and an enlarged thymus. Am J Med 85:117-121
79. Scheiff JM, Cordier AC, Haumont S (1977) Epithelial cell proliferation in thymic hyperplasia induced by triiodothyronine. Clin Exp Immunol 27:516-521
80. Ribeiro-Carvalho MM, Farias-de-Oliveira DA, Villaverde DM et al (2002) Triiodothyronine modulates extracellular matrix-mediated interactions between thymocytes and thymic microenvironmental cells. Neuroimmunomodulation 10:142-152
81. Ribeiro-Carvalho MM, Lima-Quaresma KR, Mouço T et al (2007) Triiodothyronine modulates thymocyte migration. Scand J Immunol 66:17-25
82. Yulish BS, Owens RP (1980) Thymic enlargement in a child during therapy for primary hypothyrodism. AJR Am J Roentgenol 135:157-158
83. Niendorf ER, Parker JA, Yechoor V et al (2005) Thymic hyperplasia in thyroid cancer patients. J Thorac Imaging 20:1-4
84. Michigisci T, Mizukami Y, Shuke N et al (1993) Visualization of the thymus with therapeutic doses of radioiodine in patients with thyroid cancer. Eur J Nucl Med 20:75-9
85. Montella L, Caraglia M, Abbruzzese A et al (2005) Mediastinal images resembling thymus following 131-I treatment for thyroid cancer. Monaldi Arch Chest Dis 63:114-117
86. Bazzoni N, Ambrosi B, Arosio M et al (1990) Acromegaly and thymic hyperplasia: A case report. J Endocrinol Invest 13:931-915
87. Polgreen L, Steiner M, Dietz CA et al (2007) Thymic hyperplasia in a child treated with growth hormone. Growth Horm IGF Res 17:41-46
88. Savino W, Postel-Vinay MC, Smaniotto S et al (2002) The thymus gland: A target organ for growth hormone. Scan J Immunol 55:442-452
89. de Mello-Coelho V, Gagnerault MC, Souberbielle JC et al (1998) Growth hormone and its receptor are expressed in human thymic cells. Endocrinology 139:3837-3842
90. Smaniotto S, de Mello-Coelho, Villa-Verde DM et al (2005) Growth hormone modulates thymocyte development in vivo through a combined action of laminin and CXC chemokine ligand 12. Endocrinology 146:3005-3017
91. Timsit J, Savino W, Safieh B et al (1992) Growth hormone and insulin-like growth factor-I stimulate hormonal function and proliferation of thymic epithelial cells. J Clin Endocrinol Metab 75:183-188
92. Fahy GM (2003) Apparent induction of partial thymic regeneration in a normal human subject: A case report. J Anti Aging Med 6:219-227
93. Caffey J, Sibley R (1960) Regrowth and overgrowth of the thymus after atrophy induced by oral administration of adrenocorticosteroids in human infants. Pediatrics 26:762-770
94. Doppman JL, Oldfield EH, Chrousos GP et al (1986) Rebound thymic hyperplasia after treatment of Cushing's syndrome. AJR Am J Roentgenol 147:1145-1147
95. Tabarin A, Catargi B, Chanson P et al (1995) Pseudotumors of the thymus after correction of hypercortisolism in patients with ectopic ACTH syndrome: A report of five cases. Clin Endocrinol (Oxf) 42:207-213
96. Otha K, Shichiri M, Kameya T et al (2000) Thymic hyperplasia as source of ectopic ACTH production. Endocr J 47:487-492
97. Sloper JC (1955) The pathology of the adrenals, thymus and certain other endocrine glands in Addison's disease: An analysis of 37 necropsies. Proc R Soc Med 48:625-628
98. Ferri C, Colaci M, Battolla L et al (2006) Thymus alterations and systemic sclerosis. Rheumatology (Oxford) 45:72-75

99. Pardo-Mindan FJ, Crisci CD, Serrano M et al (1980) Immunological aspects of sarcoidosis associated with true thymic hyperplasia. Allergol Immunopathol (Madrid) 8:91-96
100. Nomori H, Ishihara T, Torikata C et al (1990) A case of massive true thymic hyperplasia with non-Hodgkin's lymphoma. Chest 98:1304-1305
101. Lee Y, Moallem S, Clauss RH (1979) Massive hyperplastic thymus in a 22-month-od infant. Ann Thorac Surg 27:356-358
102. Judd RL (1987) Massive thymic hyperplasia with myoid cell differentiation. Hum Pathol 18:1180-1183
103. Nezelof C, Normand C (1986) Tumor-like massive thymic hyperplasia in childhood: A possible defect of T-cell maturation, histological and cytoenzymatic studies of three cases. Thymus 8:177-186
104. Hofmann WJ, Momburg F, Möller P et al (1988) Intra- and extrathymic B cells in physiologic and pathologic conditions. Immunohistochemical study on normal thymus and lymphofollicular hyperplasia of the thymus. Virchows Arch A Pathol Anat Histopathol 412:431-442
105. Henry K (1968) The thymus in rheumatic heart disease. Clin Exp Immunol 3:509-523
106. Middleton G (1967) The incidence of follicular structures in the human thymus at autopsy. Aust J Exp Biol Med Sci 45:189-199
107. Judd R, Bueso-Ramos C (1990) Combined true thymic hyperplasia and lymphoid hyperplasia in Graves' disease. Pediatr Pathol 10:829-836
108. Moran CA, Suster S, Gil J et al (1990) Morphometric analysis of germinal centres in nonthymomatous patients with myasthenia gravis. Arch Pathol Lab Med 114:689-691
109. Murai H, Hara H, Hatae T et al (1997) Expression of CD23 in the germinal center of thymus from myasthenia gravis patients. J Neuroimmunol 76:61-69
110. Palestro G, Tridente G, Botto Micca F et al (1983) Immunohistochemical and enzyme histochemical contributions to the problem concerning the role of the thymus in the pathogenesis of myasthenia gravis. Virchows Arch B Cell Pathol Incl Mol Pathol 44:173-186
111. Tamaoki N, Habu S, Kameya T (1971) Thymic lymphoid follicles in autoimmune diseases. II. Histological, histochemical and electron microscopic studies. Keio J Med 20:57-68
112. Bofill M, Janossy G, Willcox N et al (1985) Microenvironments in the normal thymus and the thymus in myasthenia gravis. Am J Pathol 119:462-473
113. Phillips LH, Torner JC (1996) Epidemiologic evidence for a changing natural history of myasthenia gravis. Neurology 47:1233-1238
114. Matsuda M, Dohi-Iijima N, Nakamura A et al (2005) Increase in incidence of elderly-onset patients with myasthenia gravis in Nagano Prefecture Japan. Intern Med 44:572-577
115. Wekerle H, Müller-Hermelink HK (1986) The thymus in myasthenia gravis. In Müller-Hermelink HK (ed) The human thymus. Springer-Verlag, Berlin, pp 179-206
116. Marx A, Wilisch A, Schultz A et al (1997) Pathogenesis of myasthenia gravis. Virchows Arch 430:355-364
117. Joshi VV, Oleske JM, Minnefor AB et al (1984) Pathology of suspected acquired immune deficiency syndrome in children: A study of eight cases. Pediatr Pathol 2:71-87
118. Nagane Y, Utsugisawa K, Obara D et al (2003) Dendritic cells in hyperplastic thymuses from patients with myasthenia gravis. Muscle Nerve 27:582-589
119. Emilie D, Crevon MC, Cohen-Kaminsky S et al (1991) In situ production of interleukins in hyperplastic thymus from myasthenia gravis patients. Hum Pathol 22:461-468
120. Rosenberg M, Jaúregui WO, Herrera MR et al (1986) Recurrence of thymic hyperplasia after trans-sternal thymectomy in myasthenia gravis. Chest 89:888-889
121. Schalke BC, Mertens HG, Kirchner T et al (1987) Long-term treatment with azathioprine abolishes thymic lymphoid follicular hyperplasia in myasthenia gravis. Lancet 2(8560):682
122. Kirchner T, Schalke B, Melms A et al (1986) Immunohistological patterns of non-neoplastic changes in the thymus in Myasthenia gravis. Virchows Arch B Cell Pathol Incl Mol Pathol 52:237-257
123. Ishii W, Matsuda M, Hanyuda M et al (2007) Comparison of the histological and immunohistochemical features of the thymus in young- and elderly-onset myasthenia gravis without thymoma. J Clin Neurosci 14:110-115
124. Mackay IR, Degail P (1963) Thymic "germinal centers" and plasma cells in systemic lupus erythematosus. Lancet 2(7309):667
125. Goldstein G, Abbot A, Mackay IR (1968) An electron-microscope study of the human thymus: Normal appearances and findings in myasthenia gravis and systemic lupus erithematosus. J Pathol Bacteriol 95:211-215
126. Biggart JD, Nevin NC (1967) Hyperplasia of the thymus in progressive systemic sclerosis. J Pathol Bacteriol 93:334-337
127. Burnet FM, Mackay IR (1962) Lymphoepithelial structures and autoimmune diseases. Lancet 2:1030-1033
128. Morgenstern NL, Shearn MA (1973) Thymic hyperplasia in Behçet's syndrome. Lancet 1(7801):482
129. Izumi H, Nobukawa B, Takahashi K et al (2005) Multilocular thymic cyst associated with follicular hyperplasia: Clinicopathologic study of 4 resected cases. Hum Pathol 36:841-844
130. Aarli JA, Gilhus NE, Matre R (1992) Myasthenia gravis with thymoma is not associated with an increased incidence of non-muscle autoimmune disorders. Autoimmunity 11:159-162
131. Lindner A, Schalke B, Toyka KV (1997) Outcome in juvenile-onset myasthenia gravis: A retrospective study with long-term follow-up of 79 patients. J Neurol 244:515-520
132. Pescarmona E, Rendina EA, Ricci C et al (1989) Histiocytosis X and lymphoid follicular hyperplasia of the thymus in myasthenia gravis. Histopathology 14:465-470

133. Wong KF, Chau KF, Chan JK et al (1995) Pure red cell aplasia associated with thymic lymphoid hyperplasia and secondary erythropoietin resistance. Am J Clin Pathol 103:346-347
134. Michie W, Gunn A (1966) The thyroid, the thymus and autoimmunity. Br J Clin Pract 20:9-13
135. Sandler M, Sacks G, Linde R et al (1983) The CT detection of thymic hyperplasia in association with thyrotoxicosis: Case report. Comput Radiol 7:365-368
136. Beddingfield GW, Campbell DC Jr, Hood RH Jr et al (1967) Simultaneous disorders of thyroid and thymus. Report of two cases. Ann Thorac Surg 4:445-450
137. Van Herle AJ, Chopra IJ (1971) Thymic hyperplasia in Graves' disease. J Clin Endocrinol Metab 32:140-146
138. Nicholson RL (1978) Thymic hyperplasia in thyrotoxicosis. J Can Assoc Radiol 29:264-265
139. Corridan M (1963) The thymus in hepatic cirrhosis. J Clin Pathol 16:445-447
140. Tsuchiya M, Asakura H, Yoshimatsu H (1989) Thymic abnormalities and autoimmune disease. Keio J Med 38:383-402
141. Tsuchiya M, Hibi T, Watanabe M et al (1991) Thymectomy in ulcerative colitis: A report of cases over a 13 year period. Thymus 17:67-73
142. Seemayer TA, Laroche AC, Russo P et al (1984) Precocious thymic involution manifest by epithelial injury in the acquired immune deficiency syndrome. Hum Pathol 15:469-474
143. Davis AE Jr (1984) The histopathological changes in the thymus gland in the acquired immune deficiency syndrome. Ann N Y Acad Sci 437:493-502
144. Grody WW, Fligiel S, Naeim F (1985) Thymus involution in the acquired immunodeficiency syndrome. Am J Clin Pathol 84:85-95
145. Schuurman HJ, Krone WJ, Broekhuizen R et al (1989) The thymus in acquired immune deficiency syndrome. Comparison with other types of immunodeficiency diseases, and presence of components of human immunodeficiency virus type 1. Am J Pathol 134:1329-1338
146. Linder J (1987) The thymus gland in secondary immunodeficiency. Arch Pathol Lab Med 111:1118-1122
147. Haynes BF, Hale LP (1998) The human thymus. A chimeric organ comprised of central and peripheral lymphoid components. Immunol Res 18:175-192
148. Joshi VV, Oleske JM, Saad S et al (1986) Thymus biopsy in children with acquired immunodeficiency syndrome. Arch Pathol Lab Med 110:837-842
149. Quijano G, Siminovich M, Drut R (1997) Histopathologic findings in the lymphoid and reticuloendothelial system in pediatric HIV infection: A postmortem study. Pediatr Pathol Lab Med 17: 845-856
150. Müller JG, Stahl-Hennig C, Rethwilm A et al (1991) Morphological alterations of lymph nodes and thymus during the early course of SIV infection of rhesus monkeys. Verh Dtsch Ges Pathol 75:102-107
151. Müller JG, Krenn V, Schindler C et al (1993) Alterations of thymus cortical epithelium and interdigitating dendritic cells but no increase of thymocyte cell death in the early course of simian immunodeficiency virus infection. Am J Pathol 143:699-713
152. Prevot S, Audouin J, Andre-Bougaran J et al (1992) Thymic pseudotumorous enlargement due to follicular hyperplasia in a human immunodeficiency virus sero-positive patient. Immunohistochemical and molecular biological study of viral infected cells. Am J Clin Pathol 97:420-425
153. Burke AP, Anderson D, Benson W et al (1995) Localization of human immunodeficiency virus 1 RNA in thymic tissues from asymptomatic drug addicts. Arch Pathol Lab Med 119:36-41
154. Mishalani SH, Lones MA, Said JW (1995) Multilocular thymic cyst. A novel thymic lesion associated with human immunodeficiency virus infection. Arch Pathol Lab Med 119:467-470
155. Kontny HU, Sleasman JW, Kingma DW et al (1997) Multilocular thymic cysts in children with human immunodeficiency virus infection: Clinical and pathologic aspects. J Pediatr 131:264-270
156. Avila NA, Mueller BU, Carrasquillo JA et al (1996) Multilocular thymic cysts: Imaging features in children with human immunodeficiency virus infection. Radiology 201:130-134
157. Kondo K, Miyoshi T, Sakiyama S et al (2001) Multilocular thymic cyst associated with Sjogren's syndrome. Ann Thorac Surg 72:1367-1369
158. Moran CA, Suster S (1997) Mediastinal yolk sac tumors associated with prominent multilocular cystic changes of thymic epithelium: A clinicopathologic and immunohistochemical study of five cases. Mod Pathol 10:800-803
159. Moran CA, Suster S (1995) Mediastinal seminomas with prominent cystic changes. A clinicopathologic study of 10 cases. Am J Surg Pathol 19:1047-1053
160. Liang SB, Ohtsuki Y, Sonobe H et al (1996) Multilocular thymic cysts associated with thymoma. A case report. Pathol Res Pract 192:1283-1287
161. Mroczek EC, Seemayer TA, Grierson HL et al (1987) Thymic lesions in fatal infectious mononucleosis. Clin Immunol Immunopathol 43:243-255
162. Henry K (1992) The thymus gland. In: Henry K, Symmers WSTC (eds) Thymus, lymph nodes, spleen and lymphatics. Churchill Livingstone, Edinburgh, pp 27-139
163. Nobrega C, Cardona PJ, Roque S et al (2007) The thymus as a target for mycobacterial infections. Microbes Infect 9:1521-1529

CHAPTER 6

Benign and Malignant Tumors

Cesar A. Moran

Introduction

The gamut of benign and malignant lesions that can occur in the mediastinum or thymus is wide in spectrum and beyond the scope of a chapter dealing with this rich pathology. This chapter will focus on primary mediastinal lesions with special interest in those that are more commonly seen. Although metastatic tumors to the mediastinum, in some circumstances, may mimic primary mediastinal tumors, they will be addressed in the context of the primary mediastinal lesions.

Benign Tumors

The presence of benign tumors in the mediastinal compartment can be viewed in two different aspects, namely benign cystic lesions and benign solid tumors.

Benign Cystic Lesions

Mediastinal cysts are some of the most commonly encountered benign tumors in this region. Important to note is that some of these benign cysts, although not necessarily of thymic origin, are coded under the designation of mediastinal cysts just by the fact that some gastrointestinal or upper respiratory structures are located in the mediastinal compartment. Some of these cysts will include esophageal, enteric, and bronchogenic cysts. In any of those cysts, the lining covering such structures will lead to the correct interpretation, i.e., columnar, respiratory, and squamous epithelium. However, in cases in which the lining of these cystic structures is difficult to determine, a good number of these cysts are gathered under the designation of foregut cysts. Regarding more specifically thymic cysts, the two most important are the unilocular and the multilocular thymic cyst [1, 2]. Unilocular thymic cysts are simple cysts with virtual absence of reactive or inflammatory changes. Unilocular cysts are more commonly seen in the pediatric age group, and histologically the diagnosis does not pose a problem. Multilocular thymic cysts (MTC) occur namely in adult individuals and may pose some difficulties in diagnosis.

Multilocular Thymic Cyst (MTC)

MTC is a distinctive thymic lesion probably unrelated to congenital (unilocular) thymic cyst, which has been postulated to derive from an acquired inflammatory reactive process [2]. Because of the large size and extension into adjacent structures, these lesions clinically may be confused with a malignant neoplasm.

Due to this particular fact – extension to adjacent structures – complete surgical resection is of great importance. In some cases in which complete surgical resection is not accomplished, recurrences of these lesions have been recorded [2]. To be underscored is the fact that many other tumors, either primary or metastatic to the mediastinum, may also present with MTC-like features. Thus, extensive sampling and adequate clinical information are imperative.

Histologically, MTC shows distinctive features, namely the presence of multiple cystic structures separated by areas of fibrosis, inflammatory infiltrate, and/or residual thymic tissue. The cystic structures are usually lined by squamous epithelium, which at times may show atypical squamous features and pseudoepitheliomatous hyperplasia [3, 4] mimicking a possible squamous cell carcinoma. Other areas may show dilated Hassall's corpuscles, lymphoid hyperplasia, cholesterol cleft granulomas, or even extensive areas of hemorrhage (Figs. 6.1, 6.2). Although necrosis may be present in these cysts, it is usually not extensive or the main component of these lesions.

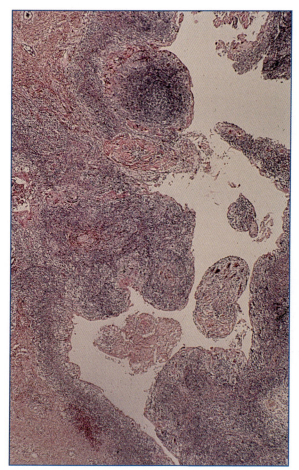

Fig. 6.1 Multilocular thymic cyst showing a cystic structure with lymphoid hyperplasia

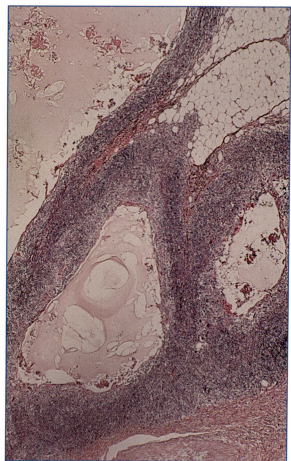

Fig. 6.2 Multilocular thymic cyst with dilated Hassall's corpuscles and lymphoid hyperplasia

Solid Benign Tumors

Sclerosing Mediastinitis

Several processes showing inflammatory and fibrosing changes in which the etiology is not determined have been grouped under the designation of idiopathic fibroinflammatory (Fibrosing/Sclerosing) lesions of the mediastinum [5]. In general, these lesions are characterized by extensive fibrosis that may involve mediastinal structures such as great vessels, pleura, pericardium, and thymus. Although, as stated before, a specific cause has not been determined, there is speculation that these lesions may obey immunological disturbances [6, 7]. The process appears to more commonly affect black people, and an analogy between sclerosing mediastinitis and keloid has been drawn [8]. Important to note is that similar lesions may also occur in the background of infectious conditions, namely fungal diseases such as histoplasma, blastomyces, etc.

Histologically, three main stages have been described in these lesions: Stage I: predominantly edematous with admixed spindle cells, inflammatory cells, and thin-walled vessels (cytologic atypia and necrosis are absent); Stage II: ill-defined lesions composed of hyalinized connective tissue with scattered inflammatory cells; and Stage III: lesions composed predominantly of dense or sclerotic fibroconnective tissue (calcifications may be present, cellularity and inflammatory cells are inconspicuous).

Thymolipoma

Thymolipoma is an unusual benign tumor of the thymus that often is reported as a peculiarity. Only a few large series of these unusual tumors have been reported [9, 10]. These tumors may occur in any individual at any age, and cases in patients younger than 10 years have been documented [9]. Patients may be completely asymptomatic or present with symptoms due to compression of the tumor in adjacent structures. No association between thymolipomas and myasthenia gravis has been documented.

Histologically, the tumors are composed of variable amounts of mature adipose tissue intermixed with remnants of thymic tissue. Hassall's corpuscles may appear dilated and calcified (Fig. 6.3).

Hemangioma

Hemangioma is a benign vascular tumor of unusual occurrence in the mediastinal region [11, 12]. These tumors can occur at any age without sex discrimination, although they are more common in younger individuals under 35 years of age. Clinically, the patients may be asymptomatic or present with symptoms related to the size of the tumors such as cough, chest pain, etc. Mediastinal hemangiomas may reach a large size of more than 10 cm in greatest diameter, and some authors consider that they do not represent true tumors but vascular malformations.

Histologically, these tumors show similar features as those occurring in soft tissues, namely capillary hemangiomas characterized by a solid proliferation of endothelial cells with dilated small vessels, while other tumors show dilated vascular spaces with inflammatory infiltrate, fibrous tissue, and smooth muscle proliferation.

Benign Neuroendocrine Tumors

The two most important tumors to be considered in this family include paraganglioma and ectopic parathyroid adenomas.

Paraganglioma

These tumors are also named aortic body tumors because of their anatomic predisposition in the aortic arch. However, these neoplasms may also occur in the posterior mediastinum [13, 14]. Although more common in the adult population, these neoplasms have been also documented in younger patients. Some patients may present with symptoms related to the functionality of the neoplasms including headache, hypertension, and sweating, while others may be asymptomatic. The tumors are usually small, but they can reach about 10 cm in diameter.

Histologically, these tumors show the classic so-called *zellballen* pattern of growth, composed of islands of larger cells with macronuclei. In some cells the nuclei are bizarre, giving the impression of a malignant neoplasm (Figs. 6.4, 6.5). However, despite the cellular atypia, mitotic activity is absent or rare. Extensive hyalinization may be seen in these cases, while in others the pattern of growth may be that of a spindle cell proliferation. In some cases, immunohistochemical studies may be necessary to corroborate the diagnosis

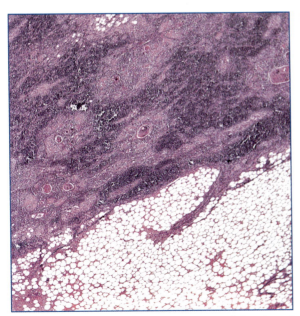

Fig. 6.3 Thymolipoma showing remnants of thymic and adipose tissue

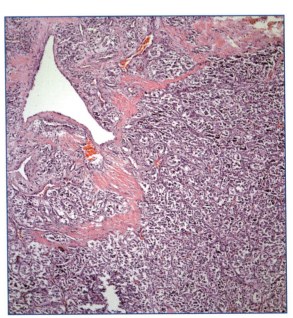

Fig. 6.4 Paraganglioma with a classic nesting pattern and dilated vascular structures

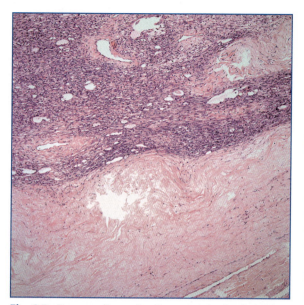

Fig. 6.5 Paraganglioma showing extensive hyalinization

and to separate these tumors from other more aggressive neuroendocrine neoplasms. Positive staining for neuroendocrine markers, such as chromogranin and synaptophysin, and negative staining for epithelial markers, such as keratin, are features of paragangliomas. S-100 protein is positive in sustentacular cells.

Mediastinal Parathyroid Adenomas

These are very unusual neoplasms. Recently, a large series showed that these tumors occurred essentially in adult individuals with abnormalities in the metabolism of calcium and phosphorus and in whom neck exploration failed to reveal an enlarge parathyroid gland [15]. The size of these tumors is rarely large, and the diagnosis is confirmed by surgical resection of the tumor.

Histologically, the tumors show the same features of parathyroid adenomas of the neck, which essentially may show oncocytic, clear cell features or a combination of both with discrete vascular spaces. Although mitotic figures may be present, they are rare. No necrosis or fibrous bands separating the cellularity are components of mediastinal parathyroid adenomas. However, in large tumors, the possibility of parathyroid carcinoma needs to be ruled out. Ectopic parathyroid carcinomas in the mediastinum have also been reported. The presence of necrosis, fibrous bands, and mitotic activity are features commonly associated with carcinomas. Immunohistochemically, parathyroid adenomas just like other neuroendocrine neoplasms, may also show positive staining with neuroendocrine markers such as chromogranin and synaptophysin. Parathyroid adenomas may also show positive staining for epithelial markers such as keratin. The use of immunohistochemical staining for parathyroid hormone is crucial in establishing a correct interpretation.

Benign Lymphoid Lesions

The most important lesion in this family is Castleman's disease. Although this condition represents mainly an enlargement of lymph nodes, the lesion in the mediastinum may resemble other more common tumors such as thymomas [16, 17]. Patients may present with symptoms of fever and hyperglobulinemia. Histologically, two variants have been described: the plasma cell variant which is characterized by the presence of sheets of mature plasma cells with areas in which remnants of lymphoid follicles may still be present, and the hyaline-vascular variant characterized by the presence of small germinal centers with a concentric arrangement, so-called onionskin. Some germinal centers may show penetration by a capillary, which has been called a lollipop appearance.

Other Unusual Benign Tumors

Although there are many benign tumoral conditions that may present as anterior mediastinal lesions, some that need to be kept in mind include adenomatoid tumors [18], Langerhans cell histiocytosis (histiocytosis X) [19], and Rosai-Dorfman's disease [20] of the mediastinum. Although these conditions are rare, they need to be considered in the differential diagnosis of tumors of unusual histology or lesions composed of histiocytes.

Malignant Tumors

The mediastinum can be the seed of a wide variety of malignant tumors of epithelial, neuroendocrine, germ cell, mesenchymal, or lymphoid origin. To facilitate their study in this chapter, they will be separated accordingly.

Thymic Epithelial Neoplasms

The two most important representatives of these tumors are thymoma and thymic carcinoma. These entities will be discussed separately.

Thymoma

Over the last decade, the study of thymomas has generated a great deal of interest, and several classification systems have been presented including an adapted World Health Organization (WHO) schema based on previously published classification systems. Interestingly, not one of the currently available systems or even the schema of the WHO has gained unanimous acceptance. Needless to say, the practical application of the WHO schema may not only be completely arbitrary but also quite difficult and problematic [21-36]. Therefore, the study of thymomas is still an evolving one. Table 6.1 depicts the most commonly used systems in the diagnosis of thymoma. Most authors believe that the single most important factor in predicting outcome in these patients is the capsular integrity of the tumor, leaving histology of the tumor as a secondary issue. Regarding the pathological staging of these tumors, the most accepted system is the one proposed by Masaoka and modified by Koga [25]. For practical purposes, the diagnosis of thymomas should include not only whether the tumor is or is not encapsulated but also the extent of invasion, if invasive, and the histological type of the tumor.

Histologically, even though there are several classifications and the schema of the WHO for thymomas, these classifications still emphasize the proportion of lymphocytes present in the tumor. There are only a few differences in some of the classification systems for the diagnosis of "mixed" thymomas. The fact is that thymomas are well known to show a wide variety of growth patterns and morphological changes. Thus, the significance of these histological classification systems will help only to properly classify some of the cases. In addition, the more histological sections one has available for review, the more likely that a great majority of thymomas will show mixed histologies, thus casting serious doubt as to the usefulness of these classifications with respect to determining outcome by histology (Figs. 6.6-6.8).

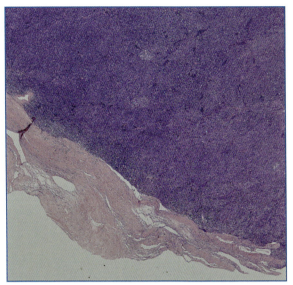

Fig. 6.6 Encapsulated Thymoma (Type B1, cortical, lymphocyte-rich)

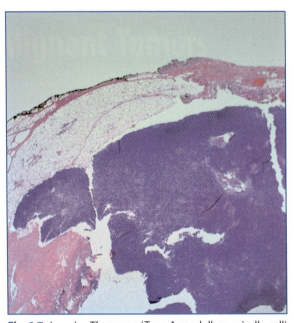

Fig. 6.7 Invasive Thymoma (Type A, medullary, spindle cell)

Table 6.1 Commonly used nomenclatures for thymomas with the respective synonym in the WHO Schema

WHO schema	Suster & Moran	Muller-Hermelink	Conventional
Type A	Thymoma	Medullary	Spindle
Type AB	Thymoma	Mixed	–
Type B1	Thymoma	Predominantly cortical	Lymphocyte-rich
Type B2	Thymoma	Cortical	Mixed
Type B3	Atypical thymoma	Well-differentiated Ca	Epithelial-rich
Type C	Thymic carcinoma	Carcinoma	–

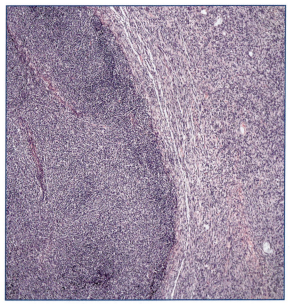

Fig. 6.8 Mixed Thymoma (Type A, B, cortical and medullary, spindle cell and lymphocyte-rich)

Thymic Carcinoma

By definition, thymic carcinoma is a tumor originating from the thymic epithelium with overtly cytologic features of malignancy and loss of organotypical features of thymic differentiation (Fig. 6.9) [37-45]. Similar to thymomas, controversy still exists regarding criteria for this tumor's diagnosis, and just the same as thymomas, thymic carcinomas may also show a wide spectrum of histopathological patterns. Thus, of significant importance in the diagnosis of thymic carcinoma is a strict clinico-radiological-pathological correlation. In other words, histologically speaking, since thymic carcinomas will display similar features as carcinomas of other origins, such a diagnosis must be based on exclusion of carcinoma elsewhere. From the morphological point of view, there is some agreement that there are two different histological variants: low-grade and high-grade thymic carcinomas (see Table 6.2).

Neuroendocrine Carcinomas

Primary neuroendocrine carcinomas (carcinoids) of the thymus are unusual and represent less than 5% of all mediastinal tumors [46-56]. Although the majority of these neoplasms follow an aggressive behavior, the prognosis may also be closely related to the degree of differentiation, and to the extent of the tumors at the time of diagnosis. The prognosis may also depend on any underlying medical disease associated with these tumors. Thymic neuroendocrine tumors can be associated with the multiple endocrine neoplasia syndrome type I (MEN-type I) as well as to other conditions including Sipple syndrome, hyperparathyroidism, ADH secretion, and Eaton-Lampert syndrome among others. The nature of these tumors leads one to the preferable designation of carcinoma rather than the ambiguous term of "carcinoid". In addition, contrary to the schema presented by the WHO in their latest version into two different categories, a three-way classification system into well (low-grade), moderately (intermediate-grade), and poorly differentiated (high-grade) neuroendocrine carcinoma is more useful, as has been proposed by others. The histological criteria for these particular diagnoses is as follows:

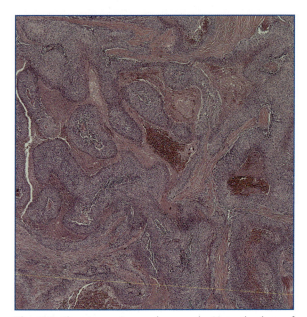

Fig. 6.9 Thymic carcinoma, low grade. Note the loss of organotypical features of thymoma

Table 6.2 Sub categorization of thymic carcinoma

Low grade carcinoma
    Well-differentiated squamous cell carcinoma
    Low-grade mucoepidermoid carcinoma
    Basaloid carcinoma

High-grade carcinoma
    Lymphoepithelioma-like carcinoma
    High-grade mucoepidermoid carcinoma
    Small cell carcinoma
    Anaplastic carcinoma
    Sarcomatoid carcinoma
    Clear cell carcinoma

- Well-differentiated (Carcinoid): organized nesting pattern, mild cellular atypia, mitotic figures, fewer than 3×10 hpf, necrosis only focal (Fig. 6.10).
- Moderately-differentiated (Atypical Carcinoid): nesting pattern alternating with sheets of neoplastic cells, moderate cellular atypia, mitotic figures more than 3 but fewer than 10×10 hpf. Necrosis, often comedo-like necrosis easily identified (Fig. 6.11).
- Poorly differentiated (small cell or large cell neuroendocrine carcinoma): loss of organized pattern, prominent cellular atypia, mitotic figures easily encountered, more than 10×10 hpf, necrosis, and hemorrhage.

It is important to note that in a limited mediastinoscopic biopsy, a definitive diagnosis regarding the classification system may be difficult, namely for the low-grade tumors. In addition, the use of immunohistochemical studies to corroborate the diagnosis is in many cases useful, as these tumors will stain positively with neuroendocrine markers, including chromogranin and synaptophysin as well as epithelial markers like keratin. The separation of these tumors into a three-way category system allows for better follow-up and perhaps for better decisions regarding additional treatment.

Neuroblastoma and Ganglioneuroblastoma

Both of these tumors are more common in the pediatric age group. However, they rarely occur in adults, and although these tumors have a predilection for the posterior mediastinum, similar cases have also been described in the anterior mediastinum in association with the thymic gland [57-59]. In a large series of these tumors in the posterior mediastinum, all the patients were under 25 years of age, and the prognosis was related to the histologic growth pattern, age, and extent of the disease at the time of diagnosis.

Histologically, the tumors may show predominance of either component, ganglioneuromatous or blastomatous. The neoplastic cellular proliferation may be arranged in a vague lobular pattern separated by thin fibroconnective tissue and composed of small cells with inconspicuous nuclei and low mitotic rate. The cells are embedded in a fibrillary background, the so-called neurophil. The presence of larger cells with ample eosinophilic cytoplasm and round prominent nuclei will determine the ganglioneuromatous component. These cells may be sparse and difficult to find, while in other cases they may be the major component of the tumor. Areas of hemorrhage, necrosis, and calcifications may be present.

Germ Cell Tumors (GCT)

These tumors are well known to occur along the midline including the anterior mediastinum. Due to their rarity, only a few comprehensive studies of these tumors are documented [57-72]. In general, mediastinal GCT may account for no more than 15% of all

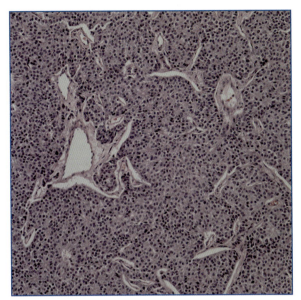

Fig. 6.10 Well differentiated neuroendocrine carcinoma (Carcinoid Tumor). Tumor shows absence of increased mitotic activity and/or necrosis

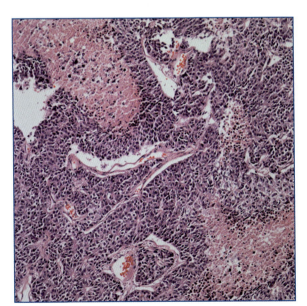

Fig. 6.11 Moderately differentiated neuroendocrine carcinoma (Atypical carcinoid). Note the presence of necrosis and nuclear atypia

mediastinal tumors. However, there are some differences in the histopathologic type and age of occurrence. For instance, seminomas are rarely seen in the pediatric age group in contrast to the occurrence of teratomatous lesions. In addition, mediastinal GCT are tumors of almost exclusive occurrence in men. Even though there are reports of non-teratomatous tumors in females, they may be exceedingly rare. The tumors that sporadically happen in female patients are teratomatous tumors. Although teratomatous tumors are more common, seminomas are not too far behind, and both of these tumors represent the most common GCT in the mediastinal compartment. Non-seminomatous and non-teratomatous tumors are rare and are below 25% in relation to other GCT.

A classification for mediastinal GCT has been proposed with only a slight change with regard to teratomatous tumors. Unfortunately, terms such as teratocarcinoma, which represent a teratoma plus embryonal carcinoma, have been used in the past as a synonym for teratomas with a malignant component. For practical purposes, the diagnosis of teratomatous lesions should include not only the malignant component present but also the percentage of it. Therefore, GCT are classified as follows:
- Mature teratoma: tumor composed of mature elements of the three distinct germinal layers, which may include intestinal epithelium, pancreas, glial tissue, etc.
- Immature teratoma: similar to mature teratoma but with an additional component of immature neuroectodermal tissue in the form of neurotubules, rosettes, and/or immature mesenchymal tissue.
- Teratomas with malignant component:
   Type I: associated with another GCT, i.e., seminoma.
   Type II: associated with another malignant epithelial neoplasm, i.e., squamous cell carcinoma.
   Type III: associated with a malignant mesenchymal component, i.e., chondrosarcoma.
   Type IV: any combination of the above.
- Seminoma.
- Yolk sac tumor (Endodermal sinus tumor).
- Choriocarcinoma.
- Combined non-teratomatous tumors (a combination of any of the above).

Seminoma

The acceptance of this neoplasm in the mediastinum dates back to the mid-1950s as a case report. In the past, similar tumors have been placed under the designation of seminomatous thymoma due to the lack of acceptance for the occurrence of GCT outside of the gonads. The tumor appears to be an exclusive tumor of men with a peak incidence in young adults. However, the tumor may also occur in older individuals. Similar syndromes, as those occurring in patients with testicular seminomas, have been described in mediastinal seminomas, including Klinefelter syndrome. Clinically, some of these patients may be asymptomatic or with symptoms related to the size of their tumor compressing adjacent mediastinal organs.

Histologically, the neoplastic cellular proliferation is composed of medium-sized cells with round nuclei and inconspicuous nucleoli, moderate eosinophilic cytoplasm, low mitotic activity, and the presence of a discrete inflammatory reaction composed of lymphocytes (Fig. 6.12). Thymic remnants, non-caseous granulomatous reaction, and cystic changes may be present in some cases. Immunohistochemical studies are commonly used to corroborate the diagnosis and include positive staining in tumor cells for placental-like alkaline phosphatase (PLAP). The tumors are also positive with epithelial markers such as epithelial membrane antigen (EMA) and low molecular weight keratin CAM5.2. More recently, CD117 (c-Kit) has been found positive in tumor cells of seminomas.

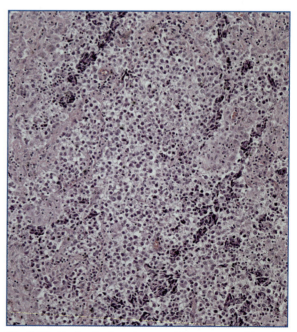

Fig. 6.12 Mediastinal seminoma with presence of the classic lymphocytic component

Non-Seminomatous Germ Cell Tumors

Yolk Sac Tumor

This tumor is the most common in this family of tumors and by far the most versatile of all. The classical presentation is that of a neoplastic cellular proliferation composed of rather small cells with scant cytoplasm, small nuclei, and inconspicuous nucleoli, with the presence of intra- and extracytoplasmic hyaline globules (Fig. 6.13). The most characteristic feature of this tumor is the presence of the so-called Schiller-Duval bodies, which are pathognomonic of this tumor. Areas of necrosis, hemorrhage, and/or high mitotic activity may be encountered in some tumors. Morphological variants including the hepatoid, intestinal, and spindle cell variant have been described. Immunohistochemically, the tumor cells may react with alpha-feto protein (AFP) as well as with keratin antibodies.

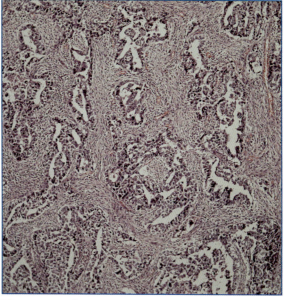

Fig. 6.14 Mediastinal embryonal carcinoma showing ill-formed glandular structures

Embryonal Carcinoma

In its pure form, this tumor is rare and often is accompanied by yolk sac tumor. Histologically, the tumor is composed of well-formed gland or abortive glandular structures composed of an embryonic type of epithelium in which the cells show a vacuolated nuclei and prominent nucleoli (Fig. 6.14). Mitotic figures are common as well as hemorrhage and necrosis. By immunohistochemistry, the tumor cells are positive for epithelial markers such as keratin and EMA as well as for AFP. Important to note is the fact that the tumor cells in embryonal carcinoma may also show positive staining for CD-30, which is a common immunohistochemical marker for anaplastic large cell lymphoma. Thus, since the setting of a mediastinal mass in a young man may be seen in both conditions, plus anaplastic large cell lymphoma may also show positive staining for EMA, it is prudent to widen the use of immunohistochemical studies to incorporate other antibodies such as keratin, AFP, or ALK-1.

Choriocarcinoma

This is the rarest of all GCT, and the histology is rather striking by the presence of two different types of cells, the multinucleated cells (syncytiotrophoblast) and the mononuclear cells (cytotrophoblast). Extensive areas of hemorrhage and necrosis are commonly seen. Immunohistochemically, the tumor cells react against antibodies for HCG as well as keratin.

Combined Non-Teratomatous GCT

Essentially, any combination can take place. Perhaps one of the most common includes the association of embryonal carcinoma and yolk sac tumor. However,

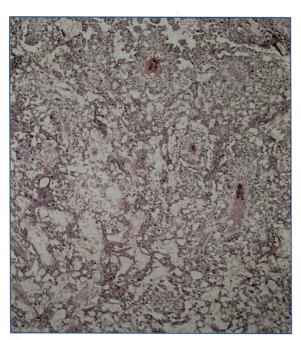

Fig. 6.13 Mediastinal yolk sac tumor showing a classic reticular pattern

yolk sac and seminoma or choriocarcinoma with yolk sac can be seen.

Mesenchymal Neoplasms

The mediastinal compartment, just like any other area in the human body, can be the site of a wide variety of mesenchymal neoplasms, which will include vascular neoplasms such as hemangioendothelioma [73], chordomas [74], rhabdomyosarcomas [75], alveolar soft part sarcomas [76], malignant cartilaginous tumors [77], liposarcomas [78], leiomyosarcomas [79], and synovial sarcoma [80]. In addition, one other tumor of mesenchymal origin that is more common in the serosal surfaces may be just as common in the mediastinal compartment, that tumor is solitary fibrous tumor. This latter neoplasm has the difficulty of mimicking histologically other neoplasms and may even share some immunohistochemical features with some of them, namely monophasic synovial sarcoma [81, 82].

The criteria used to diagnose these malignancies in the mediastinum are essentially the same as the one used for similar tumors in soft tissues. In addition, a judicious use of immunohistochemical studies is recommended in cases in which the histology is not that obvious.

Mediastinal Lymphomas

Lymphomas can be seen either as primary tumors of the mediastinum or as a secondary involvement in systemic diseases. The gamut of lymphoproliferative lesions occurring primarily in the mediastinum is wide and is represented by Hodgkin and Non-Hodgkin's lymphomas. In essence, mediastinal lymphomas could be divided into three different categories: lymphoblastic lymphoma, Hodgkin's lymphoma, and diffuse large cell lymphoma. Histologic subtypes including diffuse large cell lymphoma with sclerosis, clear cell lymphoma, "germinotropic" large cell lymphoma, anaplastic large cell lymphoma, pleomorphic large cell lymphoma, and MALT lymphoma of the thymus have been described [83-90]. The criteria used for the different diagnosis is similar to the one used for nodal lymphomas. The use of a panel of immunohistochemical studies, which would include B- and T-cell markers among others, is recommended in order to properly subcategorize these neoplasms.

References

1. Zanca P, Chuang TH, DeAvila R, Galindo DL (1965) True congenital mediastinal thymic cyst. Pediatrics 36:615-619
2. Suster S, Rosai J (1991) Multilocular thymic cyst: An acquired reactive process. Study of 18 cases. Am J Surg Pathol 15:388-398
3. Suster S, Barbuto D, Carlson G, Rosai J (1991) Multilocular thymic cysts with pseudoepitheliomatous hyperplasia. Hum Pathol 22:455-460
4. Michal M, Havlicek F (1991) Pseudo-epitheliomatous hyperplasia in thymic cysts. Histopathology 19:281-282
5. Flieder DB, Suster S, Moran CA (1997) Idiopathic fibroinflammatory (Fibrosing/Sclerosing) lesions of the mediastinum: A study of 30 cases with emphasis on morphologic heterogeneity. Mod Pathol 12:257-264
6. Sobrinho-Simoes MA, Vaz Saleiro J, Wagenvoort CA (1981) Mediastinal and hilar fibrosis. Histopathology 5:53-60
7. Kittredge RD, Nash AD (1974) The many facets of sclerosing fibrosis. AJR Am J Roentgenol 122:228-298
8. Eggleston JC (1980) Sclerosing mediastinitis. In: Fenoglio CM, Wolff M (eds) Progress in surgical pathology, vol 2. Masson, New York, p 1-17
9. Rosado-de-Christenson ML, Pugatch RD, Moran CA, Galobardes J (1994) Thymolipoma: Analysis of 27 cases. Radiology 193:121-126
10. Moran CA, Rosado-de-Christenson ML, Suster S (1995) Thymolipoma: A clinicopathologic correlation of 33 cases. Mod Pathol 8:741-744
11. McAdams HP, Rosado-de-Christenson ML, Moran CA (1994) Mediastinal hemangioma: Radiographic and CT features in 14 patients. Radiology 193:399-402
12. Moran CA, Suster S (1995) Mediastinal hemangiomas: A study of 18 cases with emphasis on the spectrum of morphological features. Hum Pathol 26:416-421
13. Moran CA, Suster S, Fishback N, Koss MN (1993) Mediastinal paragangliomas: A clinicopathologic and immunohistochemical study of 16 cases. Cancer 72:2358-2364
14. Olson JL, Salyer WR (1978) Mediastinal paraganglioma (aortic body tumor). Cancer 41:2405-2412
15. Moran CA, Suster S (2005) Primary parathyroid tumors of the mediastinum: A clinicopathologic and immunohistochemical study of 17 cases. Am J Clin Pathol 124:749-754
16. Novak L, Castro CY, Listinsky CM (2003) Multiple Langerhans cell nodules in an incidental thymectomy. Arch Pathol Lab Med 127:218-220
17. Lim R, Wittram C, Ferry JA, Shepard JA (2004) FDG PET of Rosai Dorfman disease of the thymus. AJR Am J Roentgenol 182:514
18. Keller AR, Hochholzer L, Clastleman B (1972) Hyaline-vascular and plasma cell types of giant lymph node hyperplasia of the mediastinum and other locations. Cancer 29:670-683

19. Strickler JG, Kurtin PJ (1991) Mediastinal lymphoma. Sem Diagn Pathol 8:2-13
20. Plaza JA, Dominguez F, Sustr S (2004) Cystic adenomatoid tumor of the mediastinum. Am J Surg Pathol 28:132-138
21. Moran CA, Suster S (2000) On the histologic heterogeneity of thymic epithelial neoplasms: Impact of sampling in subtyping and classification of thymomas. Am J Clin Pathol 114:760-766
22. Suster S (2006) My approach to the diagnosis of thymoma. J Clin Pathol (E-pub) May 5
23. Chalabreysse L, Roy P, Cordier JF et al (2002) Correlation of the WHO schema for the classification of thymic epithelial neoplasms with prognosis. A retrospective study of 90 tumors. Am J Surg Pathol 26:1605-1611
24. Rieker RJ, Hoegel J, Morresi-Hauf A et al (2002) Histologic classification of thymic epithelial tumors: Comparison of established classification schemes. Int J Cancer 98:900-906
25. Koga K, Matsumoto Y, Noguchi M (1994) A review of 79 thymomas: Modification of staging system and reappraisal of conventional division into invasive and non-invasive thymoma. Pathology Int 44:359-367
26. Regnad JF, Magdeleinant P, Dromer C (1996) Prognostic factors and long term results after thymoma resection: A series of 307 patients. J Thorac Cardiovasc Surg 112:376-384
27. Bernatz PE, Harrison EG, Claggett OT (1961) Thymoma: A clinicopathologic study. J Thorac Cardiovasc Surg 42:424-444
28. Bernatz PE, Khonsari S, Harrison EG (1973) Thymoma: Factor influencing prognosis. Surg Clin North Am 53:885-892
29. Marino M, Muller-Hermelink HK (1985) Thymoma and thymic carcinoma. Relation of thymoma epithelial cells to the cortical and medullary differentiation of the thymus. Virchows Arch 407:119-149
30. Kirchner T, Muller-Hermelink HK (1989) New approaches to the diagnosis of thymic epithelial tumors. Prog Surg Pathol 10:167-189
31. Quintanilla-Martinez L, Wilkins EW, Choi N, Harris N (1993) Thymoma: Histologic sub-classification is an independent prognostic parameter. Cancer 24:958-969
32. Travis WD, Brambilla E, Muller-Hermelink HK, Harris CC (2004) Pathology and genetics of tumours of the lung, pleura, thymus, and heart. In: World Health Organization Classification of Tumours, IARC Press, Lyon
33. Rosai J (1999) Histological typing of tumours of the thymus. In: World Health Organization International Histological Classification of Tumours, 2nd edn. Springer-Verlag, Berlin
34. Suster S, Moran CA (1999) Thymoma, atypical thymoma and thymic carcinoma. A novel conceptual approach to the classification of neoplasms of thymic epithelium. Am J Clin Pathol 111:826-833
35. Suster S, Moran CA (2006) Thymoma classification: Current status and future trends. Am J Clin Pathol 125:542-554
36. Suster S, Moran CA (2005) Problem areas and inconsistencies in the WHO classification of thymoma. Sem Diagn Pathol 22:188-197
37. Suster S, Rosai J (1991) Thymic carcinoma. A clinicopathologic study of 60 cases. Cancer 67:1025-1032
38. Wick MR, Scheithauer BW, Weiland LH, Bernatz PE (1982) Primary thymic carcinomas. Am J Surg Pathol 6:613-630
39. Snover DC, Levine GD, Rosai J (1982) Thymic carcinoma: Five distinctive histologic variants. Am J Surg Pathol 6:451-470
40. Suster S, Moran CA (1998) Thymic carcinoma: Spectrum of differentiation and histologic types. Pathology 30:111-122
41. Kuo TT, Chang JP, Lin FJ et al (1990) Thymic carcinomas: Histopathologic varieties and immunohistochemical study. Am J Surg Pathol 14:24-34
42. Truong LD, Mody DR, Cagle PT et al (1990) Thymic carcinoma: A clinicopathologic study of 13 cases. Am J Surg Pathol 14:151-166
43. Moran CA, Suster S (1995) Mucoepidermoid carcinoma of the thymus: A clinicopathologic study of six cases. Am J Surg Pathol 19:826-834
44. Suster S, Moran CA (1996) Primary thymic epithelial neoplasms with combined features of thymoma and thymic carcinoma. A clinicopathologic study of 22 cases. Am J Surg Pathol 20:1469-1480
45. Shimosato Y, Kameya T, Nagai K, Suemasu K (1977) Squamous cell carcinoma of the thymus. An analysis of eight patients. Am J Surg Pathol 1:109-120
46. Moran CA, Suster S (2007) Neuroendocrine carcinomas (carcinoid, atypical carcinoid, small cell carcinoma, and large cell neuroendocrine carcinoma): Current concepts. Hematol/Oncol Clin North Am 5:1-13
47. Moran CA, Suster S (2000) Neuroendocrine carcinomas (carcinoid tumor) of the thymus: A clinicopathological and immunohistochemical analysis of 80 cases. Am J Clin Pathol 114:100-110
48. Klemm KM, Moran CA (1999) Primary neuroendocrine carcinomas of the thymus. Sem Diagn Pathol 16:32-41
49. Moran CA, Suster S (2000) Thymic neuroendocrine carcinomas with combined features ranging from well-differentiated (carcinoid) to small cell carcinoma. Am J Clin Pathol 113:345-350
50. Moran CA, Suster S (1999) Spindle cell neuroendocrine carcinomas of the thymus (spindle cell thymic carcinoid): A clinicopathological and immunohistochemical study of seven cases. Mod Pathol 12:587-591
51. Moran CA, Suster S (1999) Angiomatoid neuroendocrine carcinoma of the thymus: Report of a distinctive morphological variant of neuroendocrine tumor of the thymus resembling a vascular neoplasm. Hum Pathol 30:635-639
52. Moran CA, Suster S (2000) Oncocytic neuroendocrine carcinomas of the thymus: Clinicopathological and immunohistochemical study of 22 cases. Mod Pathol 13:489-494
53. Klemm KM, Moran CA, Suster S (1999) Pigmented thymic carcinoids: A clinicopathological and immuno-

histochemical study of two cases. Mod Pathol 12:946-948
54. Suster S, Moran CA (1995) Thymic carcinoid with prominent mucinous stroma: Report of a distinctive morphological variant of thymic neuroendocrine neoplasm. Am J Surg Pathol 19:1277-1285
55. Rosai J, Higa E (1972) Mediastinal endocrine neoplasms of probable thymic origin related to carcinoid tumor. Cancer 29:1061-1074
56. Rosai J, Higa E, Davie J (1972) Mediastinal endocrine neoplasms in patients with multiple endocrine adenomatosis: A previously unrecognized association. Cancer 29:1075-1083
57. Adam A, Hochholzer L (1981) Ganglioneuroblastoma of the posterior mediastinum: A clinicopathologic review of 80 cases. Cancer 47:373-381
58. Asada Y, Marutsuka K, Mitsukawa T et al (1996) Ganglioneuroblastoma of the thymus: An adult case with syndrome of inappropriate secretion of antidiuretic hormone. Hum Pathol 27:506-509
59. Salter JE, Gibson D, Ordonez NG, Mackay B (1995) Neuroblastoma of the anterior mediastinum in an 80-year-old woman. Ultrastruc Pathol 19:305-310
60. Knapp RH, Hurt RD, Payne WS (1985) Malignant germ cell tumors of the mediastinum. J Thorac Cardiovasc Surg 89:89-82
61. Woolner LB, Jamplis RW, Kirklin JW (1955) Seminoma (germinoma) of the anterior mediastinum. N Eng J Med 252:653-657
62. Nazari A, Gagnon ED (1966) Seminoma-like tumor of the mediastinum. J Thorac Cardiovasc Surg 51:751-754
63. Moran CA, Suster S (1997) Primary germ cell tumors of the mediastinum I. Analysis of 322 cases with special emphasis on teratomatous lesions and a proposal for histopathologic classification and clinical staging. Cancer 80:681-690
64. Moran CA, Suster, Przygodsky RM, Koss MN (1997) Primary germ cell tumors of the mediastinum II. Mediastinal seminomas: A clinicopathologic and immunohistochemical study of 120 cases. Cancer 80:691-698
65. Moran CA, Suster S, Koss MN (1997) Primary germ cell tumors of the mediastinum III. Yolk sac tumor, embryonal carcinoma, choriocarcinoma, and combined non-teratomatous germ cell tumors of the mediastinum: A clinicopathologic and immunohistochemical study of 64 cases. Cancer 80:699-707
66. Moran CA, Suster S (1995) Mediastinal seminomas with prominent cystic changes. A clinicopathologic study of 10 cases. Am J Surg Pathol 19:1047-1053
67. Moran CA, Suster S (1997) Primary yolk sac tumors of the mediastinum with prominent cystic changes: Clinicopathologic study of 5 cases. Mod Pathol 10:800-803
68. Moran CA, Suster S (1997) Primary yolk sac tumors of the mediastinum with prominent hepatoid features. Am J Surg Pathol 21:1210-1214
69. Moran CA, Suster S (1997) Mediastinal choriocarcinomas. A clinicopathologic study of 8 cases. Am J Surg Pathol 21:1007-1012
70. Suster S, Moran CA, Dominguez H, Quevedo-Blanco P (1998) Germ cell tumors of the testis and mediastinum: A comparative immunohistochemical study of 100 cases. Hum Pathol 29:737-742
71. Moran CA, Suster S (1998) Primary germ cell tumors of the mediastinum: A review. Adv Anat Pathol 5:1-15
72. Dominguez H, Valdez AM, Moran CA, Suster S (2007) Germ cell tumors with sarcomatous component: A clinicopathologic and immunohistochemical study of 46 cases. Am J Surg Pathol 31:1356-1362
73. Suster S, Moran CA, Koss MN (1994) Epithelioid hemangioendothelioma of the anterior mediastinum. Clinicopathologic, immunohistochemical, and ultrastructural analysis of 12 cases. Am J Surg Pathol 18:871-881
74. Suster S, Moran CA (1995) Chordomas of the mediastinum: Clinicopathologic, immunohistochemical, and ultrastructural study of six cases presenting as posterior mediastinal masses. Hum Pathol 26:1354-1362
75. Suster S, Moran CA, Koss MN (1994) Rhabdomyosarcomas of the anterior mediastinum: Report of four cases unassociated with germ cell, teratomatous, or thymic carcinomatous components. Hum Pathol 25:349-356
76. Flieder DB, Moran CA, Suster S (1997) Primary alveolar soft part sarcoma of the mediastinum: A clinicopathological and immunohistochemical study of two cases. Histopathology 31:469-473
77. Suster S, Moran CA (1997) Malignant cartilaginous tumors of the mediastinum: Clinicopathological study of six cases presenting as extraskeletal soft tissue masses. Hum Pathol 28:588-594
78. Klimstra D, Moran CA, Koss MN, Rosai J (1995) Primary liposarcomas of the mediastinum: A study of 27 cases. Am J Surg Pathol 19:782-791
79. Moran CA, Suster S, Perino G et al (1994) Benign and malignant smooth muscle tumors of the mediastinum. Cancer 74:2251-2260
80. Suster S, Moran CA (2005) Primary synovial sarcomas of the anterior mediastinum. Am J Surg Pathol 29:569-578
81. Witkin GB, Rosai J (1989) Solitary fibrous tumor of the mediastinum. Am J Surg Pathol 13:547-557
82. Moran CA, Suster S, Koss MN (1992) The spectrum of histologic growth patterns in benign and malignant fibrous tumors of the pleura. Sem Diagn Pathol 9:169-180
83. Lichtenstein AK, Levine A, Taylor CR (1980) Primary mediastinal lymphoma in adults. Am J Med 68:509-514
84. Perrone T. Frizzera G, Rosai J (1986) Mediastinal diffuse large cell lymphoma with sclerosis. A clinicopathologic study of 60 cases. Am J Surg Pathol 10:176-191
85. Davies RE, Dorfman RF, Warnke RA (1990) Primary large cell lymphoma of the thymus: A diffuse B-cell neoplasm presenting as primary mediastinal lymphoma. Hum Pathol 21:1262-1268
86. Moller P, Lammler B, Eberlein-Gonska M (1986) Primary mediastinal clear cell lymphoma of B-cell type. Virchows Arch [A] 409:79-92

87. Suster S (1992) Large cell lymphoma with marked tropism for germinal centers. Cancer 69:2910-2916
88. Suster S, Moran CA (1990) Pleomorphic large cell lymphomas of the mediastinum. Am J Surg Pathol 20:224-232
89. Isaacswon PG, Chan KKC, Tang C (1990) Low-grade B-cell lymphoma of mucosa-associated lymphoid tissue arising in the thymus. Am J Surg Pathol 14:342-351
90. Strickler JG, Kurtin PJ (1991) Mediastinal lymphoma. Sem Diag Pathol 8:2-13

CHAPTER 7
Clinical Features of Thymus Pathology

Ghulam Khaleeq, Hakim A. Ali, Ali I. Musani

Introduction

Thymus pathology embraces a broad spectrum of features, varying from major immunologic abnormalities affecting all organ systems to minor abnormalities with limited clinical consequences. Some individuals with thymus pathology may have all the features of the disease while others may have only a few features. In this chapter we will review clinical features of common thymus pathologies. Tables 7.1 and 7.2 list the localized and systemic symptoms due to mediastinal tumors [1].

Clinical Features Due to Congenital Pathology of Thymus

The thymus and parathyroid are derived from 3rd pharyngeal pouches [2, 3]. Development of thymus is a series of epithelial/mesenchymal inductive interactions between neural crest-derived arch mesenchyme and pouch endoderm. Abnormalities during development can result in different clinical syndromes.

Table 7.1 Localizing symptoms secondary to tumor invasion of surrounding structures (taken with permission from Baum's and Crapo [1])

Involved anatomic structure	Localizing SYMPTOMS
Bronchi/trachea	Dsypnea, postobstructive pneumonia, atelectasis, hemoptysis
Esophagus	Dysphagia
Spinal cord/vertebral column	Paralysis
Recurrent laryngeal nerve	Hoarseness, vocal cord paralysis
Phrenic nerve	Diaphragmatic paralysis
Stellate ganglion	Horner syndrome
Superior vena cava	Superior vena cava syndrome

Table 7.2 Systemic syndromes secondary to primary mediastinal tumors and cysts (taken with permission from Baum's and Crapo [1])

Syndrome	Tumor
Myasthenia gravis, RBC aplasia, hypogammaglobulinemia, Good syndrome, Whipple disease, megaesophagus, myocarditis	Thymoma
Multiple endocrine adenomatosis, Cushing syndrome	Carcinoid, thymoma
Hypertension	Pheochromocytoma, ganglioneuroma, chemodectoma
Diarrhea	Ganglioneuroma
Hypercalcemia	Parathyroid adenoma, lymphoma
Thyrotoxicosis	Intrathoracic goiter
Hypoglycemia	Mesothelioma, teratoma, fibrosarcoma, neurosarcoma
Osteoarthropathy	Neurofibroma, neurilemoma, mesotheioma
Vertebral abnormalities	Enteric cysts
Fever of unknown origin	Lymphoma
Alcohol-induced pain	Hodgkin's Disease
Opsomyoclonus	Neuroblastoma

22q11.2 Deletion Syndrome

22q11.2 deletion syndrome is the commonest chromosome deletion syndrome with an incidence of 1:4,000 live births [4]. This syndrome results in variable clinical phenotypes which may differ between patients even with identical deletions. Syndromes associated with 22q11.2 deletion include:
- DiGeorge syndrome
- Velocardiofacial syndrome
- Conotruncal anomaly face syndrome
- CHARGE syndrome (coboloma, heart disease, atresia choanae, retarded growth and central nervous system development, genital hypoplasia, and ear abnormalities and/or deafness [5]) (Table 7.3).

Abnormal pharyngeal arch development results in defects in the development of the parathyroid glands, thymus, and conotruncal region of the heart. Defective thymic development can be associated with impaired immune function. Immunodeficiency is associated with T-cell deficiency and abnormalities of T-cell clonality or impairment of T-cell proliferative responses. Humoral deficiencies have also been identified in these patients. 22q11.2 deletion syndrome patients are also at increased risk of autoimmune diseases. A number of immune defects may predispose to the development of autoimmunity in these patients including increased infection, impaired development of natural T-regulatory cells and impaired thymic central tolerance [7] (Table 7.3).

Thymic Aplasia (DiGeorge Syndrome) (DGS)

DiGeorge syndrome, described in 1965, comprises abnormalities of the parathyroid glands, absence or hypoplasia of the thymus, and conotruncal abnormalities of the heart such as pulmonary atresia and severe forms of tetralogy of Fallot [8]. This rare condition affects approximately 1 in 4,000 live births [9-21]. It is caused by fetal malformation of the third and fourth branchial arches at about 7 weeks of gestation, due to abnormal cephalic migration of neural crest cells into these regions. These cells take part in the development of the skull, palate, thymus, and parathyroid glands. Abnormalities in development can result in dysmorphic facies, palatal abnormalities, and hypoparathyroidism (Table 7.4).

Table 7.3 Clinical findings in patients with chromosome 22q11.2 deletion syndrome (table taken from Kobrynski LJ et al [6] with permission from Elsevier. Data in this table is taken from references [8-18])

Cardiac anomalies	49-83%
Tetralogy of Fallot	17-22%
Interrupted aortic arch	14-15%
Ventriculoseptal defect	13-14%
Truncus arteriosus	7-9%
Hypocalcemia	17-60%
Growth hormone deficiency	4%
Palatal anomalies	69-100%
Cleft palate	9-11%
Submucous cleft palate	5-16%
Velopharyngeal insufficiency	27-92%
Bifid uvula	5%
Renal anomalies	36-37%
Absent or dysplastic	17%
Obstruction	10%
Reflux	4%
Opthalmological abnormalities	7-70%
Tortuous retinal vessels	58%
Posterior embryotoxon (anterior segment dysgenesis)	69%
Neurological	8%
Cerebral atrophy	8%
Cerebellar hypoplasia	0-4%
Dental	
Delayed eruption, enamel hypoplasia	2-5%
Skeletal abnormalities	17-19%
Cervical spine anomalies	40-50%
Vertebral anomalies	19%
Lower limb anomalies	15%
Speech Delay	79-84%
Developmental delay in infancy	75%
Developmental delay in childhood	45%
Behavior or psychiatric problems	9-50%
Attention deficit hyperactivity disorder	25%
Schizophrenia	6-30%

Clinical Features of Thymic Aplasia (DiGeorge Syndrome) (DGS)

The clinical presentation of the 22q11 deletion syndrome is highly variable. Most patients have a subset of the most common features. The presentation can be subtle and difficult to identify or more severe and easily recognized at birth. Approximately 6-10% of cases are familial; frequently, one of the parents is only recognized to carry the 22q11 deletion after a more severely affected child is diagnosed [22].

Craniofacial Anomalies

Facial Features

Typical facial dysmorphia includes hooded eyelids, auricular anomalies (could have squared off or overfolded helices, protuberant ears, preauricular tags or pits, attached lobes or small ears), a prominent nasal

Table 7.4 Clinical features of DiGeorge syndrome (taken with permission from Wurdak H et al [23])

Craniofacial anomalies	
Cleft palate	Incomplete closure of the palate
Micrognathia	Small size of the lower jaw
Ear anomalies	Typically low set, deficient vertical diameter, abnormal auricle/pinna folding
Telecanthus	Increased distance between eyes
Small mouth	Associated with hyper nasal speech
Glandular malformations	
Hypo- or aplasia of the parathyroid glands	Neonatal hypocalcaemia with tetany or seizures due to impaired calcium homeostasis
Hypo- or aplasia of the thymus	T-cell deficiency with susceptibility to infections due to impaired T-cell maturation
Cardiovascular defects	
Tetralogy of Fallot	Complex of heart malformations: (1) ventricular septal defect (2) pulmonic stenosis (3) overriding aorta (4) hypertrophy of the right ventricle
Type B interrupted aortic arch	Discontinued aortic arch between the left carotid artery and the left subclavian artery
Truncus arteriosus	Ventricles with a common arterial outflow trunk
Right aortic arch	Persistence of the bilateral system of embryonic pharyngeal arch vessels
Transposition of the great arteries	Reversed aorta and pulmonary artery, with the aorta arising from the right ventricle and the pulmonary artery receiving blood from the left ventricle
Aberrant right subclavian artery	Anomalous origin from the proximal descending aorta
Ventricular septal defects	Hole connecting the ventricles
Behavioral disorders	Variable mild to moderate
Learning difficulties Paranoid schizophrenia Major depressive illness	

root, a bulbous nasal tip with hypoplastic nasal alae, a small mouth, micrognathia, a short forehead, and some midfacial flattening (Fig. 7.1).

Palate Anomalies

Anomalies of the palate are a common problem occurring in 69-100% of patients [6]. It results in significant morbidity for these patients. Approximately 9-11% of patients have a cleft palate, while 5-16% have a submucosal cleft palate, and 5% of have a bifid uvula. The palate should be carefully examined for a bifid uvula, which can indicate the presence of a submucous cleft in the palate.

In addition to cleft palate, 27-92% [7] of patients have velopharyngeal insufficiency, which is defined as incomplete closure of the velopharyngeal valve during speech. This disorder manifests as hypernasal speech, nasal air emission, and compensatory articulation disorders. Velopharyngeal insufficiency can only be diagnosed with the emergence of speech, so the diagnosis is usually delayed.

The pathogenesis of velopharyngeal insufficiency seems to be multifactorial. Velopharyngeal

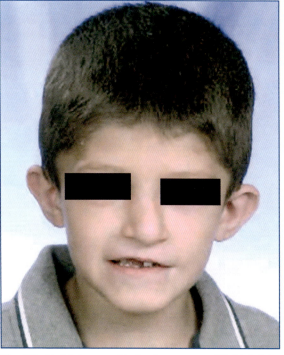

Fig. 7.1 Facial dysmorphia in chromosome 22q11.2 deletion syndrome (in this patient, a slightly bulbous nose tip and hooded eyes are the primary features) [6]

disproportion whereby the palate is too short relative to the depth of the pharynx has been observed. Neurologic or muscular velopharyngeal hypotonia can also be present. Adenoid hypoplasia is commonly observed in patients with a 22q11 deletion and can contribute to velopharyngeal insufficiency. The presence of an overt or submucous cleft palate also contributes to velopharyngeal insufficiency (Fig. 7.2).

Feeding Disorders

Feeding disorders are a common problem. Nearly 70% of patients are estimated to have nasopharyngeal reflux, characterized by reflux of liquids out of the nose because of insufficient closure of the velopharynx during swallowing. A hallmark sign of the infant with a 22q11 deletion, this symptom resolves without intervention during the toddler years and does not predict hypernasality of speech [8, 21, 24].

In addition, patients with a 22q11 deletion are commonly diagnosed with gastroesophageal reflux, esophageal dysmotility, and constipation, all of which compound their feeding disorders.

Otorhinolaryngologic Problems

Patients with a 22q11 deletion frequently have otolaryngologic disorders ranging from acquired to congenital anomalies [25]. Chronic otitis media and sinusitis are common problems, given their propensity to frequent infections. Reported congenital anomalies include laryngeal web, tracheomalacia, laryngomalacia, and tracheal compression or distortion from vascular rings.

Glandular Malformations

Hypoplasia or aplasia of the parathyroid glands results in hypoparathyroidism in a significant subset of patients. Hypocalcemia is reported in 17-60% of patients with a 22q11 deletion [7]. Studies suggest that hypoparathyroidism occurs in 13-69% of patients outside the neonatal period [26, 27]. Reports have clearly documented cases in which hypoparathyroidism recurred or occurred for the first time in later decades of life and may even be the first presenting symptom indicative of the 22q11 deletion syndrome [28, 29]. Other endocrinologic abnormalities have been reported, including growth hormone deficiency and thyroid disease.

Immunodeficiency

Patients with DGS or chromosome 22q11.2 deletions display a range of T-cell numbers and function, ranging from normal to severely deficient. In different studies nearly 80% of patients with a 22q11 deletion have demonstrated abnormalities of their immune system [5, 21, 30, 31]. "Complete" DiGeorge syndrome with total absence of the thymus and a severe T-cell immunodeficiency accounts for <0.5% of patients. The majority of patients with 22q11.2 deletion syndromes have "partial" defects with impaired thymic development rather than complete absence with variable defects in T-cell numbers. All patients with DiGeorge syndrome without the deletion have T-cell compromise. This compromise in T-cell production is due to thymic hypoplasia [32]. T-cells that successfully transit the thymus are functionally normal, and there is no intrinsic T-cell defect. The com-

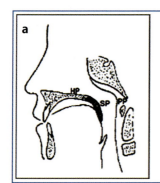 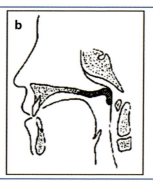 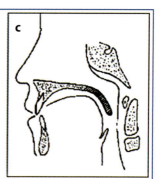

Fig. 7.2 a-c Velopharyngeal function in normal individuals and patients with velopharyngeal dysfunction [22] (taken with permission from Elsevier Limited). The velopharynx is pictured at rest (**a**), during normal phonation (**b**), and during phonation in a patient with velopharyngeal dysfunction (**c**). Note that in the patient with velopharyngeal dysfunction, the soft palate fails to move juxtaposed to the posterior pharynx and therefore allows the escape of air during phonation. HP, hard palate; PP, posterior pharynx; SP, soft palate (courtesy of Richard Kirschner, MD, Philadelphia, PA)

promise is purely in T-cell production. Patients with DiGeorge syndrome without the deletion have variable levels of circulating T-cells as do the patients with the deletion [33, 34]. Patients of both types with dramatically low circulating T-cells should be considered for a fully sibling-matched bone marrow transplant or a thymus transplant.

Chinen et al. [35] assessed the long-term T-cell populations in DiGeorge syndrome. In their cohort of 45 patients they monitored peripheral blood T-cell subsets and percentages from birth to 120 months of age. They also evaluated humoral immunity by quantification of immunoglobulin levels and testing antibody titer to recall antigens. T-cell subsets counts from patients with DiGeorge syndrome were generally lower than those of age-matched normal populations. In this study, a significant deterioration of T-cell number or function did not occur over time. Moreover, immunoglobulin deficiencies or inadequate production of specific antibodies were also not detected. Sullivan et al. [36] prospectively studied 19 patients between 1994 and 1997. They found decreased number of peripheral blood T-cells with a preserved T-cell function. The improvement in peripheral T-cell count was variable in the study. The patients with the lowest T-cell count improved the most in their first year of life.

Humoral immune deficiencies have been associated with DiGeorge syndrome. Gennery et al. [37] investigated humoral immunodeficiency in 32 patients. They measured lymphocyte subsets, immunoglobulins, IgG subclasses, specific vaccine antibodies, and autoantibodies. In their series 81% of patients (26 patients) had severe or recurrent infections, of which 13 (50%) had abnormal serum immunoglobulin measurements and 55% had an abnormal response to pneumococcal polysaccharide antigen. In a study by Smith et al. [38] they reported a 13% prevalence of immunoglobulin A (IgA) deficiency in their cohort of 32 patients. Jawad et al. [30] studied the laboratory and clinical features of immunodeficiency in their cohort of 195 patients. In their study the pattern of changes seen with aging in normal control patients were also seen in patients with chromosome 22q11.2 deletion syndrome. Recurrent infection and autoimmune disease were common in this series but had no significant relationship to specific immunologic laboratory features.

Multiple studies have demonstrated an increased incidence of autoimmune phenomenon in patients with DiGeorge syndrome. Autoimmune diseases reported in different studies include juvenile rheumatoid arthritis [39], hematologic autoimmune diseases including autoimmune cytopenias [40], idiopathic thrombocytopenia [41], and Evans syndrome [42]. Celiac disease has also been reported in patients with 22q11.2 deletion syndrome [43].

Immunodeficient conditions are frequently associated with increased rates of malignancies. T-cells and natural killer cells participate in the surveillance and killing of transformed cells. T-cell compromise in other disorders is specifically associated with lymphomas although the incidence of other malignancies may be increased. There may be an increased incidence of malignancy in DiGeorge syndrome, although larger cohort studies are needed [44, 45].

Cardiac Anomalies

Studies estimate that approximately 49-83% of patients with a 22q11 deletion have congenital heart disease [9, 21]. The most common cardiac defects include a subset of conotruncal defects (tetralogy of Fallot, interrupted aortic arch, and truncus arteriosus) and perimembranous ventricular septal defects. The term conotruncal refers to the structure of the fetal heart at an early stage in development, in which the distal portion is called the trunco-aortic sac. The aortic and pulmonary roots subsequently develop from this area, and defects in these structures are referred to as conotruncal defects. Other rare defects that are reported include hypoplastic left heart syndrome, heterotaxy syndrome, valvar pulmonary stenosis, and a bicuspid aortic valve.

Developmental and Behavioral Features

Neurocognitive, developmental, behavioral, and psychiatric disorders have been described to represent an integral component of the 22q11 deletion syndrome. A wide range of behavioral and psychiatric disorders is commonly observed in this patient population. Mean full-scale IQ scores are in the range of borderline intellectual function, but academic achievement scores are generally in the low-normal range [46]. Language skills are also typically delayed and remain impaired later in life. There is a 14% incidence of autistic spectrum disorders [47]. The incidence of schizophrenia or psychosis in chromosome 22q11.2 deletion is not well known but is reported to vary between 6% and 30% [7]. The neurocognitive, developmental, behavioral, and psychiatric disorders in 22q11 deletion syndrome are complex and need a multidisciplinary treatment approach.

Velocardiofacial syndrome, or Shprintzen's syndrome [48], comprises similar cardiac abnormalities along with cleft palate, a characteristic facies, and learning difficulty. A third syndrome, known as "conotruncal anomalies face", also linked to 22q11 syndrome has been described. These syndromes are described in detail elsewhere in the book.

Clinical Features Due to Epithelial Tumors of Thymus

Introduction

Thymoma is the most common cause of an anterior mediastinal mass in adults accounting for about 0.2-1.5% of all cancers and 20 % of mediastinal tumors. Approximately 90% of tumors of the thymus are thymomas. The remaining 10% are thymic carcinoma, carcinoid tumors, or lymphomas (Table 7.5).

Thymomas are derived from thymic epithelial cells demonstrating a spectrum of histologic patterns that encompass both epithelial and lymphocytic components in varying proportions [49]. The epithelial cells are embryologically derived from the lower portion of the third pharyngeal pouch and are believed to be responsible for the neoplastic element in thymomas. The lymphocytes associated with both the normal thymus and thymomas are predominantly immature T-lymphocytes and demonstrate TdT positivity [50]. Immunoglobulin and T-cell receptor gene studies have failed to show genotypic evidence supporting the neoplastic nature of the lymphocytic component [51].

Classification

Thymomas initially were classified according to their proportion of epithelial and lymphocytic components and the shape of epithelial cells; this classification repeatedly showed a lack of clinical relevance to patient response and survival [52-54]. This was based on a similar classification proposed by Lattes and Jonas a few years earlier [55].

Table 7.5 Tumors of the thymus

Thymoma
Thymic carcinoma
Thymic lymphoma
Thymic carcinoid
Thymic germ cell neoplasm
Thymic lipoma
Thymic cyst
Thymic myoid tumor
Thymic histiocytic tumor

Marino and Muller-Hermelink Classification (1985)

In the mid-1980s, Marino and Muller-Hermelink revised this traditional classification based on microscopic resemblance of tumor subtypes to the normal thymic epithelial cells and thymic cortex [56].

In 1989, Kirchner and Muller-Hermelink proposed a functional classification of thymomas based on the morphologic resemblance of the tumor with various compartments of the normal thymus, and five types of organotypic thymic epithelial tumors were proposed: medullary, mixed, predominantly cortical, cortical, and well-differentiated thymic carcinoma [57]. The clinical significance of the Müller-Hermelink classification system as a prognostic factor has been reported in several previous studies [58].

WHO Classification

The 1999 WHO classification of thymomas further modified the Marino classification, adding thymic carcinoma to the classification schema, simplifying the terminology, and providing prognostic relevance (Table 7.6).

This was based on the morphology of epithelial cells as well as the lymphocyte-to-epithelial cell ratio. In this system, thymomas were divided into two

Table 7.6 The definitions of World Health Organization Classification of Thymic Epithelial Tumors (taken with permission from Rosai J et al. [59])

Type	Definition
A	A tumor comprised of a homogenous population of neoplastic epithelial cells with spindle/oval shape, lacking nuclear atypia, and accompanied by few or no nonneoplastic lymphocytes
AB	A tumor in which foci with the features of type A thymoma are admixed with foci rich in lymphocytes: the segregation of two patterns can be sharp or indistinct
B1	A tumor that resembles the normal functional thymus in that it combines large expanses with an appearance practically indistinguishable from that of normal thymic cortex with areas resembling thymic medulla
B2	A tumor in which the neoplastic epithelial component appears as scattered plump cells with vesicular nuclei and distinct nucleoli among a heavy population of lymphocytes; perivascular spaces are common
B3	A tumor comprised predominantly of epithelial cells with a round or polygonal shape and exhibiting mild atypia admixed with a minor component of lymphocytes; foci of squamous metaplasia and perivascular spaces are common

groups depending on whether the neoplastic epithelial cells and their nuclei have a spindle and/or oval shape (type A) or whether these cells have a dendritic or plump (epithelioid) appearance (type B). Tumors that combine these two morphologies are designated type AB. Type B tumors were subdivided further into three subtypes designated B1, B2, and B3, respectively, on the basis of the proportional increase of the epithelial component and the emergence of atypia of the neoplastic cells. All kinds of thymic carcinomas are categorized as type C [59, 60].

In 2004 WHO revised the classification and included implementation of recurrent genetic alterations that have been identified in thymomas and thymic carcinomas. These alterations correlate with the histological WHO subtype and the clinical behavior. Another important category now included in the histological classification of thymic tumors is the group of combined thymic epithelial tumors. Combined thymic epithelial tumors are neoplasms with at least two distinct areas, each corresponding to one of the histological thymoma and/or thymic carcinoma types, including neuroendocrine carcinomas. The most frequent combination is that of a type B2 and a type B3 component. In 2004 WHO identified some new rare entities including micronodular thymoma, biphasic thymoma and hepatoid carcinomas and Carcinoma with t (15;19) translocation.

In the current classification, the term "type C thymoma" is no longer used, since now all nonorganotypic malignant epithelial neoplasms other than germ cell tumors are designated thymic carcinomas. The subtype of thymic carcinoma (e.g., squamous cell, mucoepidermoid, lymphoepithelioma-like) must be further specified. In addition, thymic neuroendocrine tumors (NEC), except for paragangliomas, are now included in the category of thymic carcinomas [61].

Other Classifications

Suster and Moran proposed the histologic grading of the tumors based on the premise that primary thymic epithelial neoplasms form part of a continuous spectrum of lesions that range from well-differentiated to moderately differentiated to poorly differentiated neoplasms.

In this proposal, the well-differentiated tumors corresponded to tumors designated by convention as thymoma, the poorly differentiated neoplasms were those conventionally designated as thymic carcinomas, and tumors showing intermediate features of differentiation were designated as atypical thymoma [62].

Kuo et al. proposed to classify thymomas simply based on their cytomorphologic features into spindle cell, small polygonal cell, mixed (spindle cell and small polygonal cell), organoid, large polygonal cell, and squamoid thymomas. Their classification was supported by the cytokeratin immunohistochemical expression [63].

Masaoka Staging [64]: Tumor staging is considered to be the most significant prognostic factor in determining patient survival. Thymoma spreads via direct extension through its capsule into adjacent structures such as lung, mediastinal soft tissue, or pleura and can metastasize distantly. The extent of capsule invasion and the involvement of thoracic and extrathoracic structures determine the stage, which is correlated to the risk of recurrence and survival. Thus, extensive tissue sampling of the resected tumor is essential to define microscopic and macroscopic invasion through the fibrous capsule. The staging system used for thymoma as proposed by Masaoka is outlined in Table 7.7.

Prognostic and Clinical Relevance of Classifications and Staging: The prognostic relevance of the staging and classification has been discussed in several studies, but it still remains to be conclusively determined. Some reports place emphasis on the clinical relevance of the WHO schema, whereas other reports display skepticism about its clinical validity.

Okumura et al. [65] studied clinical features as well as postoperative survival of patients with thymoma, but not thymic carcinoma, with reference to WHO histologic classification based on an experience with 273 patients over a 44-year period. In patients with type A, AB, B1, B2, and B3 tumors, the respective proportions of invasive tumor were 11.1%, 41.6%, 47.3%, 69.1%, and 84.6% and the respective 20-year survival rates were 100%, 87%, 91%, 59%, and 36% (Fig. 7.3).

According to the Masaoka staging system, the 20-year survival rates were 89%, 91%, 49%, 0%, and 0% in patients with Stage I, II, III, IVa, and IVb disease, respectively (Fig. 7.4).

Table 7.7 Masoaka staging system for thymomas (this material is reproduced with permission of Wiley-Liss inc., a subsidiary of John Wiley & Sons, inc. © American Cancer Statement [64])

Stage	Definition
I	Macroscopically, completely encapsulated; microscopically, no capsular invasion
IIa	Macroscopic invasion into surrounding fatty tissues or mediastinal pleura
IIb	Microscopic invasion into the capsule
III	Macroscopic invasion into the neighboring organ (i.e., pericardium, great vessels, or lung)
IVa	Pleural or pericardial dissemination
IVb	Lymphogenous or hematogenous metastases

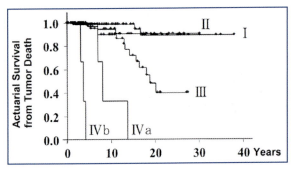

Fig. 7.3 Survival based on WHO classification (this material is reproduced with permission of Wiley-Liss inc., a subsidiary of John Wiley & Sons, inc. © American Cancer Statement [65])

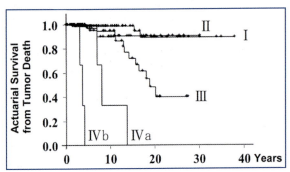

Fig. 7.4 Survival based on Masoaka staging system (this material is reproduced with permission of Wiley-Liss inc., a subsidiary of John Wiley & Sons, inc. © American Cancer Statement [64])

By multivariate analysis, the Masaoka staging system and the WHO histologic classification system were significant independent prognostic factors, whereas age, gender, association with myasthenia gravis, completeness of resection, or involvement of the great vessels were not significant independent prognostic factors. The WHO histologic classification system reflects the oncologic behavior of thymoma [65].

Many studies have found type B3 thymoma [well-differentiated thymic carcinoma (WDTC) as defined by the Müller-Hermelink classification system] to have a different behavior than other thymomas. Type B3 tumors have significant numbers (although fewer than type B1 and B2 tumors) of CD4 positive/CD8 positive, double-positive cells inside the tumor, whereas type C tumors do not. Furthermore, type B3 tumors often were associated with myasthenia gravis. For these reasons, type B3 tumors are supposed to be related functionally more to type B1 and B2 tumors. The poorer survival and the higher tumor recurrence rate in the patients with type B3 tumors compared with other types of thymomas, however, seem to indicate more careful follow-up and treatment for these patients compared with the treatment for patients with other types of thymomas. When using the WHO classification, it is critical to distinguish type B3 thymoma from other tumor types. The 15-year recurrence-free rate of the 64 patients with type A, AB, B1, and B2 thymomas was significantly higher from that of the 33 patients with type B3 thymoma [66].

Kondo et al. [67] reclassified a series of 100 thymomas resected at Tokushima University Hospital and four affiliated hospitals in Japan between 1973 and 2001 according to the WHO histologic classification and reported its clinicopathologic relationship and prognostic relevance and found the WHO histologic classification a good prognostic factor.

Another retrospective, clinicopathologic analysis of 108 patients showed on multivariate analysis that the WHO subtype (A-B2 vs. B3 vs. C) could predict the tumor-related survival, but the Masaoka stage was the most important prognostic factor affecting the postoperative survival [68]. The Masaoka staging system, WHO histologic classification, and complete resection were significant independent prognostic factors [69].

Two hundred thymomas from the Shanghai Chest Hospital with a mean follow-up time of 15 years (range, 1 to 246 months) were studied for the relevance of WHO histologic subtype and other factors [stage, therapy, and myasthenia gravis (MG)] for survival. Tumor stage was the most important determinant of survival in thymoma patients, but the WHO histologic subtype is an independent prognostic factor in Stage I and II thymomas, among which WHO type A, AB, and B1 thymomas form a low-risk group [70].

Epidemiology

The peak incidence of thymomas is between the ages of 40 and 60 years, with equal gender predilection. These neoplasms are rare in children. There is no predilection for a particular race or geographic distribution [71, 72]. A recent study indicated that in thymoma found to have capsular invasion, there is a predilection for males and Asians or Pacific islanders [73].

Thymomas are extremely rare in children, but when they occur, they present as highly aggressive tumors with a high mortality rate [74]. Among 23 patients with thymoma, Cohen and colleagues noted that 2 had received radiation for an enlarged thymus in childhood, 17 and 28 years before the diagnosis of thymoma, respectively [75].

Clinical Features

Thymomas have been recognized more often recently because of increased aggressiveness in eval-

Table 7.8 Presenting symptoms and signs of patients with thymoma

Asymptomatic
Manifestations related to local growth
Chest pain
Cough
Dyspnea
Dysphagia
Pleural effusion
Pericardial effusion
Superior vena cava syndrome
Intrathoracic hemorrhage
Endobronchial obstruction
Hemoptysis
Parathymic syndromes and related symptoms

Table 7.9 Parathymic syndromes (well recognized)

Myasthenia gravis
Red cell aplasia
Hypogammaglobulinemia
Polymyositis
Autoimmune thyroid disease
Sjogrens Syndrome

uating patients with myasthenia gravis but there are multiple other modes of presentation (Table 7.8) [76].

Asymptomatic. Two thirds of patients are asymptomatic at the time of diagnosis; an anterior mediastinal mass is discovered incidentally on the chest roentgenogram in 30-50% of cases [72].

Manifestations Related to Local Effects: The rest of the patients typically have nonspecific chest pain, cough, or dyspnea [77]. Superior vena cava syndrome, pleural effusion, and pericardial effusion have been reported and indicate invasiveness. Pleural disease can mimic mesotheliomas [78]. Pericardial involvement usually occurs at a later stage and massive pericardial effusions have been reported [79]. About 9-12 cases of primary intrapericardial thymomas have been reported [80]. Tumor involvement of the great vessels is a poor prognostic factor [81]. Thymomas with polypoid endobronchial growth have been reported in invasive cases leading to variable respiratory complaints [82, 83]. Local invasion can lead to necrosis and hemorrhage that has given rise to spontaneous hemothorax [84].

Ectopic thymus tissue can develop due to aberrant migration and later in life can cause nodules or masses and even neoplastic changes in atypical places, usually the neck [85].

Parathymic syndromes: Approximately 40-70% of thymomas have at least laboratory evidence of one or more of the two dozen systemic "parathymic" syndromes that have been recognized. Myasthenia gravis is most frequent among these, reported in 10-50% of patients with thymoma [86]. How thymoma produces myasthenia gravis is unknown, but autoantibodies to the postsynaptic acetylcholine receptor appear to explain the dysfunction of the neuromuscular junction [87] and are found in the majority of patients with myasthenia.

The other associated conditions seen in patients with thymoma include red cell aplasia, hypogammaglobulinemia, polymyositis, and (rarely) systemic lupus erythematosus, rheumatoid arthritis, thyroiditis, hyperthyroidism, and other cytopenias [88]. When an anterior mediastinal mass is present with myasthenia gravis, red cell aplasia, or hypogammaglobulinemia, the diagnosis of thymoma is essentially established. Patients with thymoma also have an increased incidence of collagen vascular disease, Whipple's disease, and malignancy elsewhere in the body [89] (Table 7.9).

The illnesses associated with thymoma are similar to those in APS-II, although the frequency of specific disorders is different. (APS-II is the more common of the immunoendocrinopathy syndromes.)

In one review of patients with thymoma, myasthenia gravis occurred in 44% of the patients, red blood cell aplasia in approximately 20%, hypoglobulinemia in 6%, autoimmune thyroid disease in 2%, and adrenal insufficiency in 1 of 423 patients. The frequency of autoimmune thyroid disease reported in patients with thymoma is probably an underestimate, given the frequency of unsuspected thyroid disease in patients with myasthenia gravis. Mucocutaneous candidiasis in adults is also associated with thymoma. In most patients, the thymoma are malignant, although temporary remissions of the autoimmune disease can occur with resection of the tumor [90] (Table 7.10).

Myasthenia Gravis: Is a common association of thymomas occurring in more than a third of patients. It will be discussed in Chap. 8.

Red Cell Aplasia: Isolated red cell aplasia may be present in 5-10% of patients with thymoma (1/3 with spindle cell). In this situation, there is an almost total absence of red cell precursors in the bone marrow and reticulocytes of the peripheral blood and a marked decrease of erythroblasts in the bone marrow.

One third of these patients also have reduced counts of both leukocytes and platelets. The exact etiology of this disorder is not known, but it has been reported to occur in patients together with MG and thymoma, which suggests an autoimmune mechanism [91]. The bone marrow is usually quite cellu-

Table 7.10 Less commonly reported parathymic syndromes

Systemic lupus erythematosus
Rheumatoid arthritis
Thyroiditis
Cytopenias
Autoimmune adrenal disease
Lichen Planus
Acute pericarditis and myocarditis
Alopecia areata
Cushing's syndrome
Hemolytic anemia
Limbic encephalopathy
Nephrotic syndrome
Panhypopituitarism
Pernicious anemia
Sarcoidosis
Scleroderma
Sensorimotor radiculopathy
Stiff-persons' syndrome
Ulcerative colitis

lar, and erythropoietin levels are typically high. An immunoglobulin G (IgG) inhibitor of erythroblastic growth has been described in the serum of some patients [92]. Thymectomy in these patients results in improvement in approximately 30% of the patients. Steroids, immunosuppressive agents and octreotide have been tried with varying degrees of success [93].

Hypogammaglobulinemia: Hypogammaglobulinemia was first reported by Good in 1954 [94]; it is seen in about 5% of the patients with thymoma. Both cellular and humoral immunity are decreased in these patients. This acquired syndrome results in extreme susceptibility to recurrent, and often serious, infections. Infections like mucocutaneous candidiasis, viral infection and P. carinii can be seen. It occurs in about 5-10% of patients with thymoma, and a thymoma is found in 10% of patients with acquired hypogammaglobulinemia [95]. There is a decrease in all major immunoglobulins, particularly IgG and IgA, and decreased eosinophils in the blood and bone marrow. A combined deficit in cell-mediated immunity can also be seen. Almost a third of patients have PRCA, too. Like those with PRCA, the age group is somewhat older (>40 years), and the thymoma is of the spindle-cell type in 75% of cases. The pathogenesis is obscure. There is a lack of pre-B-cells, B-cells, and plasma cells in the bone marrow, with decreased peripheral B-cells. Thymectomy does not result in any improvement; palliative treatment with immunoglobulins is indicated. Only occasional remissions in hypogammaglobulinemia have been seen after thymectomy.

Radiological Appearance

Radiographically thymomas are usually detected near the junction of the heart and great vessels; typically, they are round or oval with smooth or lobulated margins. Compared with thymic hyperplasia, which is typically symmetrical, thymoma usually distorts the gland's normal shape and extends to one side [96]. Computed tomography (CT) is invaluable for detecting small thymomas and assessing possible invasion of surrounding structures, such as the mediastinum, pleura, and pericardium. It can show calcifications in or at the periphery of the tumor in about 20% of cases, although they bear no relation to invasiveness. The presence of a fat plane all around the tumor is a good sign of noninvasiveness, but, conversely, fibrous adherence to surrounding structures may simulate invasion. CT can also help differentiate thymomas from vascular structures and tumors, such as aneurysms, particularly when intravenous contrast is used. As with virtually all-solid mass lesions of the mediastinum, thymoma is diagnosed with certainty only by examination of tissue. However, CT can reveal gross invasion and MRI can demonstrate the continuity of a mediastinal mass with the thymus [97] and discern invasion of vascular structures [98]. Preliminary experience with somatostatin receptor scintigraphy [99, 100] appears promising for discerning thymoma and other thymic tumors from benign thymic hyperplasia.

Prognosis

Thymomas are neoplastic, but most have relatively benign biologic behavior. Patients whose tumors are fully encapsulated can expect survival equal to that of the general population. Invasive tumors have a poorer prognosis, with 50-77% 5-year and 30-55% 10-year survival [101, 102]. Recurrence after resection occurs in nearly a third of patients [101].

The presence of a thymoma-associated systemic syndrome has traditionally been regarded as a poor prognostic sign. However, with improvements in perioperative management of patients with myasthenia gravis, the adverse effect of parathymic manifestations on the prognosis of patients with thymoma appears to be offset by the earlier diagnosis of thymoma discovered because of myasthenic symptoms [101, 103]. Karnofsky performance status has also been found to be a predictor of prognosis [104].

Treatment

Thymoma may respond to hormonal therapy [105], but are usually managed by resection via a median sternotomy approach or via video-assisted thoracoscopic surgery. Most authors favor removal of as much tumor mass as possible, even when it invades surrounding tissues. Adjunctive treatment with postoperative radiotherapy is provided [106]; the addition of preoperative or adjuvant chemotherapy appears promising. Thymectomy may also improve symptoms in some patients with myasthenia gravis.

Thymic Carcinoma

Thymic carcinomas are epithelial neoplasms of the thymus that are characterized by a high degree of cytologic atypia. These tumors, unlike thymomas, express highly aggressive behavior and should thus be classified separately. Thymic carcinoma is a histologically malignant process that invades locally and frequently metastasizes [107]. The prognosis depends on the histologic grade and the anatomic stage and is generally poor. Resection and combined chemotherapy and radiation therapy are advocated. Thymic carcinoma includes a heterogeneous group of neoplasms, of which more than half are undifferentiated carcinomas. Other tumor subtypes seen include squamous cell carcinoma, spindle cell carcinoma, lymphoepithelioma-like carcinoma, mucoepidermoid carcinoma, basaloid carcinoma, clear cell carcinoma, and adenoid cystic tumor [108, 109] (Table 7.11).

Cellular Subtypes of Thymic Carcinoma

Unlike their thymoma counterpart, thymic carcinomas lack immature T-lymphocytes and are TdT negative [110]. Additionally, thymic carcinomas express the cytokeratin marker CD5, which is helpful in distinguishing these tumors from nonthymic epithelial malignancies [111].

These tumors usually present in adult men and are seen only rarely in children. Symptoms include weight loss, shoulder discomfort, cough, and dyspnea. Paraneoplastic syndromes generally are not associated with thymic carcinoma. Well-differentiated thymic carcinoma has been reported in association with myasthenia gravis [110]. The spindle cell variety is generally an aggressive subtype, with mortality rates of up to 50% within 5 years reported [112, 113]. There is increasing evidence that Epstein-Barr virus (EBV) might play a role in the development of a lymphoepithelioma-like carcinoma of the thymus gland, as is seen in nasopharyngeal carcinomas. EBV nuclease antigen has been detected in tumorous cells, and Southern blot analysis has demonstrated the EBV viral genome in the cells of thymic lymphoepithelioma-like carcinoma [114]. Although EBV-associated lymphoepitheliomas of the nasopharynx are often treated successfully, the thymic counterpart appears to have a poor prognosis, probably because of delayed diagnosis. Other forms of thymic carcinoma are rare. Computed tomography usually shows an anterior mediastinal mass infiltrating along the pleura or mediastinum with necrosis or calcification [115].

Thymic carcinomas are aggressive and highly lethal tumors. Generally, well-differentiated squamous carcinoma, low-grade mucoepidermoid carcinoma, and basaloid thymus carcinoma have a more favorable prognosis. The other types are more aggressive. Usually, these patients present with advanced-stage disease and are candidates for multimodality treatment, including surgery, radiation therapy, and chemotherapy [116]. The combination of cisplatin, vinblastine, and bleomycin as used in the treatment of germ cell tumors has been applied to these neoplasms.

Ectopic Thymic Cancers

In some very rare cases, however, thymus cells may be ectopic, which means existing in a location in which they are not normally found. The most likely place for ectopic thymus cells is in the neck near the thyroid gland as a result of abnormal migration during fetal development. During fetal development, the cells that make up the thymus migrate down to the mediastinum. In very rare cases, some of this tissue fails to migrate, forming in the neck.

Thymic Lymphoma

Lymphomas, along with thymomas, are the most common tumors of the thymus. Hodgkin's disease is, as a rule, of the nodular sclerosis type, and it was for-

Table 7.11 Cellular subtypes of thymic carcinoma

Keratinizing squamous cell carcinoma
Nonkeratinizing squamous cell carcinoma
Lymphoepithelioma-like carcinoma
Adenosquamous carcinoma
Mucoepidermoid carcinoma
Clear-cell carcinoma
Papillary adenocarcinoma
Adenocarcinoma not otherwise specified
Basaloid carcinoma
Sarcomatoid carcinoma

merly considered to be a granulomatous thymoma [117]. It is frequently confined to the thymus. Although any lymphoma, including Burkitt's lymphoma, may arise in the thymus, the lymphoblastic type in children typically involves the mediastinum in a third of cases and is of T-cell origin.

Interestingly, the thymus is also a common site for mediastinal Hodgkin's lymphoma, and normal thymic tissue may enlarge following chemotherapy for lymphoma (a process termed *thymic rebound*), mimicking recurrence of the primary disease [118]. Primary thymic lymphomas are less common, and their prognosis is linked with early treatment.

Rios et al. [119] reviewed 10 primary thymic lymphomas – four Hodgkin's and six non-Hodgkin's [4 primary mediastinal B lymphomas (PMBLs) and 2 lymphoblastic T lymphomas]. Most of the patients were females, with a mean age of 23 +/-10 years. The initial diagnostic suspicion in the Hodgkin's lymphomas was thymoma in 2 cases and lymphoma in the other 2. All of them underwent surgery, including an intraoperative biopsy, which was completed with a thymectomy in the two in which thymoma was reported. They were treated with radio- and chemotherapy. The response was partial in 2 cases, and treatment was completed with a bone marrow transplant (one died and the other had active disease). The non-Hodgkin's lymphomas were large tumors and of short evolution. All of them received surgery, with an intraoperative biopsy in four and a thymectomy in two. They were treated with chemotherapy, with associated radiotherapy in two. The response was total in three, with two recurring, who are in complete remission after a BMT. In the other three the response was partial. PTLs are uncommon but aggressive, principally the non-Hodgkin's lymphomas. The main treatment is radio- and chemotherapy, with associated bone marrow transplantation in selected cases.

Extranodal marginal-zone B-cell lymphoma (MZBL) of mucosa-associated lymphoid tissue (MALT) arising in the thymus is rare with 20-25 cases reported, predominantly Asian. Inagaki et al. investigated 15 cases of thymic MALT lymphoma to systematically characterize its clinical, histopathological, and molecular features. There was a marked female predilection (male:female = 1:4), with a mean age of 55 years at diagnosis. There was a strong association with autoimmune disease, especially Sjögren's syndrome. Thirteen of 15 cases expressed immunoglobulin (Ig) A phenotype; IgA expression in thymic MALT lymphoma was in striking contrast with the IgM phenotype observed in most of the Sjögren's syndrome-associated MZBLs and MALT lymphomas at other sites. Thymic MALT lymphoma may represent a distinct subgroup of MALT lymphoma characterized by an apparent predilection for Asians, a strong association with autoimmune disease, frequent presence of cysts, consistent plasma cell differentiation, tumor cells expressing IgA phenotype, and consistent lack of API2-MALT1 gene fusion [120]. Sixty-eight percent of these patients had autoimmune diseases or hyperglobulinemia [121].

Clinical Features Due to Neuroendocrine Tumors of Thymus

Neuroendocrine tumors arising in thymus are extremely rare with approximately 200 cases reported in the literature [122]. They accounted for 4% of anterior mediastinal tumors in one series [123]. The median age at diagnosis ranged from 40 to 58 years, and men predominate in all series (67-91%) [122, 124-126].

Classification of Thymic Neuroendocrine Tumors

Thymic carcinoids are identical to well-differentiated neuroendocrine carcinoma of foregut derivation [125]. These are potentially malignant tumors and often develop distant metastases, sometimes after long intervals [125, 126]. There has been no satisfactory classification system to predict its progression. Table 7.12 lists the proposed classification for thymic neuroendocrine tumors (Table 7.12).

Table 7.12 TNM classification of thymic neuroendocrine tumors (this material is reproduced with permission of Wiley-Liss inc., a subsidiary of John Wiley & Sons, inc. © American Cancer Statement [127])

Classification	Description
T1	Macroscopically completely encapsulated and microscopically no capsular invasion
T2	Macroscopic adhesion or invasion into surrounding fatty tissue or mediastinal pleura, macroscopic invasion into capsule
T3	Invasion into neighboring organs, such as pericardium, great vessels, and lung
T4	Pleural or pericardial dissemination
N0	No lymph node metastasis
N1	Metastasis to anterior mediastinal lymph nodes
N2	Metastasis to intrathoracic lymph nodes, except for anterior mediastinal lymph nodes
N3	Metastasis to extrathoracic lymph nodes
M0	No hematogenous metastasis
M1	Hematogenous metastasis

Histologic Grading of Thymic Neuroendocrine Tumors

Thymic neuroendocrine tumors are subclassified into three groups according to histologic grade. Grade 1 thymic neuroendocrine tumors are composed of round to polygonal cells exhibiting little pleomorphism. Mitoses are rare. Grade 2 tumors show mild to moderate cellular pleomorphism with one or two mitotic figures per 20 high-power fields (×400). Grade 3 tumors have a higher degree of cellular pleomorphism and a higher nuclear to cytoplasmic ratio than grade 2 tumors. Mitoses were identified more easily, with six to eight mitoses per 10 high-power fields (×400) [124].

Tiffet et al. [122] had twelve patients in their series. The median age was 58 years (age range, 35 to 78 years). Eight of 12 patients (66.6%) were men. Four patients were asymptomatic and had their tumor discovered on a routine chest radiograph. Seven patients presented with local symptoms related to the mediastinal mass ranging from cough and chest pain to superior vena cava syndrome and hoarseness. One patient presented with lethargy, weight loss, and polyuria due to ectopic adrenocorticotrophic hormone (ACTH) secretion. Two patients were diagnosed with multiple endocrine neoplasia, type 1 (MEN-1). Chest CT scans in this series showed an anterior mediastinal mass that appeared to be homogeneous in five patients and heterogeneous with central necrosis and cystic degeneration in four patients. Only three tumors were well circumscribed, with the other nine tumors showing invasion into the surrounding tissue. No tumors showed calcification. Bronchoscopy was performed in 8 patients, and the findings were normal in 7 patients. In 1 patient bronchoscopy revealed extrinsic compression of the left main bronchus.

Fukai et al. [124] had 15 patients in their series. The median age was 50 years (age range 19 to 73 years). Ten (66.7%) of 15 patients were male. Two patients presented with Cushing's syndrome while 1 patient presented with myasthenia gravis. In the patient with myasthenia gravis the computed tomographic scans revealed a large cystic mass in the right lobe of the thymus and a small homogenous solid mass in the left lobe of the thymus. Microscopically, the cystic tumor was found to be thymoma, and the solid tumor was a thymic neuroendocrine carcinoma. Computed tomographic scan was successful in revealing the lesions in all patients. Total resection was possible in 13 (86.7%) of 15 patients in this series. Distant metastases developed in 10 (76.9%) of 13 patients who received total resection. Of these 10 patients, 6 died of distant metastases 5 to 25 months after recurrence. Cushing's syndrome on clinical presentation was associated with a poorer prognosis with early metastasis.

De Montpreville et al. [125] had fourteen patients in their series. There were 3 women and 11 men with an age range from 35 to 71 years. Twelve patients presented with local symptoms while two patients were asymptomatic on presentation. Commonest symptoms included chest pain, dyspnea, superior vena caval (SVC) syndrome and dysphonia. Other symptoms included cough, left recurrent laryngeal nerve paralysis, and weight loss. One patient had a multiple endocrine neoplasia syndrome; another had neurofibromatosis. One patient had Cushing's syndrome that appeared secondarily and was related to metastases.

Other rare presentations of thymic neuroendocrine tumors include recurrent pericarditis [128].

Differential Diagnosis of Thymic Neuroendocrine Tumors

The thymic neuroendocrine tumors should be differentiated from other mediastinal neuroendocrine neoplasms [129]. A metastasis, especially from a bronchopulmonary carcinoid tumor, must be clinically excluded. Mediastinal parathyroid adenomas and nonsecreting mediastinal parathyroid carcinoma can be considered in the differential diagnosis of thymic carcinoid tumor with malignant behavior. Mediastinal paraganglioma [130] can be distinguished from carcinoid tumors by its lack of immunoreactivity for cytokeratin. Nonneuroendocrine mediastinal neoplasms, which can histologically be confused with carcinoid tumors, are infrequent thymomas without any lymphoid component. Immunohistochemical negativity for neuroendocrine markers can permit accurate diagnosis in these cases.

Thymic Neuroendocrine Tumors and Thymic Epithelial Tumors

The thymic carcinoid tumors represent a specific entity that is separated from the other malignant epithelial thymic tumors, namely, thymomas and thymic carcinomas. There are several elements that suggest that thymic carcinoid tumors can be compared with the group of thymic carcinomas. The thymic carcinomas are rare and not associated with immunologic disorders such as myasthenia gravis. These carcinomas have a propensity to produce lymph node and extrathoracic metastases [107, 112]. Such clinical features are shared with thymic carcinoid tumors and clearly distinguish these tumors from the more common and less aggressive thymomas. Furthermore, the prognosis in patients with thymic carcinoid tumors is close to the survival rate (33.3% at 5 years) reported for thymic carcinomas [112].

In summary, thymic carcinoid tumors present with a variety of clinical onsets, and behave as malignant tumors; they have a distinctive histologic and immunohistologic appearance. These neoplasms can either be asymptomatic, associated with symptoms related to local growth, or part of a MEN syndrome and can produce endocrinopathy, especially Cushing's syndrome. Operation is the most effective treatment and complete resection offers the best hope for long-term survival [125].

Clinical Features Due to Immune Dysfunction in Thymus Pathology

Clinical features due to immunologic dysfunction of the thymus are discussed in other sections of the chapter. Clinical features due to myasthenia gravis are discussed in detail in Chap. 8.

Clinical Features Due to Infections Affecting the Thymus

Thymus plays a unique role in T-cell development and susceptibility to infection in its absence. In addition to its role in T-cell development, thymus can be directly or indirectly involved in infections.

Thymus and Human Immunodeficiency Virus

The acquired immune deficiency syndrome (AIDS) was recognized in 1981, when five unusual cases of Pneumocystis carinii pneumonia (PCP) occurring in young homosexual men from Los Angeles were reported to the Centers for Disease Control and Prevention (CDC) [131]. The depletion in numbers and function of T-helper cells further suggested that a lymphotropic agent might be responsible. Indeed, a human T-lymphotropic retrovirus that was immunologically related to human T-cell leukemia virus type I (HTLV-I) was detected in lymph node tissue from a French patient who was at risk for AIDS [132]. Thymus pathology has been described in children affected with human immunodeficiency virus (HIV). The pathologic changes in thymus are related with direct viral invasion and subsequent involution of the gland [133]. Joshi et al. described three types of lesion in thymus occurring in children affected with HIV.

1. Precocious involution with depletion of lymphocytes and microcystic dilatation of Hassall corpuscles.
2. Disinvolution, which is an aberrant form of involution with reduction or complete absence of Hassall corpuscles.
3. Thymitis, which is characterized by lymphocytic infiltration of thymic cortex and medulla.

HIV Infection Presenting with Multiloculated Thymic Cysts

Leonidas et al. [134] reported 3 patients with HIV infection presenting with multiloculated thymic cysts. Clinical features in these patients included parotitis, sinusitis, generalized lymphadenopathy and lymphocytic interstitial pneumonitis (LIP). All these masses were found on chest radiography. Two out of the 3 patients had their masses resected, all 3 patients were doing well at the time of the series publication.

Avila et al. [135] reported four patients with HIV infection and multiloculated thymic cysts. Surgical biopsy of the lesions revealed follicular hyperplasia and diffuse plasmacytosis with no evidence of neoplasia or infection.

Thymus in Early and Late HIV-1 Infection

In early HIV infection, the lymphoid infiltrate of the thymic perivascular space is increased compared to normal thymus while in late HIV infection, the HIV-1 infected thymus is prematurely atrophic with changes that are similar to, but more exaggerated than, normal atrophic thymus [136, 137].

Role of the Thymus in Immune Reconstitution in HIV Infection

Haynes et al. [138] studied the role of adult thymus in T-cell reconstitution in patients with HIV-1 infection. They had two groups of patients. In the first group, they evaluated mediastinal tissue from 7 adult patients who died of complications of HIV-1 infection for the presence of thymus, for inflammation, and for areas of active thymopoiesis. In the second group, they studied three thymectomized patients with HIV-1 infection to determine directly the effect of loss of the thymus on the clinical course of HIV-1 infection and on the ability to respond to HAART (Highly active antiretroviral therapy) with rises in CD4$^+$ T-cells. In their study they found minimal contributions of the thymus to maintenance or reconstitution of the peripheral pool of T-cells in the adult HIV-1-infected patients. In their first group of patients it was revealed that 5 of 7 (71%) patients had either no thymus or no areas of thymopoiesis, demonstrating that no contribution to the peripheral T-cell pool was being made by the thymus in those subjects at the time of death. In the second group they found that thymectomy did not preclude long-term survival or prevent the presence or rise of naive-phenotype peripheral T-cells after HAART. However further studies did not confirm this thymic impairment. A study by Sopper et al. [139] in the simian immunodeficiency virus, (SIV)-infected rhesus monkeys showed that while absolute numbers of CD4+ T-cells are decreased in peripheral blood, there was a global increase in proliferation and in absolute CD4+ T-cell numbers in all lymphoid organs during the asymptomatic phase of the infection. An increase in T-cell numbers in lymphoid organs combined with the high T-cell turnover induced by the virus during the asymptomatic phase of HIV infection suggests that the thymus plays an important role in T-cell homeostasis during the asymptomatic phase of HIV-1 infection. Similarly, studies have shown that thymus plays a major role in immune reconstitution in patients on HAART [140, 141].

Tuberculosis of Thymus

Tuberculosis usually involves mediastinal lymph nodes. Thymic tuberculosis represents remnants of post primary localized mediastinal lymphadenitis. Only a few cases of thymic tuberculosis have been reported in the literature [142-144]. These lesions are usually mistaken for neoplasia, but after resection on pathology there is inflammatory reaction, with accumulation of granulomas formed by giant cells in thymic tissue.

In a study by Nobrega et al. [145] in the mouse model, using aerogenic or intravenous routes of infection, they showed that the thymus was consistently colonized by *Mycobacterium tuberculosis*, *Mycobacterium avium* or *Mycobacterium bovis*. When compared to organs such as the liver and spleen, the bacterial load reaches a plateau at later time-points after infection, while in contrast to the spleen and the lung no granuloma were found in the thymus of mice infected with *M. tuberculosis* or *M. avium*. Since T-cell differentiation depends, to a large extent, on the antigens encountered within the thymus, infection of this organ might alter the host's immune response to infection. Further studies are awaited to address the significance of these findings.

Conclusions

Thymus pathology consists of heterogenous groups of diseases. These diseases, although rare, can present with myriad symptoms. The most common thymus pathology is thymoma. Thymic neoplasms have been recognized more often recently because of increased aggressiveness in evaluating patients with myasthenia gravis. This chapter reviews the clinical manifestations of common thymus pathologies.

References

1. Crapo JD, Glassroth J, KarlinskyJ et al (2004) Baum's textbook of pulmonary diseases. Lippincott Williams & Wilkins, Philadelphia, PA
2. Assarsson E, Chambers BJ, Hogstrand K et al (2007) Severe defect in thymic development in an insertional mutant mouse model. J Immunol 178:5018-5027
3. Boehm T, Bleul CC (2007) The evolutionary history of lymphoid organs. Nat Immunol 8:131-135
4. Devriendt K, Fryns JP, Mortier G et al (1998) The annual incidence of DiGeorge/velocardiofacial syndrome. J Med Genet 35:789-90
5. Sullivan KE, Jawad AF, Randall P et al (1998) Lack of correlation between impaired T cell production, immunodeficiency, and other phenotypic features in chromosome 22q11.2 deletion syndromes. Clin Immunol Immunopathol 86:141-146
6. Kobrynski LJ, Sullivan KE (2007) Velocardiofacial syndrome, DiGeorge syndrome: The chromosome 22q11.2 deletion syndromes. Lancet 370:1443-1452
7. McLean-Tooke G, Spickett P, Gennery AR (2007) Immunodeficiency and autoimmunity in 22q11.2 deletion syndrome. Scand J Immunol 66:1-7
8. McDonald-McGinn DM, Kirschner R, Goldmuntz E et al (1999) The Philadelphia story: The 22q11.2 deletion: Report on 250 patients. Genet Couns 10:11-24
9. Ryan AK, Goodship JA, Wilson DI et al (1997) Spectrum of clinical features associated with interstitial chromosome 22q11 deletions: A European collaborative study. J Med Genet 34:798-804

10. Gerdes M, Solot C, Wang PP et al (1999) Cognitive and behavior profile of preschool children with chromosome 22q11.2 deletion. Am J Med Gene 85:127-133
11. Moss EM, Batshaw ML, Solot CB et al (1999) Psychoeducational profile of the 22q11.2 microdeletion: A complex pattern. J Pediatr 134:193-198
12. Swillen A, Devriendt K, Legius E et al (1997) Intelligence and psychosocial adjustment in velocardiofacial syndrome: A study of 37 children and adolescents with VCFS. J Med Gene 34: 453-458
13. Wang PP, Woodin MF, Kreps-Falk R et al (2000) Research on behavioral phenotypes: Velocardiofacial syndrome (deletion 22q11.2). Dev Med Child Neurol 42: 422-427
14. Weller E, Weller R, Jawad A et al (1999) Psychiatric diagnoses in children with velocardiofacial syndrome, American Academy of Child and Adolescent Psychiatry, Chicago
15. Vantrappen G, Devriendt K, Swillen A et al (1999) Presenting symptoms and clinical features in 130 patients with the velo-cardio-facial syndrome. The Leuven experience, Genet Coun 10:3-9
16. Yan W, Jacobsen LK, Krasnewich DM et al (1998) Chromosome 22q11.2 interstitial deletions among childhood-onset schizophrenics and "multidimensionally impaired". Am J Med Genet 81:41-43
17. Motzkin B, Marion R, Goldberg R et al (1993) Variable phenotypes in velocardiofacial syndrome with chromosomal deletion. J Pediatr 123:406-410
18. Shprintzen RJ, Goldberg R, Golding-Kushner KJ et al (1992) Late-onset psychosis in the velo-cardio-facial syndrome. Am J Med Genet 42:141-142
19. Lischner HW, Dacou C, DiGeorge AM (1967) Normal lymphocyte transfer (NLT) test: Negative response in a patient with congenital absence of the thymus. Transplantation 5:555
20. Botto LD, May K, Fernhoff PM, Correa A et al (2003) A population-based study of the 22q11.2 deletion: Phenotype, incidence, and contribution to major birth defects in the population. Pediatrics 112:101-107
21. McDonald-McGinn DM, LaRossa D et al (1997) The 22q11.2 deletion: Screening, diagnostic workup, and outcome of results; report on 181 patients. Genet Test 1:99-108
22. Goldmuntz E (2005) DiGeorge Syndrome: New Insights. Clinics in Perinatology 32:963-978
23. Wurdak H, Ittner LM, Sommer L (2007) DiGeorge syndrome and pharyngeal apparatus development. Bioessays 28:1078-1086
24. Eicher PS, McDonald-McGinn DM, Fox CA et al (2000) Dysphagia in children with a 22q11.2 deletion: Unusual pattern found on modified barium swallow. J Pediatr 137:158-164
25. Dyce O, McDonald-McGinn D, Kirschner RE et al (2002) Otolaryngologic manifestations of the 22q11.2 deletion syndrome. Arch Otolaryngol Head Neck Surg 128:1408-1412
26. Brauner R, Le Harivel de Gonneville A, Kindermans C et al (2003) Parathyroid function and growth in 22q11.2 deletion syndrome. J Pediatr 142:504-508
27. Taylor SC, Morris G, Wilson D et al (2003) Hypoparathyroidism and 22q11 deletion syndrome. Arch Dis Child 88:520-522
28. Scire G, Dallapiccola B, Iannetti P et al (1994) Hypoparathyroidism as the major manifestation in two patients with 22q11 deletions. Am J Med Genet 52:478-482
29. Greig F, Paul E, DiMartino-Nardi J et al (1996) Transient congenital hypoparathyroidism: Resolution and recurrence in chromosome 22q11 deletion. J Pediatr 128:563-567
30. Jawad AF, McDonald-McGinn DM, Zackai E et al (2001) Immunologic features of chromosome 22q11.2 deletion syndrome (DiGeorge syndrome/velocardiofacial syndrome). J Pediatr 139:715-723
31. Sullivan KE (2004) The clinical, immunological, and molecular spectrum of chromosome 22q11.2 deletion syndrome and DiGeorge syndrome. Curr Opin Allergy Clin Immunol 4:505-512
32. DiGeorge AM (1968) Congenital absence of the thymus and its immunological consequences: Concurrance with congenital hypothyroidism. Birth Defects 4:116-121
33. Barrett DJ, Ammann AJ, Wara DW et al (1981) Clinical and immunologic spectrum of the DiGeorge syndrome. J Clin Lab Immunol 6:1-6
34. Bastian J, Law S, Vogler L et al (1989) Prediction of persistent immunodeficiency in the DiGeorge anomaly. J Pediatr 115:391-396
35. Chinen J, Rosenblatt HM, Smith EO et al (2003) Long-term assessment of T-cell populations in DiGeorge syndrome. J Allergy Clin Immunol 111:573
36. Sullivan KE, McDonald-McGinn D, Driscoll DA et al (1999) Longitudinal analysis of lymphocyte function and numbers in the first year of life in chromosome 22q11.2 deletion syndrome (DiGeorge syndrome/velocardiofacial syndrome). Clin Diagn Lab Immunol 6:906
37. Gennery AR, Barge D, O'Sullivan JJ et al (2002) Antibody deficiency and autoimmunity in 22q11.2 deletion syndrome. Arch Dis Child 86:422
38. Smith CA, Driscoll DA, Emanuel BS et al (1998) Increased prevalence of immunoglobulin A deficiency in patients with the chromosome 22q11.2 deletion syndrome (DiGeorge syndrome/velocardiofacial syndrome). Clin Diagn Lab Immunol 5:415
39. Davies K, Stiehm ER, Woo P, Murray KJ (2001) Juvenile idiopathic polyarticular arthritis and IgA deficiency in the 22q11 deletion syndrome. J Rheumatol 28:2326-2334
40. Davies JK, Telfer P, Cavenagh JD et al (2003) Autoimmune cytopenias in the 22q11.2 deletion syndrome. Clin Lab Haematol 25:195-197
41. Lawrence S, McDonald-McGinn DM, Zackai E, Sullivan KE (2003) Thrombocytopenia in patients with chromosome 22q11.2 deletion syndrome. J Pediatr 143:277-278
42. Kratz CP, Niehues T, Lyding S et al (2003) Evans syndrome in a patient with chromosome 22q11.2 deletion syndrome: A case report. Pediatr Hematol Oncol 20:167-172

43. Digilio MC, Giannotti A, Castro M et al (2003) Screening for celiac disease in patients with deletion 22q11.2 (DiGeorge/velo-cardio-facial syndrome). Am J Med Genet 121A:286-288
44. Scattone A, Caruso G, Marzullo A et al (2003) Neoplastic disease and deletion 22q11.2: A multicentric study and report of two cases. Pediatr Pathol Mol Med 22:323-341
45. McDonald-McGinn DM, Reilly A, Wallgren-Pettersson C et al (2006) Malignancy in chromosome 22q11.2 deletion syndrome (DiGeorge syndrome/velocardiofacial syndrome). Am J Med Genet A 140:906
46. Simon TJ, Bearden CE, Moss EM et al (2002) Cognitive development in VCFS. Prog Pediatr Cardiol 15:109-117
47. Fine SE, Weissman A, Gerdes M et al (2005) Autism spectrum disorders and symptoms in children with molecularly confirmed 22q11.2 deletion syndrome. J Autism Dev Disord 35:70
48. Shprintzen RJ, Goldberg RB, Lewin ML et al (1978) A new syndrome involving cleft palate, cardiac anomalies, typical facies, and learning disabilities: Velo-cardio-facial syndrome. Cleft Palate J 15:56
49. Dadmanesh F, Sekihara T, Rosai J (2001) Histologic typing of thymoma according to the new World Health Organization classification. Chest Surg Clin N Am 11:407-420
50. Ito M, Taki T, Miyake M et al (1988) Lymphocyte subsets in human thymoma studied with monoclonal antibodies. Cancer 61:284-287
51. Chan WC, Zaatari GS, Tabei S et al (1984) Thymoma: An immunohistochemical study. Am J Clin Pathol 82:160-166
52. Bernatz PE, Harrison EG, Clagett OT (1961) Thymoma: A clinicopathologic study. Thorac Cardiovasc Surg 42:424-444
53. Gray GF, Gutowsk III WT (1979) Thymoma. A clinicopathologic study of 54 cases. Am J Surg Pathol 3:235-249
54. Pescarmona E, Rendina EA, Venuta F et al (1990) The prognostic implication of thymoma histologic subtyping. A study of 80 consecutive cases. Am J Clin Pathol 93:190-195
55. Lattes R, Jonas S (1957) Pathological and clinical features in 80 cases of thymoma. Bull N Y Acad Med 33:145-147
56. Marino M, Muller-Hermelink HK (1985) Thymoma and thymic carcinoma. Relation of thymoma epithelial cells to the cortical and medullary differentiation of thymus. Virchows Arch A Pathol Anat Histopathol 407:119-149
57. Kirchner T, Muller-Hermelink HK (1989) New approaches to the diagnosis of thymic epithelial tumors. Prog Surg Pathol 10:167-189
58. Quintanilla-Martinez L, Wilkins EW Jr, Choi N, Efird J et al (1994) Thymoma. Histologic subclassification is an independent prognostic factor. Cancer 74:606-617
59. Rosai J, Sobin LH (1999) Histological typing of tumours of the thymus. WHO, International histologic classification of tumors. Springer-Verlag, Berlin
60. Chalabreysse L, Roy P, Cordier JF et al (2002) Correlation of the WHO schema for the classification of thymic epithelial neoplasms with prognosis: A retrospective study of 90 tumors. Am J Surg Pathol 26:1605-1611
61. Ströbel P, Marx A, Zettl A, (2005) Thymoma and thymic carcinoma: An update of the WHO Classification 2004. Surg Today 35:805-811
62. Suster S, Moran CA (2006) Thymoma classification: Current status and future trends. Am J Clin Pathol 125:542-554
63. Kuo T (2000) Cytokeratin profiles of the thymus and thymomas: Histogenetic correlations and proposal for a histological classification of thymomas. Histopathology 36:403
64. Masaoka A, Monden Y, Nakahara K et al (1981) Follow-up study of thymomas with special reference to their clinical stages. Cancer 48:2485-2492
65. Okumura MD, Ohta M, Tateyama H (2002) A clinical study of 273 patients. Cancer 94:624-632
66. Sonobi S, Miyamoto H, Ozumi H (2005) Clinical usefulness of the WHO histological classification of thymoma. Ann of Thorac Cardiovasc Surg 11:367-373
67. Kondo K, Yoshizawa K et al (2004) WHO histologic classification is a prognostic indicator in thymoma. Ann Thorac Surg 77:1183-1188
68. Kim DJ, Yang WI, Choi SS et al (2005) Prognostic and clinical relevance of the World Health Organization schema for the classification of thymic epithelial tumors: A clinicopathologic study of 108 patients and literature review. Chest 127:755-761
69. Rena O, Papalia E, Maggi G et al (2005) World Health Organization histologic classification: An independent prognostic factor in resected thymomas. Lung Cancer 50:59-66
70. Chen G, Marx A, Wen-Hu C (2002) New WHO histologic classification predicts prognosis of thymic epithelial tumors. A clinicopathologic study of 200 thymoma cases from China. Cancer 95:420-429
71. Thomas CR, Wright CD, Loehrer PJ (1999) Thymoma: State of the art. J Clin Oncol 17:2280-2289
72. Patterson GA (1992) Thymomas. Semin Thorac Cardiovasc Surg 4:39-44
73. Engels EA, Pfeiffer RM (2003) Malignant thymoma in the United States: Demographic patterns in incidence and associations with subsequent malignancies. Int J Cancer 105:546-551
74. Spigland N, Di Lorenzo M, Youssef S et al (1990) Malignant thymoma in children: A 20-year review. J Pediatr Surg 25:1143-1146
75. Cohen DJ, Ronnigen LD, Graeber GM et al (1984) Management of patients with malignant thymoma. J Thorac Cardiovasc Surg 87:301
76. Sperling B, Marschall J, Kennedy R (2003) Thymoma: A review of the clinical and pathological findings in 65 cases Can J Surg 46:37-42
77. Morgenthaler TI, Brown LR, Colby TV et al (1993) Thymoma. Mayo Clin Proc 68:1110-1123

78. Moran CA, Travis WD, Rosado-de-Christenson M et al (1992) Thymomas presenting as pleural tumors. Report of eight cases. Am J Surg Pathol 16:138
79. Nishimura T, Kondo M, Miyazaki S et al (1982) Two-dimensional echocardiographic findings in cardiovascular involvement by invasive thymoma. Chest 81:752-754
80. McAllister HA, Fenoglio JJ (1978) Atlas of tumor pathology. Tumors of the cardiovascular system. Second series, fascicle 15. Armed Forces Institute of Pathology, Washington DC
81. Blumberg D, Burt ME, Bains MS et al (1998) Thymic carcinoma: Current staging does not predict prognosis. J Thorac Cardiovasc Surg 115:303-9
82. Abiko M, Sato T, Shiono S et al (1999) A case of invasive thymoma displaying endobronchial extension. J Jpn Soci Bronch 21:289-293
83. Sakuraba M, Sagara Y, Tamura A (2005) A case of invasive thymoma with endobronchial growth. Ann Thorac Cardiovasc Surg 11(2):114-116
84. Wright C, Wain C (2006) Acute presentation of thymoma with infarction or hemorrhage. Ann Thorac Surg 82:1901-1904
85. Jung JI, Kim HH, Park SH (1999) Malignant ectopic thymoma in the neck: A case report. Am J Neuroradiol 20:1747-1749
86. Silverman NA, Sabiston DC Jr (1980) Mediastinal masses. Surg Clin North Am 60:757-777
87. Lennon VA, Lambert EH (1980) Myasthenia gravis induced by monoclonal antibodies to acetylcholine receptors. Nature 285:238-240
88. Souadjian JV, Enriquez P, Silverstein MN et al (1974) The spectrum of diseases associated with thymoma. Coincidence or syndrome? Arch Intern Med 134:374-379
89. Shields TW (1991) Thymic tumors. In: Shields TW (ed) Mediastinal surgery. Lea & Febiger, Philadelphia
90. Hayashi A, Shiono H, Okumura M (2007) Thymoma accompanied by lichen planus. Interact Cardiovasc Thorac Surg
91. Bailey RO, Dunn HG, Rubin AM et al (1988) Myasthenia gravis with thymoma and pure red blood cell aplasia. Am J Clin Pathol 89:687-693
92. Krantz SB (1990) Pure red cell aplasia. In: Givel JC, Merlini M, Clarke DB, Dusmet M (eds) Surgery of the thymus. Pathology, associated disorders and surgical technique. Springer-Verlag, Berlin
93. Palmieri G, Lastoria S, Colao A et al (1997) Successful treatment of a patient with a thymoma and pure red-cell aplasia with octreotide and prednisone. N Engl J Med 336:263
94. Good RA (1954) Agammaglobulinemia: A provocative experiment of nature. Bull Univ Minn Hosp 26:1
95. Rosenberg JC (1993) Neoplasms of the mediastinum. In: DeVita Jr VT, Hellman S, Rosenberg SA (eds) Cancer. Principles and practice of oncology, 4th edn. JB Lippincott, Philadelphia
96. Rosado de Christenson ML, Galobardes J, Moran CA (1992) Thymoma: Radiologic-pathologic correlation. Radiographics 12:151-168
97. Kiyosue H, Miyake H, Komatsu E, Mori H (1994) MRI of cervical masses of thymic origin. J Comput Assist Tomogr 18:206-208
98. Sakai F, Sone S, Kiyono K et al (1992) MR imaging of thymoma: Radiologic-pathologic correlation. AJR Am J Roentgenol 158:751-756
99. Lastoria S, Vergara E, Palmieri G et al (1998) In vivo detection of malignant thymic masses by indium-111-DTPA-D-Phel-octreotide scintigraphy. J Nucl Med 39:634-639
100. Liu RS, Yeh SH, Huang MH et al (1995) Use of fluorine-18 fluorodeoxyglucose positron emission tomography in the detection of Thymoma: A preliminary report. Eur J Nucl Med 22:1402-1407
101. Lewis JE, Wick MR, Scheithauer BW et al (1987) Thymoma: A clinicopathologic review. Cancer 60:2727-2743
102. Blumberg D, Port JL, Weksler B et al (1995) Thymoma: A multivariate analysis of factors predicting survival. Ann Thorac Surg 60:908-913
103. Kohman LJ (1997) Controversies in the management of malignant thymoma. Chest 112:296S-300S
104. Gripp S, Hilgers K, Wurm R (1998) Thymoma: Prognostic factors and treatment outcomes. Cancer 83:1495-1503
105. Kurup A, Loehrer PJ Sr (2004) Thymoma and thymic carcinoma: Therapeutic approaches. Clin Lung Cancer 6:28-32
106. Curran WJ Jr, Kornstein MJ, Brooks JJ, Turrisi AT 3rd (1988) Invasive thymoma: The role of mediastinal irradiation following complete or incomplete surgical resection. J Clin Oncol 6:1722-1727
107. Hsu CP, Chen CY, Chen CL et al (1994) Thymic carcinoma: Ten years' experience in twenty patients. J Thorac Cardiovasc Surg 107:615-620
108. Walker AN, Mills SE, Fechner RE (1990) Thymomas and thymic carcinomas. Semin Diagn Pathol 7:250-265
109. Ritter JH, Wick MR (1999) Primary carcinomas of the thymus gland. Semin Diagn Pathol 16:18-31
110. Chung DA (2000) Thymic carcinoma – Analysis of nineteen clinicopathological studies. Thorac Cardiovasc Surg 48:114-119
111. Hishima T, Fukayama M, Fujisawa M et al (1994) CD5 expression in thymic carcinoma. Am J Pathol 145:268-275
112. Suster S, Rosai J (1991) Thymic carcinoma. A clinicopathologic study of 60 cases. Cancer 67:1025-1032
113. Wick MR, Scheithauer BW, Weiland LH et al (1982) Primary thymic carcinomas. Am J Surg Pathol 6:613-630
114. Leyvraz S, Henle W, Chahinian AP et al (1985) Association of Epstein-Barr virus with thymic carcinoma. N Engl J Med 312:1296-1299
115. Lee JD, Choe KO, Kim SJ et al (1991) CT findings in primary thymic carcinoma. J Comput Assist Tomogr 15:429-433
116. Thomas CR, Wright CD, Loehrer PJ (1999) Thymoma: State of the art. J Clin Oncol 17:2280-2289
117. Wick MR, Rosai J (1990) Neuroendocrine, germ cell, and nonepithelial tumors. In: Givel JC, Merlini M,

Clarke DB, Dusmet M (eds) Surgery of the thymus. Pathology, associated disorders and surgical technique. Springer-Verlag, Berlin
118. Burns DE, Schiffman FJ (1993) Beguiled by the gallium: Thymic rebound in an adult after chemotherapy for Hodgkin's disease. Chest 104:1916-1919
119. Rios A, Torres J, Roca MJ (2006) Primary thymic lymphomas. Rev Clin Esp 206:326-331
120. Inagaki H, Chan JK, Ng JW et al (2002) Primary thymic extranodal marginal-zone B-cell lymphoma of mucosa-associated lymphoid tissue type exhibits distinctive clinicopathological and molecular features. Am J of Path 160:1435-1443
121. Shimizu K, Ishii G, Nagai K et al (2005) Extranodal Marginal Zone B-cell Lymphoma of Mucosa-associated Lymphoid Tissue (MALT Lymphoma) in the Thymus: Report of Four Cases. Japanese Journal of Clinical Oncology 35:412-416
122. Tiffet O, Nicholson AG, Ladas G et al (2003) A clinicopathologic study of 12 neuroendocrine tumors arising in the thymus. Chest 124:141-146
123. Wick MR, Scott RE, Li CY et al (1980) Carcinoid tumor of the thymus: A clinicopathologic report of seven cases with a review of the literature. Mayo Clin Proc 55:246-254
124. Fukai I, Masaoka A, Fujii Y et al (1999) Thymic neuroendocrine tumor (thymic carcinoid): A clinicopathologic study in 15 patients. Ann Thorac Surg 67:208-211
125. De Montpreville VT, Macchiarini P, Dulmet E (1996) Thymic neuroendocrine carcinoma (carcinoid): A clinicopathologic study of fourteen cases. J Thorac Cardiovasc Surg 111:134-141
126. Economopoulos G, Lewis J Jr, Lee M et al (1990) Carcinoid tumors of the thymus. Ann Thorac Surg 50:58-61
127. Yamakawa Y, Masaoka A, Hashimoto T et al (1991) A tentative tumor-node-metastasis classification of thymoma. Cancer 68:1984-1987
128. Gelfand E, Basualdo C, Callaghan J (1981) Carcinoid tumor of the thymus associated with recurrent pericarditis. Chest 79:350-351
129. Wick MR, Rosai J (1991) Neuroendocrine neoplasms of the mediastinum. Semin Diagn Pathol 8:35-51
130. Moran CA, Suster S, Fishback N, Koss MN (1993) Mediastinal paragangliomas: A clinicopathologic and immunohistochemical study of 16 cases. Cancer 72:2358-2364
131. Pneumocystis pneumonia – Los Angeles, 1981 (1996) MMWR Morb Mortal Wkly Rep 30:250-252
132. Barre-Sinoussi F, Chermann JC, Rey F et al (1983) Isolation of a T-lymphotropic retrovirus from a patient at risk for acquired immune deficiency syndrome (AIDS). Science 220:868-871
133. Joshi VV (1991) Pathologic changes associated with HIV infection in children. In: Pizzo PA, Wilfred CM (eds) Pediatric AIDS. Williams & Wilkins, Baltimore
134. Leonidas J, Berdon W, Valderrama E et al (1996) Human immunodeficiency virus infection and multilocular thymic cysts. Radiology 198:377-379
135. Avila N, Mueller B, Carrasquillo J et al (1996) Multilocular thymic cysts: Imaging features in children with human immunodeficiency virus infection. Radiology 201:130-134
136. Haynes BF, Hale LP, Weinhold KJ et al (1999) Analysis of the adult thymus in reconstitution of T lymphocytes in HIV-1 infection. J Clin Invest 103:453-460
137. Haynes BF, Hale LP (1998) The human thymus: A chimeric organ comprised of central and peripheral lymphoid components. Immunol Res 3:175-92
138. Haynes BF, Hale LP, Weinhold KJ et al (1999) Analysis of the adult thymus in reconstitution of T lymphocytes in HIV-1 infection. J Clin Invest 103:921
139. Sopper S, Nierwetberg D, Halbach A et al (2003) Impact of simian immunodeficiency virus (SIV) infection on lymphocyte numbers and T-cell turnover in different organs of rhesus monkeys. Blood 101:1213-1219
140. Autran B, Carcelain G, Li TS et al (1997) Positive effects of combined antiretroviral therapy on CD4+ T cell homeostasis and function in advanced HIV disease. Science 277:112-116
141. Zhang ZQ, Notermans DW, Sedgewick G et al (1998) Kinetics of CD4+ T cell repopulation of lymphoid tissues after treatment of HIV-1 infection. Proc Natl Acad Sci U S A 95:1154-1159
142. Duprez A, Cordier R, Schmitz P (1962) Tuberculoma of the thymus. First case of surgical excision. J Urol Nephrol 44:115-120
143. Simmers TA, Jie C, Sie MC (1997) Thymic tuberculosis: A case report. Neth J Med 51:87-90
144. FitzGerald JM, Mayo JR, Miller RR et al (1992) Tuberculosis of the thymus. Chest 102:1604-1605
145. Nobrega C, Cardona PJ, Roque S et al (2007) The thymus as a target for mycobacterial infections. Microbes Infect 9:1521-1529

CHAPTER 8
Thymus and Myasthenia Gravis. Pathophysiological and Clinical Features

Loredana Capone, Riccarda Gentile, Rudolf Schoenhuber

The History of Myasthenia Gravis

In 1672 Thomas Willis published a book, "De anima brutorum" in which he wrote about "a woman who temporarily lost her power of speech and became mute as a fish" [1]. This has been interpreted as being the first written description of myasthenia gravis (MG). Others give credit to Wilks for the first report of disease in 1877, characterized as a bulbar palsy without anatomic lesion [2]. The first reasonably complete accounts were those of Erb in 1878 and Goldflam in 1893 [3, 4] and for many years thereafter, the disorder was referred to as the Erb-Goldflam syndrome. Jolly was the first to use the name myasthenia gravis in 1895 and to demonstrate the "myasthenic reaction" of muscle repeatedly stimulated by Faradism [5], introducing the basic criteria of instrumental techniques of MG diagnosis, the repetitive nerve stimulation, elaborated later by Desmedt [6].

The beneficial effect of physostigmine on myasthenic symptoms was discovered in 1934 by Mary Walker, who supposed also that the neuromuscular junctions (NMJ) were the focus of the disease [7]. Dale, Nobel Prize winner of 1936, showed acetylcoline (ACh) as neurotransmitter at the NMJ and the anticholinesterase activity of physostigmine [8]. The association of MG with thymic tumors and hyperplasia was recognized in 1901 by Carl Weigert, who described a myasthenic patient with a thymic mass [9] and in 1911 the first thymectomy was carried out by Sauerbruch in a female MG patient [10]. In 1949 Castleman and Norris reported a series of patients with thymic hyperplasia and thymoma related to MG [11].

The autoimmune nature of MG was defined by Patrick, Lindstrom, Fambrough, and Lennon in the early 1970s [12-14]. Research later showed the presence of ACh-receptor (AChR) antibodies in serum of patients affected by MG and the production of CD4+ and CD8+ cells in cases with thymomas [15].

The Epidemiology of Myasthenia Gravis

MG is an uncommon disease; estimated annual incidence is 2.5 to 20 per million. Prevalence is 50 to 400 cases per million, higher above 40 years. Lifetime risk is 500 per million. The female-to-male ratio is said classically to be 6:4, but as the population has aged, the incidence is now equal in males and females [16]. MG presents at any age, with a bimodal pattern of onset: female incidence peaks in the third decade of life, whereas male incidence peaks in the sixth or seventh decade. Mean age of onset is 28 years in females and 42 years in males. Transient neonatal MG occurs in infants of myasthenic mothers who acquire receptor antibodies via placental transfer of IgG. Some of these infants may suffer from transient neonatal myasthenia due to effects of these antibodies. Rare, nonimmune mediated forms, collectively referred to as congenital MG, may be the result of mutations that adversely affect neuromuscular transmission. Recent advances in treatment and care of critically ill patients have resulted in marked decrease in the mortality rate. The rate is now 3-4%, with principal risk factors being age older than 40 years, short history of severe disease, and thymoma. Previously, the mortality rate was as high as 30-40%.

The Pathophysiology of Myasthenia Gravis

ACh Receptor Structure

AChRs are located at peak of muscular synaptic folds. Their concentration is 10,000 per μm^2. The nicotinic AChRs consist of five polypeptide subunits clustered around the central receptor channel. Nine α subunits have been cloned, along with four β subunits. In the NMJ, δ and γ subunits also have been identified. The γ subunit is replaced by an ϵ subunit in the adult muscle. In adult skeletal muscle there are $\alpha 1$, $\alpha 1$, $\beta 1$, δ, and ϵ subunits, in fetal muscle $\alpha 1$, $\alpha 1$, $\beta 1$, δ, and γ. In extraocular muscles, some fibers contain both adult and fetal AChRs. The amino acid sequence for the α subunits consists of a glycolipid region (which contains the ACh binding site and a sulphydryl groups) with four hydrophobic regions that span the membrane.

The ACh binding site is a dimer formed by 3 or more peptide loops on the α subunit (principal component) and 2 loops on the adjacent subunit (complementary component). Their activity is binding to both sites needed for the channel to open and binding to only one site to prevent channel activation. The main immunogenic region of the AChR is the extracellular N-terminal of the polypeptide component in the α1 subunit. Structural proteins clustered at NMJs (rapsyn) and the muscle-Specific Kinase (MuSK) receptor (receptor tyrosine kinase) are involved in MG-AChR antibodies negative and in congenital MG. Other muscle membrane structural proteins are involved in different autoimmunological disorders and muscular structural pathologies (muscular dystrophies).

ACh Receptor Physiology

Nicotinic receptors are found in a variety of tissues, including the autonomic nervous system, the neuromuscular junction, and the brain of vertebrates. The high quantities of receptors in these tissues and the use of neurotoxins from snake venom (e.g., cobra venom) that bind specifically to the nicotinic receptor aided the purification of the receptor protein. Agonists such as ACh, carbamylcholine, and nicotine produce the physiological responses associated with nicotinic cholinergic activation. ACh produces an influx of sodium through a ligand-gated ion channel. ACh and carbamylcholine also stimulate muscarinic receptors and therefore should be considered mixed cholinergic agonists. Alpha-Bungarotoxin binds to the α and β subunits and probably blocks both the channel and the acetylcholine binding site. Local anesthetics and other compounds such as phencyclidine bind to the receptor, apparently at the site of the sodium channel and modulate the binding of acetylcholine to the active site. Local anesthetics also prevent ion conductance through a direct action at the channel. The sodium channel and the channel for the nicotinic AChR have some similar properties (in both structure and sensitivity to drug action) and may have a common genetic origin. When an ACh molecule binds to the α subunits of AChR, the AChR undergoes a 3-dimensional conformational change that opens the channel and results in increased sodium conductance, causing a local depolarization. The local depolarization spreads to an action potential or leads to muscle contraction when summed with the action of other receptors. Nicotinic receptors possess a relatively low affinity for ACh at rest. The affinity for ACh is increased during activation (through an allosteric mechanism which increases the likelihood of another molecule of acetylcholine binding to the other α subunit). At high concentrations of ACh, the affinity for ACh becomes higher and the receptor subsequently becomes desensitized. The ionophore (ion channel) is open during the active state and local anesthetics may bind to the open channel.

Physiology of Neuromuscular Transmission

Motor nerve impulses (action potentials) traveling down from the motor neurons through the motor fibers of peripheral nerve terminals cause the skeletal muscle fibers at which they terminate to contract. The junction between the motor axon terminal and a muscle fiber (motor endplate) is called the neuromuscular or myoneural junction. The terminals of motor axons contain thousands of vesicles filled with ACh. When an action potential reaches the axon terminal, hundreds of these vesicles discharge their ACh onto a specialized area of postsynaptic membrane on the fiber. This area contains a cluster of transmembrane channels that are opened by ACh and let sodium ions diffuse in. The interior of a resting muscle fiber has a resting potential of about −95 mV. The influx of sodium ions reduces the charge, creating an end plate potential. If the end plate potential reaches the threshold voltage (approximately −50 mV), sodium ions flow in with a rush and an action potential is created in the fiber. The action potential sweeps down the length of the fiber just as it does in an axon. No visible change occurs in the muscle fiber during (and immediately following) the action potential. This period, called the latent period, lasts from 3-10 ms. Before the latent period is over, the enzyme acetylcholinesterase breaks down the ACh in the NMJ at a speed of 25,000 molecules per second, the sodium channels close, and the field is cleared for the arrival of another nerve impulse. The resting potential of the fiber is restored by an outflow of potassium ions. The brief (1-2 ms) period needed to restore the resting potential is called the refractory period.

Presynaptic Steps Leading to Neurotransmitter Release

The arrival of action potentials and invasion of nerve terminals causes depolarization. In many neurons only 10-20% of action potentials trigger transmitter release. With repetitive trains of action potentials at 3 Hz, the number of transmitter vesicles released per potential declines with time, but at faster impulse rates, the number of transmitter vesicles released per potential may increase for a time. Depolarization of nerve terminals activates voltage-gated calcium channels (VGCCs). Channels are located in active zones, each containing two parallel arrays of VGCCs activating fast and slow neurotransmitter release. Calcium enters through activated VGCCs at the peak of the action potential and ends before the terminal is fully repolarized. Vesicle pathways are initiated by calcium entry via calcium ions sensor (synaptotagmins). Then vesicles move toward and interact with the membrane of the presynaptic terminal (docking) and become competent (priming) for fusion-pore opening calcium ions-induced, related to fast transmitter release. SNAREs (SNAP receptors) are membrane-associated proteins and are components of the fusion mechanism in synaptic exocytosis. Vesicle-associated SNAREs (v-SNARE) interact with target membrane SNAREs (t-SNARE). Synaptic vesicles SNAREs are synaptobrevin and vesicle-associated membrane protein (VAMP). Presynaptic plasma membrane SNAREs are syntaxin 1 and SNAP 25. Fast release is calcium ions triggered, synchronous, phasic, induced rapidly. Sensor protein is synaptotagmin 1 and concentration is high. Slow release is calcium ions triggered, asynchronous, continues for more than 1 sec and increases the rate of spontaneous ACh release. Sensor protein is synaptotagmins 3 or 7. Concentration is low and spontaneous release occurs at rest. Probability of fusion-pore opening after action potential is variable and depends on the tension and composition of participating membranes. Action potentials arrivals in motor terminals produce the release of ACh from 10 to 200 vesicles. Each vesicle contains 5,000 to 20,000 ACh molecules. The neurotransmitter is actively transported into the synaptic vesicles, driven by the vacuolar protein proton pump, a peripheral complex (V1) including ATPase activity that generates electrochemical gradient and drives neurotransmitter uptake. Transporters subtypes are glutamate (3 types) monoamines, GABA and glycine. Membrane potential and proton gradient contribute to uptake. Vesicle pools in the presynaptic terminal are readily releasable (20%) and reserve (80%). Resting vesicles are not present at the NMJ and the vesicle transport process involves cytoskeletal-associated proteins. Vesicles are transported through cytoplasm and clustered at active zones. After single stimulus a rapid release occurs, mildly slowed with increased number of vesicles released. Repetitive stimulation causes a prominent slowing of the endocytosis rate. Most vesicles recycle directly without passing through an endosomal intermediate. Related molecules are synaptojanin inositol 5-phosphatase, amphiphysin, dynamin, and clathrin. Other regulatory proteins are synapsins 1, 2, and 3 which link vesicles to the cytoskeleton. Reduced expression causes reduced synaptic vesicles distal to active zones and synaptic fatigue, probably regulating the reserve pool of vesicles needed for sustained synaptic transmission.

The Role of AChR Antibodies in MG

Immunogenic mechanisms play important roles in the pathophysiology of MG. Supporting clinical observations include the presence of associated autoimmune disorders in patients suffering from MG (e.g., autoimmune thyroiditis, systemic lupus erythematosus, rheumatoid arthritis). Moreover, infants born of myasthenic mothers can develop a transient myasthenia-like syndrome [17]. Patients with MG will have a therapeutic response to various immunomodulating therapies including plasmapheresis, corticosteroids, intravenous immunoglobulin (IVIg), other immunosuppressants, and thymectomy. Anti-AChR antibody is found in approximately 80-90% of patients with MG. Experimental observations supporting an autoimmune etiology of MG include the induction of a myasthenia-like syndrome in mice by injecting a large quantity of immunoglobulin G (IgG) from MG patients (passive transfer experiments), demonstration of IgG and complement at the postsynaptic membrane in patients with MG and induction of a myasthenia-like syndrome in rabbits immunized against AChR by injecting them with AChR. The exact mechanism of loss of immunologic tolerance to AChR, a self-antigen, is not understood. MG can be considered a B-cell-mediated disease, as antibodies (a B-cell product) against AChR are responsible for the disease [18]. However, the importance of T-cells in the pathogenesis of MG is becoming increasingly apparent. Antibody response in MG is polyclonal. In an individual patient, antibodies are composed of different subclasses of IgG. Binding of AChR antibodies to AChR results in impairment of neuromuscular transmission in several ways: accelerate internalization and degradation of AChR molecules, complement-mediated destruction of junctional folds of the postsynaptic membrane, block of the binding of ACh to AChR, decrease of the number of AChRs at the NMJ, damage of the junctional folds on the postsynaptic membrane and resultant decrease in available surface area for insertion of newly synthesized AChRs [19].

MuSK Antibodies

Patients without anti-AChR antibodies are recognized as seronegative MG (SNMG). Forty to fifty percent of patients with SNMG have antibodies against receptor MuSK [20]. MuSK is a receptor tyrosine kinase that plays a critical role in postsynaptic differentiation of AChRs and it mediates agrin-dependent AChR clustering and NMJ formation during development. MuSK antibody-positive MG may have a different cause and pathologic mechanism than AChR antibodies-positive disease [20]. MuSK antibodies are generally not present in those with well-established ocular MG, but they have been detected in a few cases [21]. Although nearly half of patients with SNMG will have MuSK antibodies, those with seropositive MG (SPMG) do not have antibodies to MuSK in most studies to date [22]. MuSK antibodies appear to be much less common in some SNMG populations [21, 23]; one consistent finding is that patients with SNMG and MuSK antibodies have a much lower frequency of thymic pathology than patients with SPMG [24]. Since they are seronegative, the group of patients with MuSK antibodies is not associated with the presence of underlying thymoma. In addition, thymic hyperplasia is frequent in SPMG, but this pathology is much less frequent in the MuSK-positive group. In the appropriate clinical setting (lack of AChR antibodies and typical clinical features), MuSK testing can clarify the diagnosis and perhaps direct treatment [25, 26]. However, the initial management of clinically apparent myasthenia should be the same for patients with or without AChR antibodies; this would change only if future studies find additional therapeutic differences related to MuSK status. Patients with SNMG who are MuSK positive share most of the clinical manifestations of generalized SPMG [22], with more frequent clinical aspects: symptoms occur at any age, patients are predominantly female presenting an oculobulbar form with diplopia, ptosis, and dysarthria, not purely ocular MG. There is a restricted "myopathic" form with prominent respiratory and/or proximal weakness, especially neck extension. Not related to thymic pathology (thymoma), thymectomy plays an uncertain role. Less responsiveness to acetylcholinesterase inhibitors is reported in many but not all patients [24]. They show a good responsiveness to plasma exchange and immunosuppression, with the possible exception of azathioprine.

Other Antibodies

Antistriated muscle antibodies are heterogeneous with specificity against striated muscle proteins. They are present in 30% of patients with myasthenia, but in 80% of those with thymoma [27]. These antibodies may be a useful marker for thymoma in those patients between 20 and 50 years of age. In this cohort, thymoma can be found in 60% of patients with antistriated muscle antibodies, but in less than 2% of those without these antibodies [27]. The false-positive rate (striational antibodies present without thymoma) is about 10%, but it rises to 50% in those over age 50. Under age 20, the likelihood of thymoma is low. Measurement of other skeletal muscle protein antibodies may potentially be more helpful than striational antibodies in predicting the presence of a thymoma and assessing disease prognosis [28]. One study demonstrated that antibodies to titin, an intracellular muscle protein, were found in 95% of patients with MG and thymoma but also 50% of those without thymoma. The positive predictive value of these antibodies was only 39%, but the negative predictive value was 99% [29]. Assays for antibodies to the ryanodine receptor had a lower sensitivity (70%) but a greater specificity (95%) and positive predictive value (70%). CT scanning for thymoma, in comparison, had a sensitivity, positive predictive value, and negative predictive value of 73%, 49%, and 65%, respectively. These antibodies to titin and/or ryanodine are found primarily in late-onset MG. In this population of patients, along with SPMG, the presence of these antibodies may raise the clinical suspicion of thymoma. Alternatively, the absence of anti-titin antibodies makes the presence of thymoma unlikely. Some data suggest that the presence of these antibodies predicts more severe disease and an unsatisfactory outcome after thymectomy [29, 30].

The Thymus and the Origin of Autoimmunity in MG

The majority of patients with SPMG have thymic abnormalities: hyperplasia in 60-70% and thymoma in 10-12% [18]. The thymus is the central organ in T-cell-mediated immunity, and thymic abnormalities such as thymic hyperplasia or thymoma are well recognized in myasthenic patients [11, 18] and it was proposed that the AChR expressed on thymic myoid cells is the original autosensitizing antigen and the thymic changes in MG are primary events in the autoimmune pathogenesis of the disease [31-33]. Others [34-36] suggest that the hyperplastic features in MG thymus are secondary phenomena; the AChR-specific T-cells are selectively trapped and restimulated in the thymus after prior sensitization elsewhere and thymic myoid cells can be targeted by these T-cells or the antibodies that they evoke. Antigen presentation by thymic cells via MHC class II molecules may be abnormal in patients with myasthenia. In particular, overexpression of cathepsin V, one of the enzymes responsible for cleaving the invariant chain that occupies the antigen presenting cleft of the MHC type II molecule, has been noted in the thymic tissue of patients with myasthenia and thymoma [37]. Increased production of this enzyme is present in the frankly neoplastic thymic tissue as well as in areas of inflamed gland (thymitis). Expression of mRNA and cathepsin V protein are not increased in the thymic tissue of patients with thymomas who do not have myasthenia. Other than the important role of the cathepsins in antigen processing cells, a link between enzyme overexpression and autoantibody production is unclear. It has been postulated that the availability of AChR in the thymus may play a role in pathogenesis of myasthenia. It is possible, for example, that the myoid cells are altered by viral illness involving the thymus; the proximity to antigen presenting cells and helper T-cells then facilitates the production of an immunologic response [18]. Another possibility is molecular mimicry; both herpes viruses and bacteria show cross-reactivity with AChR antibodies [38]. It seems likely that genetic factors also contribute to the pathogenesis of myasthenia gravis. Certain HLA types have been associated with myasthenia, including HLA-B8, DRw3, and DQw2 [39]. MuSK antibody-positive myasthenia is associated with haplotypes DR14 and DQ5 [40]. In addition, patients with myasthenia frequently have other immune-mediated diseases, such as systemic lupus erythematosus, rheumatoid arthritis, Graves' disease, and thyroiditis, and a family history of autoimmune disorders. It is not clear why some patients with thymoma develop myasthenia while others do not. The subtype of thymoma may be important; the development of myasthenia was significantly associated with mixed thymomas, but not with thymomas of the cortical type [41]. Among patients with MG, the presence of antititin antibodies is predictive of a thymic epithelial tumor (sensitivity 69-80% and specificity 90-100%) [29]. Patients who have late onset MG without thymoma may also have titin or ryanodine receptor antibodies. There is some suggestion that these antibodies may be associated with worse prognosis [30]. Because AChR antibodies levels do not clearly correlate with MG severity, investigators have continued to search for additional factors (e.g., other muscle antibodies, secondary cytokines, chemokines) that might positively correlate with the disease.

Clinical Course of MG

At onset MG is characterized by weakness increased by exertion. Symptoms may fluctuate throughout the day, but they are most commonly worse later in the day or evening, particularly after exercise. Early in the disease, the symptoms may be absent upon awakening. Often as the disease progresses, the symptom-free periods are lost; symptoms are continuously present but fluctuate from mild to severe. When present, this fluctuation in symptoms is an important feature that can distinguish MG from other disorders that also may present with weakness, such as myopathy or motor neuron disease. Presenting symptoms often involve extraocular muscle (EOM): diplopia or ptosis are present initially in 50% of patients [26, 42, 43] and occur during the course of illness in 90% [42, 43]. Bulbar muscle weakness is also common, along with weakness of head extension and flexion. Weakness may involve limb musculature with myopathic-like proximal weakness greater than distal muscle weakness. Systemic weakness is present at onset in 35%; isolated limb muscle weakness occurs in fewer than 10% of patients; respiratory failure as the presenting symptom is rare [16] Table 8.1.

Patients progress insidiously from mild to more severe disease over weeks to months. Weakness tends to spread from the ocular to facial, to bulbar muscles and then to truncal and limb muscles. On the other hand, symptoms may remain limited to the EOM and eyelid muscles for years. Rarely, patients with severe, generalized weakness may not have associated ocular muscle weakness. The disease remains ocular in only 16% of patients. About 87% of patients generalize within 13 months after onset. In patients with generalized disease, the interval from onset to maximal weakness is less than 36 months in 83% of patients [36, 42, 44]. Intercurrent illness (infections, thyroid dysfunction), pregnancy, emotional stress, and medications can exacerbate weakness, quickly precipitating a myasthenic crisis and rapid respiratory failure (Table 8.2).

Spontaneous remissions are rare and long, and complete remissions are even less common. Most remissions with treatment occur during the first 3 years of disease. To assess the clinical severity of symptoms and to control the results of treatment the Medical Scientific Advisory Board (MSAB) of the Myasthenia Gravis Foundation of America (MGFA) formed a Task Force in May 1997 and created the MGFA Clinical Classification (Table 8.3).

Table 8.1 Presenting symptoms of myasthenia gravis and the major considerations in the differential diagnosis

Presenting symptoms (Frequency)	Other disorders to consider
Ocular (50%)	Brainstem and cranial nerve lesions (including Horner's syndrome), thyroid ophthalmopathy, oculopharyngeal muscular dystrophy, chronic external ophthalmoplegia (mitochondrial disease)
Bulbar (15%)	Brainstem and multiple cranial nerve lesions, motor neuron disease, obstructive or malignant lesion of the nasal and oropharynx
Limb weakness (<5%)	Motor neuron disease, chronic inflammatory demyelinating polyneuropathy (CIDP) and other motor neuropathies, multiple radiculopathies, Lambert-Eaton myasthenic syndrome, myopathies
Isolated neck (uncommon)	Motor neuron disease, inflammatory myopathy, paraspinous myopathy
Isolated respiratory (rare)	Motor neuron disease, acid maltase deficiency, polymyositis
Distal limb (rare)	Motor neuron disease, CIDP and other motor neuropathies, distal myopathies

Table 8.2 Medications that can affect MG

Antibiotics	Neomycin, Streptomycin, Gentamycin, Colisitins, Telithromycin (exacerbation within 2 hours of administration), Kanamycin, anecdotal reports for Tobramycin; Amikacin; Polymyxin B; Tetracyclines; Lincomycin; Clindamycin; Erythromycin; Ampicillin; Fluoroquinolones (Norfloxacin, Ofloxacin, Pefloxacin)
Antirheumatic drugs	Prednisone (high dose: onset within days after administration), Chloroquine
NMJ blockers	Curare, Nondepolarizing agents (Vecuronium), Botulinum toxin
Other	Quinidine, Procainamide, Procaine, Magnesium, β-blockers, Phenytoin. Anecdotal reports for Verapamil; Trimethaphan; Trimethadione; Lithium; Chlorpromazine; Trihexyphenidyl; D,L-carnitine; Bretylium; Emetine; Lactate; Methoxyflurane; Contrast agents; Citrate anticoagulant; Trasylol; Gabapentin

Table 8.3 MGFA clinical classification

Class I	Any ocular muscle weakness May have weakness of eye closure All other muscle strength is normal
Class II	Mild weakness affecting other than ocular muscles May also have ocular muscle weakness of any severity
Class IIa	Predominantly affecting limb, axial muscles, or both May also have lesser involvement of oropharyngeal muscles
Class IIb	Predominantly affecting oropharyngeal, respiratory muscles, or both May also have lesser or equal involvement of limb, axial muscles, or both
Class III	Moderate weakness affecting other than ocular muscles May also have ocular muscle weakness of any severity
Class IIIa	Predominantly affecting limb, axial muscles, or both May also have lesser involvement of oropharyngeal muscles
Class IIIb	Predominantly affecting oropharyngeal, respiratory muscles, or both May also have lesser or equal involvement of limb, axial muscles, or both
Class IV	Severe weakness affecting other than ocular muscles May also have ocular muscle weakness of any severity
Class IVa	Predominantly affecting limb and/or axial muscles May also have lesser involvement of oropharyngeal muscles
Class IVb	Predominantly affecting oropharyngeal, respiratory muscles, or both May also have lesser or equal involvement of limb, axial muscles, or both

Defined by intubation, with or without mechanical ventilation, except when used during routine postoperative management. The use of a feeding tube without intubation places the patient in class IVb.
Physical variability in weakness can be significant and clearly demonstrable findings may be absent

Principles of Diagnostic Testing for MG

Diagnosis of MG, as a general rule, is based upon a characteristic history and physical examination, and two positive diagnostic tests, preferably serological (search for serum anti-AChR antibodies) and electrodiagnostic testing (repetitive nerve stimulation studies). Diagnostic investigations of MG should usually include both.

Bedside Tests

The Tensilon test and ice pack test should, in large part, be considered an extension of the neurologic examination rather than laboratory tests.

Edrophonium (Tensilon) Test

The Tensilon test may be readily performed at the bedside. It is not as sensitive, or specific, as the serological and electrophysiological studies. It works inhibiting acetylcholinesterase and prolongs the presence of neurotransmitter ACh in the NMJ, enhancing muscle strength. The action lasts for a few minutes. This test is not specific for MG; it may be positive in other NMJ disorders. Initially 2 mg of edrophonium is administered intravenously as a test dose, monitoring heart rate, because bradycardia or ventricular fibrillation may develop. After observing for about 2 min, if no clear response develops, up to 8 additional mg of edrophonium is injected. Cholinergic side effects of edrophonium may include increased salivation and lacrimation, mild sweating, flushing, urgency, and perioral fasciculations. Atropine should be readily available to reverse effects of edrophonium in case of homodynamic instability. The test is positive if after 30-45 sec after injection muscle strength improves for up to 5 min. The test requires objective improvement in muscle strength; subjective or minor responses, such as reduction of a sense of fatigue, should not be over interpreted. Sensitivity for MG is relatively low (60%) compared to other diagnostic tests. False positive results can occur in patients with Lambert-Eaton syndrome (LEMS), amyotrophic lateral sclerosis, or even localized, intracranial mass lesions and positive testing does not necessarily predict response to a longer-acting anti-AChE drug.

Ice Pack Test

In the ice pack test, a bag (or surgical glove) is filled with ice and placed on the closed lid for one minute. Since it is based on the physiologic principle of improving neuromuscular transmission at lower muscle temperatures, the eyelid muscles are the most easily cooled by the application of ice. The ice is then removed and the extent of ptosis is immediately assessed. The sensitivity appears to be about 80% [45, 46] in those with prominent ptosis. The predictive value of the test has not yet been established. The ice pack test can be used in patients with ptosis, particularly those in whom the Tensilon test is considered too risky. It is not helpful for those with extraocular muscle weakness.

Simpson Test

Testing the eyelids for fatigability can be done by asking the patient to open and close their lids several times or gaze upward for an extended time. Increased drooping is a sign of fatigue.

The phenomenon of "enhanced" ptosis can be demonstrated in patients with bilateral ptosis by elevating and maintaining the more ptotic eyelid in a fixed position. The opposite eyelid slowly falls and may close completely [47].

Cogan's lid twitch sign may be seen when the patient first looks down for a short period and then makes a saccade back to primary position. The upper eyelid elevates excessively during this upward saccade, sometimes causing a transient lid retraction, and then twitches in nystagmoid fashion or slowly droops back to a ptotic position. This is interpreted as transient improvement in lid strength after rest of the levator in down gaze, followed by droop in the primary position as the levator fatigues [48].

Electrophysiologic Confirmation

Electrodiagnostic studies are an important supplement to the immunologic studies and may also provide confirmation of the diagnosis of myasthenia. Repetitive nerve stimulation (RNS) studies and single-fiber electromyography (SFEMG) have a diagnostic sensitivity in generalized myasthenia of about 75% and 95%, respectively [44, 49].

RNS studies, due to their wide availability, are the most frequently used electrodiagnostic test for MG. The test is performed by placing the recording electrode over the endplate region of a muscle and stimulating the motor nerve to that muscle. It is important to sample distal and proximal muscles to maximize the yield. Distal muscles are technically easier, but they have a lower diagnostic sensitivity. If possible, clinically weak muscles should be included as well. To maximize the sensitivity, the muscles tested should be warm, and acetylcholinesterase inhibitors should be held for 12 h before the study. The nerve is electrically stimulated 10 times at low rates (3 Hz). The compound muscle action potential (CMAP) amplitude is recorded from the electrodes over the muscle after electrical stimulation of the nerve. In normal muscles, there is no change in CMAP amplitude with repetitive nerve stimulation. In MG there may be a progressive decline in the CMAP amplitude with the first four to five stimuli (a decremental response). An RNS study is considered positive if the decrement is greater than 20%. The RNS study is performed at rest and after exercise. In the exercise protocol, the patient is asked to exercise the muscle maximally for 15-30 seconds. A train of stimuli is performed immediately after exercise. A repair of the CMAP decremental response (a smaller percent decrement compared with the decrement seen at rest) is commonly seen, reflecting postexercise or postactivation facilitation. An additional train of stimuli is delivered at 1, 3, and 5 min after exercise. This may result in a larger decrement than seen at rest, termed postexercise or postactivation exhaustion. This exercise protocol may increase the sensitivity of RNS by an additional 5-10%. RNS studies are positive in about 75% of patients with generalized myasthenia, if recordings are made from proximal (usually trapezius and orbicularis oculi), as well as distal muscles. RNS studies are positive in approximately 50% of patients with ocular MG [44, 49]. A decremental response is not specific for MG. Decrements may be seen in other disorders of neuromuscular transmission (LEMS or botulism) and motor neuron disease. These disorders should not cause electrodiagnostic confusion when combined with studies looking for presynaptic disorders of neuromuscular transmission and standard needle electromyography.

SFEMG is more technically demanding than RNS and is less widely available, but it is the most sensitive diagnostic test for MG. A specialized needle electrode with a 25 μm recording window and the low frequency filters set at 500 Hz allows simultaneous recording of the action potentials of two muscle fibers innervated by the same motor axon. The variability in time of the second action potential relative to the first is called "jitter". Any disorder, such as MG, that reduces the safety factor of transmission at the neuromuscular junction will produce increased jitter. To maximize the sensitivity a limb and facial muscle may be studied. SFEMG is positive in greater than 95% of those with generalized myasthenia. In ocular MG, it ranges from 90 to 95% [44, 49]. Abnormal jitter is not specific for MG. It may be abnormal in motor neuron disease, polymyositis, peripheral neuropathy, LEMS, and other neuromuscular disorders. However, it is specific for a disorder of neuromuscular transmission when no other abnormalities are seen on standard needle EMG examination. The exception may be in differentiating patients suspected of ocular MG from those with Kearns-Sayre syndrome (KSS) causing chronic progressive external ophthalmoplegia (CPEO). The approximate diagnostic sensitivity of the confirmatory tests in myasthenia is shown in Table 8.4.

Associated Conditions

Thymic Tumors and Other Malignancies

The thymus is intimately involved in the pathogenesis of MG; 75% of patients with myasthenia have thymic abnormalities. Thymic hyperplasia is most common (85%), but various tumors (primarily thymoma) are present in up to 15% [50]. The thymic tumors are usually noninvasive cortical thymomas, but invasive thymic carcinoma can occur. Imaging of the mediastinum (by either computed to-

Table 8.4 Approximate sensitivity of the confirmatory tests for myasthenia gravis (percent positive)

	Generalized myasthenia	Ocular myasthenia
Acetylcholine receptor antibodies	80-85	55
MuSK antibodies (in seronegative myasthenia)	40-50	0
Repetitive nerve stimulation	75	50
Single fiber electromyography	92-99	85-95

mography or MRI) is an important component of the evaluation of any patient with MG. The detection, or absence, of striational antibodies and antibodies directed against titin and the ryanodine receptor may be helpful in predicting the presence (or absence) of thymoma (see above). MG can be considered a paraneoplastic effect of thymoma, but not of extrathymic tumors. Nonetheless, myasthenia has been associated with extrathymic tumors, such as small cell lung cancer and Hodgkin lymphoma [51]. It is uncertain from these studies whether this co-occurrence represents a true association. The data do not warrant an extensive search for malignancy, other than thymoma, in myasthenics, even in older patients.

Autoimmune Disorders

Autoimmune thyroid disease is quite common (3-8%) in patients with MG. Thus, screening for thyroid abnormalities should also be part of the initial evaluation.

Although less common than thyroid disease, rheumatoid arthritis and systemic lupus erythematosus (SLE) are more often associated with MG than in age-matched patients without MG. The clinician should be alert to the possibility of coexistent rheumatoid arthritis and SLE and perform the appropriate serologic studies and evaluation, if there are suggestive historical or examination features of these disorders.

Differential Diagnosis of MG

The differential diagnosis of MG includes conditions that mimic ocular myasthenia (like thyroid ophthalmopathy, KSS, brainstem and motor cranial nerve pathology) and conditions that mimic generalized MG like generalized fatigue ("tiredness"), motor neuron disease, LEMS, botulism, penicillamine-induced myasthenia, congenital myasthenic syndromes. Further studies to exclude other diseases in the differential diagnosis of MG are indicated in selected patients. For those with ocular or bulbar symptoms, an MRI of the brain is appropriate. CT scanning of the orbits is helpful in the differential diagnosis of ocular MG and thyroid ophthalmopathy [52, 53]. In cases of possible multiple cranial nerve abnormalities, examination of the cerebrospinal fluid for abnormal cells and cytology is usually necessary.

References

1. Willis T (1672) De anima brutorum quae hominis vitalis ac sensitiva est (exercitationes duae). Ric Davis, Oxford
2. Wilks S (1877) On cerebritis, hysteria and bulbar paralysis, as illustrative of arrest of function of the cerebrospinal centres. Guys Hosp Rep 22:7-55
3. Erb W (1879) Zur Casuistik der bulbaren Lähmungen. Über einen neuen, wahrscheinlich bulbaren Symptomencomplex. Arch Psychiatr Nervenkr 9:336-350
4. Goldflam S (1893) Über einen scheinbar heilbaren bulbärparalytischen symptomenkomplex mit beteiligung der extremitäten. Dtsch Z Nervenheilk 4:312-352
5. Jolly F (1895) Über Myastenia gravis pseudoparalytica. Berl Klin Wochenschr 32:1-7
6. Desmedt JE (1973) The neuromuscular disorder in myasthenia gravis. In: Desmedt JC (ed) New developments in electromyography and clinical neurophysiology. Karger, Basel, pp 241-304
7. Walker MB (1934) Treatment of myasthenia gravis with physostigmine. Lancet 1:1200-1201
8. Dale HH, Feldberg W, Vogt M (1936) Release of acetylcholine at voluntary motor nerve endings. J Physiol 86:353-380
9. Weigert C (1901) Pathologisch-anatomischer beitrag zur erb'schen krankheit (Myasthenia gravis). Neurol Centr Bl 20:597-601
10. Sauerbruch F, Schumacher ED (1911) Technik der Thoraxchirurgie. Julius Springer, Berlin
11. Castleman B, Norris EH (1949) The pathology of the thymus in myasthenia gravis. A study of 35 cases. Medicine 28:27-58
12. Patrick S, Lindstrom J (1973) Autoimmune response to acetylcholine receptor. Science 180:871-872
13. Fambrough DM, Drachman DB, Santyamurti S (1973) Neuromuscular junction in myasthenia gravis: Decreased acetylcholine receptors. Science 182:293-295
14. Lennon VA, Lindstrom JM, Seybold ME (1976) Experimental autoimmune myasthenia gravis: Cellular and humoral immune responses. Ann N Y Acad Sci 274:283-299
15. Buckley C, Douek D, Newsom-Davis J (2001) Immature long lived CD4+ and CD8+ cells are generated by the Thymoma in myasthenia gravis. Ann Neurol 50:64-72
16. Vincent A, Palace J, Hilton-Jones D (2001) Myasthenia gravis. Lancet 357(9274):2122-2128
17. Papazian O (1992) Transient neonatal myasthenia gravis. J Child Neurol 7:135-141
18. Drachman DB (1994) Myasthenia gravis. N Engl J Med 330:1797-1810
19. Engel AG, Arahata K (1987) The membrane attack complex of complement at the endplate in myasthenia gravis. Ann N Y Acad Sci 05:326-332
20. Hoch W, McConville J, Helms S et al (2001) Auto-antibodies to the receptor tyrosine kinase MuSK in patients with myasthenia gravis without acetylcholine receptor antibodies. Nat Med 7:365-368

21. Hanisch F, Eger K, Zierz S (2006) MuSK-antibody positive pure ocular myasthenia gravis. J Neurol 253:659-660
22. Sanders DB, El-Salem K, Massey JM et al (2003) Clinical aspects of MuSK antibody positive seronegative MG. Neurology 60:1978-1980
23. Romi F, Aarli JA, Gilhus NE (2005) Seronegative myasthenia gravis: Disease severity and prognosis. Eur J Neurol 12:413-418
24. Verma PK, Oger JJ (1992) Seronegative generalized myasthenia gravis: Low frequency of thymic pathology. Neurology 42:586-589
25. Zhou L, McConville J, Chaudhry V et al (2004) Clinical comparison of muscle-specific tyrosine kinase (MuSK) antibody-positive and -negative myasthenic patients. Muscle Nerve 30:55-60
26. Meriggioli MN, Sanders DB (2004) Myasthenia gravis: Diagnosis. Semin Neurol 24:31-39
27. Sanders DB, Massey JM (2002) The diagnostic utility of anti-striational antibodies in myasthenia gravis. Neurology 58:A229
28. Voltz RD, Albrich WC, Nagele A et al (1997) Paraneoplastic myasthenia gravis: Detection of anti-MGT30 (titin) antibodies predicts thymic epithelial tumor. Neurology 49:1454-1457
29. Chen XJ, Qiao J, Xiao BG, Lu CZ (2004) The significance of titin antibodies in myasthenia gravis-correlation with thymoma and severity of myasthenia gravis. J Neurol 251:1006-1011
30. Romi F, Skeie GO, Gilhus NE, Aarli JA (2005) Striational antibodies in myasthenia gravis: Reactivity and possible clinical significance. Arch Neurol 62:442-446
31. Wekerle H, Ketelsen UP (1977) Intrathymic pathogenesis and dual genetic control of myasthenia gravis. Lancet 1(8013):678-680
32. Kirchner T, Hoppe F, Schalke B, Müller-Hermelink HK (1988) Microenvironment of thymic myoid cells in myasthenia gravis. Virchows Arch B54:295-302
33. Marx A, Wilisch A, Schultz A et al (1997) Pathogenesis of myasthenia gravis. Virchows Arch 430:355-364
34. Utsugisawa K, Nagane Y, Tohgi H (2000) Marked increase in CD44- highly positive cells in hyperplastic thymuses from patients with myasthenia gravis. Muscle Nerve 23:507-513
35. Roxanis I, Micklem K, Willcox N (2001) True epithelial hyperplasia in the thymus of early-onset myasthenia gravis patients: Implications for immunopathogenesis. J Neuroimmunol 112:163-173
36. Sommer N, Willcox N, Harcourt GC, Newsom-Davis J (1990) Myasthenic thymus and thymoma are selectively enriched in acetylcholine receptor reactive T cells. Ann Neurol 28:312-319
37. Tolosa E, Li W, Yasuda Y et al (2003) Cathepsin V is involved in the degradation of invariant chain in human thymus and is overexpressed in myasthenia gravis. J Clin Invest 112:517-526
38. Schwimmbeck PL, Dyrberg T, Drachman DB, Oldstone MB (1989) Molecular mimicry and myasthenia gravis. An autoantigenic site of the acetylcholine receptor alpha-subunit that has biologic activity and reacts immunochemically with herpes simplex virus. J Clin Invest 84:1174-1180
39. Carlsson B, Wallin J, Pirskanen R et al (1990) Different HLA DR-DQ associations in subgroups of idiopathic myasthenia gravis. Immunogenetics 1:285-290
40. Niks EH, Kuks JB, Roep BO et al (2006) Strong association of MuSK antibody-positive myasthenia gravis and HLA-DR14-DQ5. Neurology 66:1772-1774
41. Wilisch A, Gutsche S, Hoffacker V et al (1999) Association of acetylcholine receptor alpha-subunit gene expression in mixed thymoma with myasthenia gravis. Neurology 52:1460-1466
42. Grob D, Arsura EL, Brunner NG, Namba T (1987) The course of myasthenia gravis and therapies affecting outcome. Ann N Y Acad Sci 505:472-499
43. Oosterhuis HJ (1989) The natural course of myasthenia gravis: A long term follow up study. J Neurol Neurosurg Psychiatry 52:1121-1127
44. Weinberg DH, Rizzo JF 3rd, Hayes MT et al (1999) Ocular myasthenia gravis: Predictive value of single-fiber electromyography. Muscle Nerve 22:1222-1227
45. Sethi K, Rivner MH, Swift TR (1987) The ice pack test for myasthenia gravis. Neurology 37:1383-1385
46. Golnik KC, Pena R, Lee AG, Eggenberger ER (1999) An ice test for the diagnosis of myasthenia gravis. Ophthalmology 106:1282-1286
47. Gorelick PB, Rosenberg M, Pagano RJ (1981) Enhanced ptosis in myasthenia gravis. Arch Neurol 31:531
48. Cogan D (1965) Myasthenia gravis: A review of the disease and a description of lid twitch as a characteristic sign. Arch Ophthalmol 74:217-221
49. Oh SJ, Kim DE, Kuruoglu R et al (1992) Diagnostic sensitivity of the laboratory tests in myasthenia gravis. Muscle Nerve 15:720-724
50. Castleman B (1966) The pathology of the thymus gland in myasthenia gravis. Ann N Y Acad Sci 135:496-505
51. Fujita J, Yamadori I, Yamaji Y et al (1994) Myasthenia gravis associated with small-cell carcinoma of the lung. Chest 105:624-625
52. Langmann A, Lindner S, Koch M, Diez J (2004) Okuläre myasthenie: Eine diagnostische und therapeutische Herausforderung-eine Übersicht. Klin Monatsbl Augenheilkd 221:77-86
53. Barohn RJ (2003) Standards of measurements in myasthenia gravis. Ann N Y Acad Sci 998:432-439

CHAPTER 9
Radiologic Diagnosis: X-ray, CT and MRI

Matteo Zanichelli, Manuela Gozzi, Mario Bertolani

Background

The name *thymus* comes from the Latin derivation of the Greek *thymos*, meaning "warty excrescence"; however, since thymos also means "soul" or "spirit", the ancient Greeks believed the thymus gland to be the seat of the soul [1-3].

Galen of Pergamum (130-200 AD), being the first to observe that the thymus was somehow proportionally largest during infancy and dwindled in size with aging [4], referred to the thymus as "the organ of mystery", a definition that persisted for almost two millennia, during which the thymus was believed to be the organ of purification of the nervous system, a protective thoracic cushion, and a center of regulation of fetal and neonatal respiration.

Implications for Imaging of Thymic Embryology

The thymus originates from the third and fourth branchial pouch and contains elements of derivation from all three germ layers [5-7].

The two symmetrical structures merge on the median line and finally migrate to the anterior mediastinum; up until week 9 the thymus is an exclusively epithelial structure but from week 10 lymphoid cells migrate from the liver and the marrow into the thymus which becomes lobulated. Cortical (lymphocyte) and medullary (epithelial) development is completed after 14-16 weeks. Neck-to-anterior mediastinum development and migration explains the presence of tissue of thymic origin, which can also grow into a thymoma, in ectopias along the entire path of migration of the thymus, although it is most often placed in the neck base.

The Normal Thymus

In infants and children up to 5 years of age the thymus has a four-sided shape, with biconvex lateral contours.

The thymus is a bilobated gland of triangular shape and straighter margins, located in the anterior portion of the superior mediastinum; in adults it extends above the sternal manubrium up to the IV costal cartilage [8].

The morphology of the normal thymus is highly diverse, most especially in children and young adults.

The thymus achieves its maximum size related to body weight before birth (sometimes being larger than the heart) and its maximum absolute size at puberty; thereafter its growth comes to an end.

Thymus involution starts at puberty, through volume reduction and adipose infiltration leading to an almost complete atrophy: epithelial cells disappear and there remain few lymphocytes against a background of adipose tissue.

The normal thymus at CT and MRI has been broadly studied [9-13].

At CT, the thymus has a homogeneous density and is usually viewed anteriorly from the aortic trunk and the origin of the large vessels; the left lobe is usually slightly larger than the right one; agenesia of one lobe is, instead, a rare occurrence.

At CT, the gland is best measured through thickness of the lobes on a plane perpendicular to the long axis of the gland. The maximum normal thickness is 18 mm before age 20 and 13 mm thereafter.

Baron has examined over 150 CT scans of subjects with a normal thymus: thickness decreases with aging, from 1.1 cm in the 6- to 19-year age bracket to 0.5 mm over 50 years of age, with a standard deviation of 0.4 and 0.27 cm, respectively.

At MRI, the thymic parenchyma has a homogeneous signal, with an intermediate T1 signal that increases with age proportionally with adipose infiltration [14-15]; in T2-weighted sequences the signal of the thymus is high at all ages.

Echotomographic Aspect of the Thymus in Infants and Children

In infants the thymus can be accurately examined via a suprasternal and parasternal echotomographic approach up to the age of 2 years [16-17], though some authors maintain that it can be correctly studied in children up to 8 years of age [18-20].

Normally, it has smooth margins and the shape of a triangle or of a tent in longitudinal scans whereas in transverse scans it is trapezoid or bilobated in shape; it lies in the anterior mediastinum and extends downwards to reach the heart (more rarely the diaphragm); an inferior cervical extension of the thymus is not a rare occurrence.

The large vessels, the vena cava, the aorta, the pulmonary artery, and sometimes also the supra-aortic trunks, surrounded by the thymus, are easily identifiable.

The thymic tissue has a homogeneously hypoechogenous aspect, with echogenicity similar to that of the liver but less than that of the thyroid and does not cause compression of the large vessels [21]; instead, neoplasms or lymphadenomegaly are less homogeneous.

Table 9.1 Thymic masses

Thymic neoplasms
    Benign or invasive thymoma
    Carcinoma
    Thymolipoma
    Lymphoma, in particular Hodgkin lymphoma
    Carcinoids (some of which secreting ACTH)
    Germ-cell tumors
Thymic cysts
    Simple cysts
    Multilocular cysts
    Cystic neoplasms
        Thymoma
        Lymphoma
        Germ-cell tumors
Thymic hyperplasia
    "True" rebound hyperplasia from:
        Chemotherapy
        Corticosteroid therapy
        Radiotherapy
        Stress
        Cushing Syndrome treatment
        Bone marrow transplantation
    Lymphoid hyperplasia associated to:
        Myasthenia gravis
        Systemic lupus erythematosus (SLE)
        Sclerodermia
        Rheumatoid arthritis
        Nodose polyarteritis
        Behçet's Disease
        Hashimoto thyroiditis
        Addison's Disease
        Auto-immune hemolytic anemia
        Thyreotoxicosis
        Graves' Disease

The Diseased Thymus

Thymic Hyperplasia

Thymic hyperplasia involves an increase in the age-related volume of the organ as a result of an increase in cells with normal histologic architecture (true hyperplasia) or of the lymphocyte component only (lymphoid hyperplasia) [22, 23].

True hyperplasia and lymphoid hyperplasia can be accompanied by a number of pathological conditions and imaging is not enough to tell one form from the other in that both show a symmetric and diffuse enlargement of the thymus (Table 9.1).

It would appear that true thymic hyperplasia results from a rebound with the volume of the thymus being restored to normal in response to the end of stressful factors such as chemotherapy, radiotherapy, steroid therapy, and burns that can induce glandular atrophy [24].

Thymic atrophy occurs in up to 90% of patients who have received chemotherapy for malignant extra-thoracic neoplasms [25].

Normally, at the end of therapy the gland resumes a morphology similar to that it had before treatment; however, in some cases there may be, in particular in young patients and most especially in children, a rebound hyperplasia (i.e., an increase by over 50% of the baseline volume) [26].

Rebound hyperplasia occurs more frequently 3 to 8 months (average 4.2 months) after the end of chemotherapy and the onset is quicker in young patients [27].

Lymphoid hyperplasia is not a rare occurrence in a normally-sized thymus and is accompanied by a number of immunopathic diseases like myasthenia gravis (MG), systemic lupus erythematosus (SLE), sclerodermia, rheumatoid arthritis, polyarteritis nodosa, Behçet's Disease, Hashimoto thyroiditis, Addison's Disease, autoimmune hemolytic anemia, thyreotoxicosis, and Graves' Disease [28-34].

Thymic hyperplasia can only rarely be appreciated and evaluated at plain chest X-ray, most especially in adults; instead, CT scan allows for a good evaluation of the transverse diameter of the thymus, which must be lower than 1.8 cm in normal subjects up to 20 years of age and lower than 1.3 cm in adults over 20 years of age (Fig. 9.1).

Usually, at CT, the hyperplastic gland retains a symmetric and regular shape, with smooth contours, has a homogeneous density, and models itself on the adjacent mediastinal structures without having a mass effect [35].

In patients receiving chemotherapy for malignant neoplasms that can metastasize to the thymus, differential diagnosis should consider an increase in the size of the thymus as a result of secondarisms. Diagnostic elements are symptoms related to a neoplastic relapse or the presence of a mediastinal mass which, in light of its symmetry, morphology, and density, does not show the characteristics of a normal hyperplasia and which compresses surrounding structures [36].

Equally challenging can be the differential diagnosis between thymic hyperplasia and thymoma, which has major therapeutical consequences, and relies upon clinical symptoms and the identification of a well-defined thymic mass.

In difficult cases, Chemical-Shift MRI (Fig. 9.2) can be helpful in suggesting a possible hyperplasia in the presence of adipose tissue with an abatement of the signal in images in phase opposition; this technique can also be used for the differential diagnosis between thymic hyperplasia and neoplastic involvement of the thymus [37].

Thymic Cysts

Thymic cysts are rare mediastinal lesions, accounting for as little as 1-2% of all anterior mediastinal masses, and can be congenital or acquired.

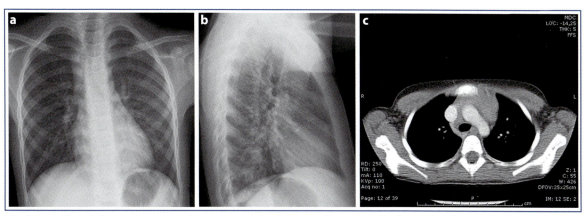

Fig. 9.1a-c Thymic hyperplasia. An enlargement of the right superior mediastinal marginal line can be detected in a PA (**a**) projection of chest X-ray and not in the LL projection (**b**). **c** Hypodense, homogeneous formation with smooth contours in the antero-superior mediastinum found at CT

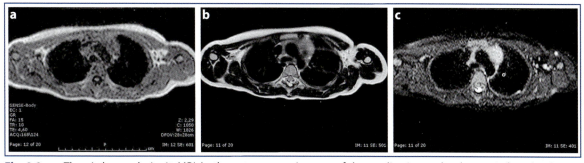

Fig. 9.2a-c Thymic hyperplasia. At MRI, in the antero-superior part of the mediastinum, the thymus is found to be enlarged, homogeneously isointense in the weighted T1 sequence (**a**) and hyperintense in the weighted T2 sequence (**b**) and STIR (**c**)

Congenital Thymic Cysts

These occur most frequently in pediatric patients and most likely result from remnants of the thymus-pharyngeal duct [38-42].

As a rule, they are asymptomatic and are an incidental finding. Sometimes they cause dyspnea and only rarely thoracic pain following bleeding or infection [43].

Usually they are uniloculated, with small and thin walls, even though large cysts have been reported.

At plain X-ray, congenital thymic cysts cannot be distinguished from other nonlobulated thymic masses, including thymoma; thin wall calcifications are a rare occurrence [44-46].

At CT (Fig. 9.3), congenital thymic cysts are masses with homogeneous hydric density, very thin walls, occasionally with thin, soft-tissue septa inside; rarely they can be denser due to their being filled with proteinaceous material, in which case they mimic a solid lesion though without contrast-enhancement [47].

In some cases the diagnostic process can usefully be completed with MRI (Fig. 9.4): indeed, cysts usually have a low signal in T1 and a high signal in T2; however, where there is a bleeding inside, the MRI detects an increase in the signal, including in T1-weighted sequences [48, 49].

Acquired Thymic Cysts

Usually, these occur inside infective (HIV), inflammatory or neoplastic foci or are related to prior thoracotomic surgery [50-53].

Amongst malignant neoplasms that can be associated to acquired thymic cysts, mention should be made of Hodgkin lymphoma, seminoma, thymoma, and thymic carcinoma [54, 55].

Acquired cysts located in an area where a Hodgkin lymphoma develops can be connected to a cystic degeneration unrelated to therapy or secondary to radio- or chemotherapy (in which case, most of them are benign cystic formations).

At CT, acquired thymic cysts are usually multilocular, with variable size and wall thickness and can contain hemorrhage or calcifications which result in a nonhomogeneous density of the cyst.

Thymic Neoplasms

Primary thymic tumors originate from the different tissues that compose the thymus: thymomas and thymic carcinomas are thymic tumors of epithelial origin with different histologic aspects and different biological behavior; other thymic neoplasms include thymolipomas, neuroendocrine tumors, lymphomas (most especially Hodgkin lymphoma), and tumors of the germ line.

Thymomas

Thymomas are the most common primary neoplasm of the anterior mediastinum in adults, though in 10% of cases they can result from ectopic foci.

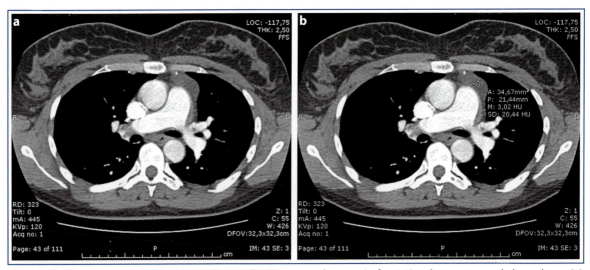

Fig. 9.3a,b Thymic cyst. At CT, in the anterior mediastinum, regular-margin formation, homogeneously hypodense (**a**), with hydric density (**b**) and without contrast enhancement

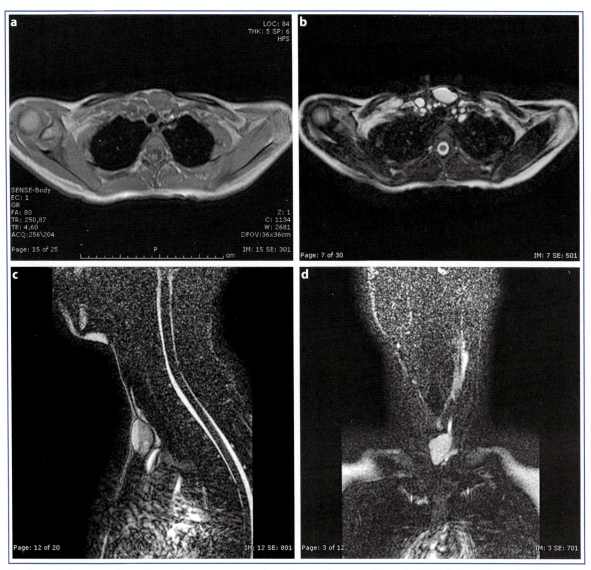

Fig. 9.4a-d Congenital thymic cyst from a remnant of the thymo-pharyngeal duct. At MRI, lobulated formation, isointense in the weighted T1 sequence (**a**) and hyperintense in the weighted T2 sequence in the various spatial planes (**b-d**)

The highest incidence is in patients over 40, with no gender differences, while they are a rare occurrence in pediatric patients.

Most thymomas are found at routine X-rays in asymptomatic patients, while only a smaller proportion of patients have thoracic pain or cough due to compression of the airways.

Thymomas can also accompany a paraneoplastic syndrome with MG [56-58], hypogammaglobulinemia, and aplasia of the red-cell line [59, 60]; in this regard, in case of MG, a CT can usefully be performed to exclude a thymoma, including in patients with negative X-rays.

At chest X-ray (Fig. 9.5), thymoma is a capsulated mass, well marked off from surrounding tissues, roughly spherical and more or less lobulated; typically, it develops anteriorly relative to the aortic arch and is unilateral [61].

At CT, it often appears in the form of multilobulated masses originating from one or both lobes of the thymus and distorting the normal contour of the thymus; they can be homogeneous or heterogeneous due to the presence of cystic areas of necrosis and thin, linear calcifications in the periphery of the thymoma or inside it [62].

At MRI (Fig. 9.6), thymomas are hypo-isointense

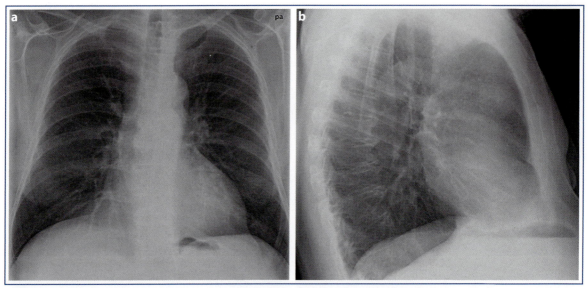

Fig. 9.5a,b PA and LL in patient with thymoma. The mass in the anterior mediastinum is shown in the LL radiogram (**b**) as a slightly opaque formation with a thin and discontinuous radioopaque calcific rim

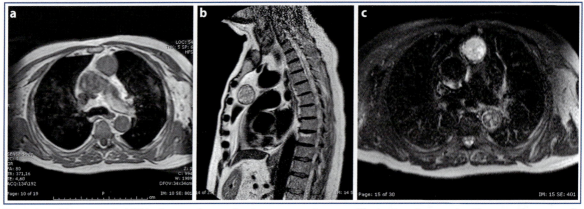

Fig. 9.6a-c Thymoma. At MRI, in the anterior mediastinum, expansive round formation characterized by smooth, even walls and hypointense content in the weighted T1 sequence (**a**) and nonhomogeneous in the weighted T2 sequence (**b**) and STIR (**c**) with small, intralesional liquid areolas

in T1 and hyper-intense in T2 with an often nonhomogeneous aspect due to the presence of cystic, necrotic, and hemorrhagic areas and, frequently, with fibrous septa inside [63] (Table 9.2).

The prognosis of thymomas depends on whether they are invasive or noninvasive [64].

From a histological point of view, no characteristics of malignancy have been observed that correlate to a precise biological behavior of this tumor; likewise, its size does not correlate to the degree of invasiveness [65].

In "noninvasive" thymomas, the entire neoplasm is inside the capsule, with no extracapsular spreading.

Even though CT and MR are capable of highlighting invasive aspects, under- or overestimation can occur and final staging can only be established through surgery and anatomopathology [66].

An "invasive" behavior can be diagnosed via imaging in the presence of: infiltrating, poorly defined margins; well-defined invasion of the vessels and of the vascular wall; irregular interface with the adjacent pulmonary parenchyma and diffusion to the homolateral pleura.

Pleural diffusion appears in the form of isolated pleural nodulations rather than a diffuse thickening

Table 9.2 Imaging of thymoma

Location (in order of frequency of occurrence) 　(Prevascular) antero-superior mediastinum 　Cardio-phrenic angle 　Neck Chest X-ray 　Mediastinal mass 　Smooth or lobulated margins 　Often unilateral 　Calcifications CT and MRI 　Variable-density soft tissue mass 　Cystic spaces 　Calcifications 　Invasive (aspect similar to that of thymic carcinoma) 　　Poorly defined, with lobulated or infiltrating margins 　　Oval shape 　　Invasion of the mediastinal fat, of the large vessels and of the thoracic wall 　　Adjacent lung parenchyma 　　Focal or diffuse pleural masses 　　Expansion to the abdomen through the diaphragmatic hiatus

of the pleura (differential diagnosis with mesothelioma) [67].

Since large thymomas can also expand to the abdomen (Fig. 9.7) through the diaphragmatic hiatus, the upper abdomen should be included in CT staging [68-70].

Ectopic Thymomas

Cervical ectopic thymomas are a rare occurrence, which appear as a mass in the thoracic inlet dislocating the trachea and which can be mistaken for a mass originating from the thyroid; they occur more frequently in females than in males and usually do not cause myasthenic symptoms [71, 72].

Thymic Carcinomas

Thymic carcinomas account for approximately 20% of malignant tumors of the thymus in adults [73].

They are highly malignant [74, 75] with signs of local invasion and seeding to loco-regional lymph nodes and metastases to the lungs, the liver, the encephalus, and the bones.

Usually, these tumors are not accompanied by paraneoplastic syndromes and the prognosis is adverse, despite therapy, in most cases [76, 77].

Usually, these are large masses, associated, often also at onset, to intrathoracic lymphadenomegaly and pleural and pericardial involvement.

At CT, these neoplasms are heterogeneous, with necrosis and calcifications, poorly defined margins showing a diffuse involvement of the pleura, the pericardium, and the mediastinum rather than isolated foci like in isolated thymoma [78].

At MRI (Fig. 9.8), they show an intermediate signal intensity in T1 and a high intensity in T2 with areas where the signal can be very heterogeneous due to necrosis and hemorrhage [79].

Thymolipomas

These are rare and benign thymic neoplasms accounting for 3-9% of all thymic tumors.

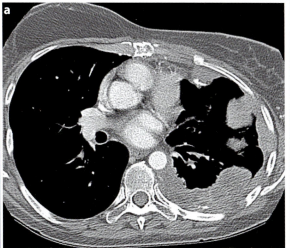 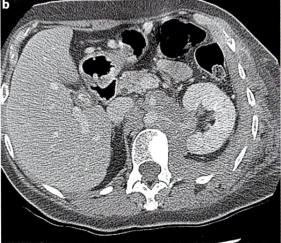

Fig. 9.7a,b Thymoma with pleuric (**a**) and retro-peritoneal (**b**) diffusion. Nodular thickening of the pleura similar to a mesothelioma with retrocrural extraperitoneal extension and extension along the left postero-lateral abdominal wall

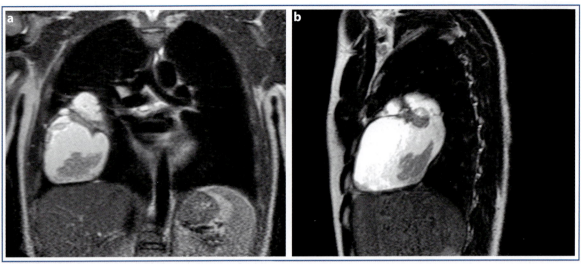

Fig. 9.8a,b Thymoma with a mainly cystic aspect, incidentally found after a trauma. The weighted T2 coronal (a) and sagittal (b) MR scans show a small solid component as part of a mainly cystic mediastinal mass

They occur in a broad age range and in both genders, though most frequently in young adults.

As a rule they are asymptomatic, grow slowly, and are an occasional finding.

There have been cases of thymolipomas accompanied by MG, Graves' Disease, aplastic anemia, and hypogammaglobulinemia like in the case of thymomas [80].

Histologically, they are composed of mature adipose tissue and areas of normal or involuted thymic tissue; transformation into a thymosarcoma is an exceptionally rare occurrence. They are predominantly located in the anterior, superior, or inferior mediastinum, can become significantly large and, being soft, adapt to the surrounding tissues, thus mimicking cardiomegalia, atelectasia, or inferior or superior lobar consolidation or diaphragmatic supraelevation in the presence of an infrapulmonary component [81].

CT scan shows a mediastinal mass, starting from the thymus, which surrounds adjacent structures and adapts to them; density is the same as adipose tissue though with speckling due to the presence of denser areas, often elongated or frankly linear resulting from remnants of thymic tissue or septa.

MRI documents a mediastinal mass with a high signal in T1-dependent images with hypo-intense areas the meaning of which is similar to the hyperdense structures at CT [82].

Thymic Lymphomas

Lymphomatous involvement of the thymus is often found as part of a more generalized disease, most frequently Hodgkin lymphoma [83].

Thymic involvement is often associated to an involvement of the lymph nodes of the mediastinum, while the isolated form is surely more rare an occurrence.

At plain X-ray, thymic lymphoma appears as a unilateral or bilateral mass of the anterior mediastinum, often well marked off.

At CT, it is possible to appreciate a diffuse enlargement of the thymus or the presence of one or multiple nonhomogeneous thymic masse(s) with cystic areas of focal necrosis [84].

Differential diagnosis between a thymic lymphoma and a normal thymus in young patients or rebound thymic hyperplasia in pediatric patients and young adults is not easy in that neither CT nor MR provide univocal answers, though a certain heterogeneity of the signal at MR appears to be suggestive of a neoplasm.

Neuroendocrine Tumors of the Thymus

These are rare tumors, the potential malignancy of which is largely variable; histologically they range from benign forms (thymic carcinoids) to highly malignant forms (small-cell tumor of the thymus) [85-87].

Amongst these, thymic carcinomas occur predominantly in males in their 40s-50s and are accompanied in roughly half of the cases by hormonal disorders, including the Cushing Syndrome which results from the production of adrenocorticotropic hormones.

At plain X-ray, neuroendocrine tumors appear as masses of the anterior mediastinum with well-defined contours and internal calcifications.

At CT and MRI, these masses are typically large, nonhomogeneous, with signs of local infiltration [88].

References

1. Jacobs MT, Frush DP, Donnelly LF (1999) The right place at the wrong time: Historical perspective of the relation of the thymus gland and pediatric radiology. Radiology 210:11-16
2. Haubrich WS (1997) Medical meanings. American College of Physicians, Philadelphia, p 225
3. Skinner HA (1961) Origin of medical terms, 2nd edn. Williams & Wilkins, Baltimore, p 404
4. May MT (1968) Galen on the usefulness of the parts of the body. Cornell University Press, Ithaca, NY, p 30
5. Shimosato Y, Mukai K (1997) Tumors of the thymus and related lesions. In: Shimosato Y, Mukai K (eds) Atlas of tumor pathology: Tumors of the mediastinum, fasc 21, ser 3. Armed Forces Institute of Pathology, Washington, DC, pp 158-168
6. Lele SM, Lele MS, Anderson VM (2001) The thymus in infancy and childhood: Embryologic, anatomic, and pathologic considerations. Chest Surg Clin N Am 11:233-253
7. Suster S, Rosai J (1990) Histology of the normal thymus. Am J Surg Pathol 14:284-303
8. Baron RL, Lee JK, Sagel SS, Peterson RR (1982) Computed tomography of the normal thymus. Radiology 142:121-125
9. Moore AV, Korobkin M, Olanow W et al (1983) Age-related changes in the thymus gland: CT-pathologic correlation. AJR Am J Roentgenol 141:241-246
10. Francis IR, Glazer GM, Bookstein FL, Gross BH (1985) The thymus: Reexamination of age-related changes in size and shape. AJR Am J Roentgenol 145:249-254
11. De Geer G, Webb WR, Gamsu G (1986) Normal thymus: Assessment with MR and CT. Radiology 158:313-317
12. Siegel MJ, Glazer HS, Wiener JI, Molina PL (1989) Normal and abnormal thymus in childhood: MR imaging. Radiology 367-371
13. Erasmus JJ, McAdams HP, Donnelly LF (2000) MR imaging of mediastinal masses. Magn Reson Imaging Clin N Am 8:59-89
14. Boothroyd AE, Hall-Craggs MA, Dicks-Mireaux C (1992) The magnetic resonance appearances of the normal thymus in children. Clin Radiol 42:378-381
15. Molina PL, Siegel MJ, Glazer HS (1990) Thymic masses on MR imaging. AJR Am J Roentgenol 155:495-500
16. Harris VJ, Ramilic J, White H (1980) The thymic mass as a mediastinal dilemma. Clin Radiol 31:263-269
17. Oh KS, Weber AL, Borden S (1971) Normal mediastinal mass in late childhood. Radiology 101:625-628
18. Lemaitre L, Marconi V, Avni F, Remy J (1987) The sonographic evaluation of normal thymus in infants and young children. Eur J Radiol 7:130-136
19. Han BK, Babcock DS, Oestneich AE (1989) Normal thymus in infancy: Sonographic characteristics. Radiology 170:471-474
20. Adam EJ, Ignotus PI (1993) Sonography of the thymus in healthy children: Frequency of visualization, size, and appearance. AJR Am J Roentgenol 161:153-155
21. Carty H (1990) Ultrasound of the normal thymus in infants: A simple method of resolving a clinical dilemma. Br J Radiol 63:737-738
22. Mendelson DS (2001) Imaging of the thymus. Chest Surg Clin N Am 11:269-293
23. Armstrong P (2000) Mediastinal and hilar disorders. In: Armstrong P, Wilson AG, Dee P, Hansell DM (eds) Imaging of the diseases of the chest, 3rd edn. Mosby, London, pp 789-892
24. Choyke PL, Zeman RK, Gootenberg JE et al (1987) Thymic atrophy and regrowth in response to chemotherapy: CT evaluation. AJR Am J Roentgenol 149:269-272
25. Hendrickx P, Dohring W (1987) Thymic atrophy and regrowth in response to chemotherapy: CT evaluation. AJR Am J Roentgenol 149:269-272
26. Abildgaard A, Lien HH, Fossa SD (1989) Enlargement of the thymus following chemotherapy for non-seminomatous testicular cancer. Acta Radiol 30:259-262
27. Levine GD, Rosai J (1978) Thymic hyperplasia and neoplasia: A review of current concepts. Hum Pathol 9:495-515
28. Franken EA (1969) Radiologic evidence of thymic enlargement in Graves' disease. Radiology 91:20-22
29. Wortsman J, McConnachie P, Baker JR Jr (1988) Immunoglobulins that cause thymocyte proliferation from a patient with Graves' disease and an enlarged thymus. Am J Med 85:117-121
30. Rosenow EC 3rd, Hurley BT (1984) Disorders of the thymus. A review. Arch Intern Med 144:763-770
31. Nicolaus S, Muller NL, Li DK (1996) Thymus in myasthenia gravis: Comparison of CT and pathologic findings and clinical outcome after thymectomy. Radiology 201:471-474
32. Brown LR, Muhm JR, Sheedy PF 2nd (1983) The value of computed tomography in myasthenia gravis. AJR Am J Roentgenol 140:31-35
33. Batra P, Herrman C Jr, Mulder D (1987) Mediastinal imaging in myasthenia gravis: Correlation of chest radiography, CT, MR and surgical findings. AJR Am J Roentgenol 148:515-519
34. Fon GT, Bein ME, Mancuso AA (1982) Computed tomography of the anterior mediastinum in myasthenia gravis. A radiologic-pathologic correlative study. Radiology 142:135-141
35. Baron RL, Lee JK, Sagel SS (1982) Computed tomography of the abnormal thymus. Radiology 142:127-134
36. Cohen M, Hill CA, Cangir A (1980) Thymic rebound after treatment of childhood tumors. AJR Am J Roentgenol 135:151-156
37. Takahashi K, Inaoka T, Murakami N et al (2003) Characterization of the normal and hyperplastic thymus on chemical-shift MR imaging. AJR Am J Roentgenol 180:1265-1269
38. Mikal S (1974) Cervical thymic cyst. Arch Surg 109:558-562
39. Fielding JF, Farmer AW, Lindsay WK, Conen PE (1963) Cystic degeneration in persistent cervical thymus: A report of four cases in children. Can J Surg 6:178-185

40. Simons JN, Robinson DW, Masters FW (1964) Cervical thymic cyst. Am J Surg 108:578-582
41. Lewis MR (1962) Persistence of the thymus in the cervical area. J Pediatr 61:887-893
42. Barrick B, O'Kell RT (1969) Thymic cysts and remnant cervical thymus. J Pediatr Surg 4:355-358
43. Chalaoui J, Samson L, Robillard P (1990) Cases of the day. General. Benign thymic cyst complicated by hemorrhage. RadioGraphics 10:957-958
44. Sltzer RA, Mills DS, Baddock SS (1968) Mediastinal thymic cyst. Dis Chest 53:186-196
45. Graeber GM, Thompson LD, Cohen DJ (1984) Cystic lesion of the thymus. An occasionally malignant cervical and/or anterior mediastinal mass. J Thorac Cardiovasc Surg 87:295-300
46. Sirivella S, Gielchinsky I, Parsonet V (1995) Mediastinal thymic cyst: A report of three cases. J Thorac Cardiovasc Surg 110:1771-1772
47. Gouliamos A, Striggaris K, Lolas C (1982) Thymic cyst. J Computed Assist Tomograf 6:172-174
48. Merine DS, Fishman EK, Zerhouni EA (1988) Computed tomography and magnetic resonance imaging diagnosis of thymic cyst. J Computed Tomogr 12:220-222
49. Murayama S, Murakami J, Watanabe H (1995) Signal intensity characteristics of mediastinal cysts masses on T1-weighted MRI. J Computed Tomogr 19:188-191
50. Leonidas JC, Berdon WE, Godine L (1996) Human immunodeficiency virus infection and multilocular thymic cysts. Radiology 198:377-379
51. Mishalani SH, Lones MA, Said JW (1995) Multilocular thymic cyst: A novel thymic lesion associated with human immunodeficiency virus infection. Arch Pathol Lab Med 119:467-470
52. Jaramillo D, Perez-Atayde A, Griscom T (1989) Apparent association between thymic cysts and prior thoracotomy. Radiology 172:207-209
53. Cuasay RS, Fernandez J, Spagna P, Lemole GM (1976) Mediastinal thymic cyst after open heart surgery. Chest 70:296-298
54. Baron RL, Sagel SS, Baglan RJ (1981) Thymic cysts following radiation therapy for Hodgkin's disease. Radiology 141:593-597
55. Lindfors KL, Meyer JE, Dedrick CG et al (1985) Thymic cysts in mediastinal Hodgkin's disease. Radiology 156:37-34
56. Port JL, Ginsberg RJ (2001) Surgery for thymoma. Chest Surg Clin N Am 11:421-437
57. Lewis JE, Wick MR, Scheithauer BW et al (1987) Thymoma: A clinicopathologic review. Cancer 60:2727-2743
58. Lennon VA, Lambert EH, Leiby KR et al (1991) Recombinant human acetylcholine receptor alpha-subunit induces chronic experimental autoimmune myasthenia gravis. J Immunol 146:2245-2248
59. Rosenow EC 3rd, Hurley T (1984) Disorders of the thymus: A review. Arch Intern Med 144:763-770
60. Masaoka A, Hashimoto T, Shibata K et al (1989) Thymomas associated with pure red cell aplasia: Histologic and follow-up studies. Cancer 64:1872-1878
61. Rosado-de-Christenson ML, Galobardes J, Moran CA (1992) Thymoma: Radiologic-pathologic correlation. Radio Graphics 12:151-168
62. Jeong YJ, Lee KS, Kim J et al (2004) Does CT of thymic epithelial tumors enable us to differentiate histologic subtypes and predict prognosis? AJR Am J Roentgenol 183:283-289
63. Sakai F, Sone S, Kiyono K et al (1992) MR imaging of thymoma: Radiologic-pathologic correlation. AJR Am J Roentgenol 158:751-756
64. Tomiyama N, Johkoh T, Mihara N et al (2002) Using the World Health Organization classification of thymic epithelial neoplasms to describe CT findings. AJR Am J Roentgenol 179:881-886
65. Han J, Lee KS, Yi CA et al (2003) Thymic epithelial tumors classified according to a newly established WHO scheme: CT and MR findings. Korean J Radiol 4:46-53
66. Quintanilla-Martinez L, Wilkins EW Jr, Ferry JA, Harris NL (1993) Thymoma: Morphologic subclassification correlates with invasiveness and immunohistologic features – A study of 122 cases. Hum Pathol 24:958-969
67. Zerhouni EA, Scott WW Jr, Baker RR et al (1982) Invasive thymomas: Diagnosis and evaluation by computed tomography. J Comput Assist Tomogr 6:92-100
68. Scatarige JC, Fishman EK, Zerhouni EA, Siegelman SS (1985) Transdiaphragmatic extension of invasive thymoma. AJR Am J Roentgenol 144:31-35
69. Jose B, Yu AT, Morgan TF, Glicksman AS (1980) Malignant thymoma with extrathoracic metastasis: A case report and review of the literature. J Surg Oncol 15:259
70. Airan B, Sharma R, Iyer KS et al (1990) Malignant thymoma presenting as intracardiac tumor and superior vena caval obstruction. Ann Thorac Surg 50:989-999
71. Lewis MR (1962) Persistence of the thymus in the cervical area. J Pediatr 61:887-893
72. Batsakis JG (1979) Tumors of the head and neck: Clinical and pathological considerations, 2nd ed. Williams & Wilkins, Baltimore, pp 233-239
73. Strollo DC, Rosado de Christenson ML, Jett JR (2002) Primary mediastinal malignant germ cell neoplasms: Imaging features. Chest Surg Clin N Am 12:645-658
74. Kirchner T, Schalke B, Buchwald J et al (1992) Well-differentiated thymic carcinoma: An organo-typical low-grade carcinoma with relationship to cortical thymoma. Am J Surg Pathol 16:1153-1169
75. Suster S, Moran CA (1999) Thymoma, atypical thymoma, and thymic carcinoma: A novel conceptual approach to the classification of thymic epithelial neoplasms. Am J Clin Pathol 111:826-833
76. Blumberg D, Burt ME, Bains MS et al (1998) Thymic carcinoma: Current staging does not predict prognosis. J Thorac Cardiovasc Surg 115:303-309
77. Rios A, Torres J, Galindo PJ et al (2002) Prognostic factors in thymic epithelial neoplasms. Eur J Cardiothorac Surg 21:307-313
78. Lee JD, Choe KO, Kim SJ (1991) CT findings in primary thymic carcinoma. J Computed Assisted Tomogr 15:429-433

79. Kushihashi T, Fujisawa H, Munechika H (1996) Magnetic resonance imaging of thymic epithelial tumors. Crit Rev Diagn Imaging 37:191-259
80. Benton C, Gerard P (1966) Thymolipoma in a patient with Graves' disease: Case report and review of the literature. J Thorac Cardiovasc Surg 51:428-433
81. Rosado-de-Christenson ML, Pugatch RD, Moran CA, Galobardes J (1994) Thymolipoma: Analysis of 27 cases. Radiology 193:121-126
82. Matsudaira N, Hirano H, Itou S et al (1994) MR imaging of thymolipoma. Magn Reson Imaging 12:959-961
83. Isaacson PG, Chan JKC, Tang C, Addis BJ (1990) Low-grade B-cell lymphoma of mucosa-associated lymphoid tissue arising in the thymus: A thymic lymphoma mimicking myoepithelial sialadenitis. Am J Surg Pathol 14:342-335
84. Werneck KE, Vassallo P, Rutsch F et al (1991) Thymic involvement in Hodgkin disease: CT and sonographic findings. Radiology 181:375-383
85. Wick MR, Scott RE, Li CY, Carney JA (1980) Carcinoid tumor of the thymus: A clinicopathologic report of seven cases with a review of the literature. Mayo Clin Proc 55:246-254
86. Economopoulos GC, Lewis JW Jr, Lee MW, Silverman NA (1990) Carcinoid tumors of the thymus. Ann Thorac Surg 50:58-61
87. Rosai J, Higa E (1972) Mediastinal endocrine neoplasm of probable thymic origin related to carcinoid tumor: Clinicopathologic study of 8 cases. Cancer 29:1061-1074
88. Lowenthal RM, Gumpel JM, Kreel L et al (1974) Carcinoid tumour of the thymus with systemic manifestations: A radiological and pathological study. Thorax 29:553-558

CHAPTER 10
PET Features

Bruno Bagni, Antonella Franceschetto, Alessandra Casolo, Marina Cucca

Background Information and Definitions

Positron emission tomography (PET) [1] is a tomographic technique of nuclear medicine in which a computer-generated image of local radioactive tracer distribution in tissues is produced through the detection of annihilation photons emitted when radionuclides introduced into the body decay and release positrons. PET with 18F-fluorodeoxyglucose (18F-FDG) uses a radio-labeled analog of glucose to image relative glucose metabolic rates in various tissues. Because glucose metabolism is increased in many malignancies, 18F-FDG PET is a sensitive method for detecting, staging, and monitoring the effects of therapy of many tumors. Computed tomography (CT) is a tomographic imaging technique that uses an X-ray beam to produce anatomic images. This anatomic information is used to detect and help to determine the location and extent of malignancies. Combined PET/CT devices provide both the metabolic information from PET and the anatomic information from CT in a single examination. As shown in some clinical experiences, the information obtained by PET-CT appears to be more accurate in evaluating patients with known or suspected malignancies than does the information obtained from either PET or CT separately and interpreted side by side.

A PET/CT scanner is an integrated device containing both a CT scanner and a PET scanner with a patient table, and is capable of obtaining a CT scan and a PET scan. If a patient does not move between the scans, the reconstructed PET and CT images will be spatially registered.

PET/CT coregistration is the process of aligning PET and CT images for the purposes of combined image display (fusion) and image analysis.

PET/CT fusion is the combined display of registered PET and CT image sets. Superimposed data typically are displayed with the PET data color coded to the CT data in gray scale.

PET/CT acquisitions can include the whole body, an extended portion of the body, or a limited portion of the body.

18F-FDG PET and CT are proven diagnostic procedures. Although techniques for registration and fusion of images obtained from separate PET and CT scanners have been available for several years, the readily apparent and documental advantages of having PET and CT in a single device have resulted in the rapid dissemination of this technology in the medical community. PET using 18F-FDG plays an important role in the evaluation of cancer. Although highly sensitive for the detection of malignancy, 18F-FDG uptake in physiological and benign processes is well documented. Recognition of unusual patterns of 18F-FDG biodistribution is important in order to avoid misinterpretation of PET images. For instance, areas of increased symmetrical 18F-FDG uptake in the cervical region and the shoulder girdle have been suggested to represent activated brown adipose tissue, rather than physiological activity in tense muscles.

201Thallium-chloride (201Tl) was the first radiopharmaceutical used for the detection of tumors, especially tumors of the thyroid and the lung. 201Tl was also a thymoma seeking-reagent, referring to cases of mediastinal thymoma. 201Tl also showed high accumulation in an unusual thymoma which had developed from the undescended thymus [2].

Differentiation of Normal and Hyperplastic Thymus from Malignant Involvement

In the evaluation of malignancy with 18F-FDG, a potential pitfall in the assessment of the anterior mediastinum is mistaking normal uptake within the thymus from disease such as adenopathy or local invasion by tumor. The thymus can be infiltrated to a number of mediastinal neoplasms, involved by metastatic disease, and most commonly by lymphoma (Figs. 10.1, 10.2) [3-7].

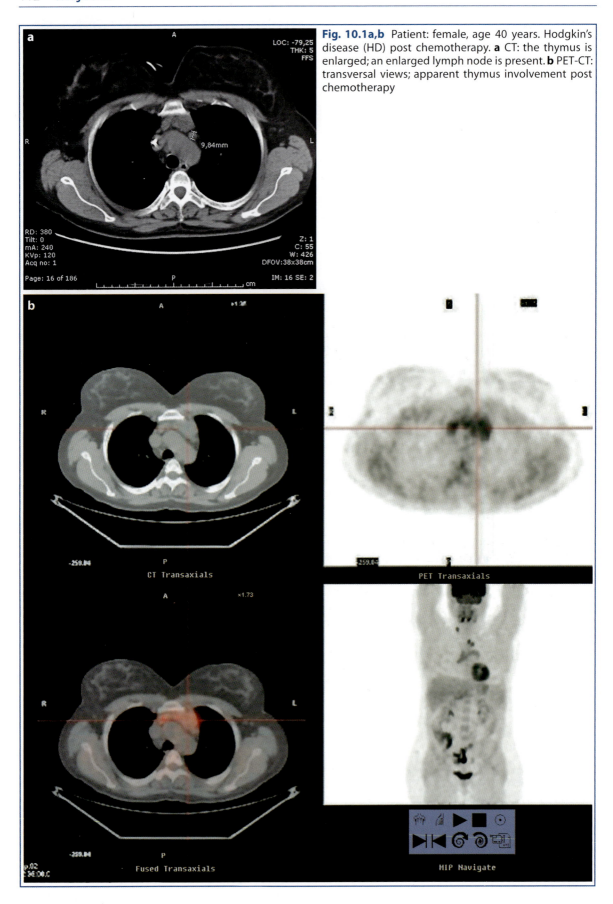

Fig. 10.1a,b Patient: female, age 40 years. Hodgkin's disease (HD) post chemotherapy. **a** CT: the thymus is enlarged; an enlarged lymph node is present. **b** PET-CT: transversal views; apparent thymus involvement post chemotherapy

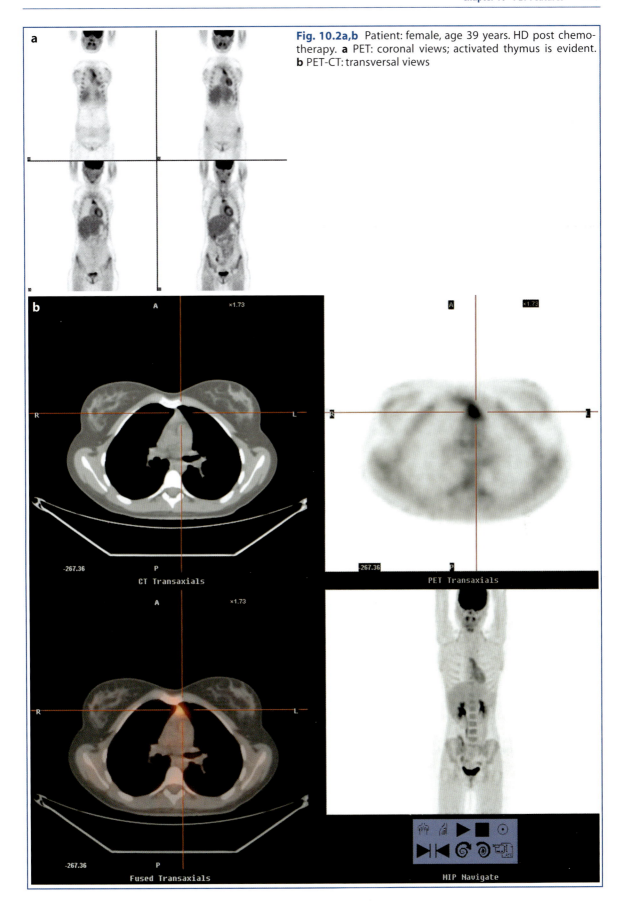

Fig. 10.2a,b Patient: female, age 39 years. HD post chemotherapy. **a** PET: coronal views; activated thymus is evident. **b** PET-CT: transversal views

The rate of thymic involvement by mediastinal Hodgkin's disease has been reported to be 70%. Even in the absence of lymphomatous infiltration, thymic enlargement may coexist with lymphoma and may be present in patients with intrathoracic Hodgkin's disease. Increased uptake within the thymus may also be due to a primary thymic malignancy such as a thymoma or thymic carcinoma. Therefore, understanding the PET appearance of physiologic thymic uptake, the appearance of thymic malignancy, and the potential distinctions between the two is essential. Normal thymic appearance is one of the key elements of assessing the thymus with 18F-FDG PET realizing which subsets of patients typically exhibit thymic 18F-FDG uptake. In general, it is accepted that the thymus can be seen at CT in every pediatric patient (Fig. 10.3). In early reports on the physiologic thymic uptake of 18F-FDG, some authors extrapolated from their experience with CT and hypothesized that thymic uptake could be a normal finding in patients under the age of 20 years [7-10]. Thymic uptake was classified as "normal" on the basis of morphologic features, size, and contour at 18F-FDG PET. Same authors suggest that metabolic activity in the thymus ceases at puberty, which is the point at which the thymus undergoes fatty infiltration and involution [11]. Subsequent studies, however, have shown that physiologic thymic uptake can be seen in patients well beyond puberty. One study examined thymic uptake at 18F-FDG PET in 94 patients ranging from 18 to 29 years of age and found that 32 of these patients exhibited normal physiologic thymic uptake. The criteria for "normal" in these patients included a normal thymus identified at CT, absence of clinical symptoms of thymus-related disease, and absence of mediastinal tumor at follow-up ranging from 6 to 69 months [12, 13]. It also found a correlation between the degree of thymic uptake and the attenuation of the thymus at CT, supporting the idea that the disappearance of thymic uptake is related to the degree of fatty infiltration of the thymus. A recent study confirmed physiologic thymic 18F-FDG uptake in adult patients with histologically normal thymic tissue and thymic enlargement at CT [14].

Although it is evident that both pediatric patients and, more rarely, adult patients can exhibit normal physiologic thymic uptake of 18F-FDG, the subset of patients who undergo chemotherapy deserves particular attention (Figs. 10.4, 10.5); thus thymic hyperplasia follows chemotherapy, especially in young patients treated for testicular malignancy or malignant lymphoma.

The phenomenon of thymic hyperplasia following chemotherapy is particularly important to recognize in young adults, in whom the thymus may not be visualized. In a study, Brink et al. [15] found an increased 18F-FDG uptake in 73% of the children with malignancy prior to chemotherapy and in 75% of the children with malignancy following chemotherapy (Fig. 10.6). However, they also found an increased uptake in 5% of the adults with lymphoma following chemotherapy. None of the adults with lymphoma prior to chemotherapy exhibited increased thymic uptake. These findings support the idea that, although thymic uptake may be a normal finding in children, it may also be expected in young adults after therapy.

A case of increased thymic uptake in a 54-year-old woman following radioiodine ablation of a follicular thyroid carcinoma was also reported.

Differentiation of thymic uptake from malignancy may be made in part on the basis of morphologic features. Characteristics of the thymus derive from experience with CT imaging [16]. In patients under the age of 5 years, the thymus is generally quadrilateral. As the patient ages, the thymus becomes more triangular with concave or straight margins and should be triangular in configuration by the age of 15 years in most patients [17].

Although PET does not offer the same resolution as CT or magnetic resonance (MR) imaging, the appearance of physiologic thymic uptake at PET is characteristic. The thymus appears as a triangular retrosternal region of increased uptake, a finding that corresponds to the bilobed configuration of the thymus [18]. In questionable cases, correlation with findings at cross-sectional imaging modalities such as CT or MR imaging may better delineate the contour of the pertinent region; this is easily reached with PET-CT.

18F-FDG PET provides information regarding the metabolic rate of thymic tissue. Several investigators have examined the relationship between the rate of glucose metabolism and the presence of thymic neoplasia or mediastinal malignancy using standardized uptake value (SUV) to measure 18F-FDG uptake. SUVs have gained wide acceptance as a method of assessing 18F-FDG uptake by tissue, despite the fact that they may be affected by various factors, including time elapsed between 18F-FDG injection and imaging, the patient's body fat content, body weight, and serum glucose level, and use of a maximum pixel value versus an average pixel value for the region of interest. The available data indicate that SUVs may have a limited role in the differentiation of a normal thymus from thymic neoplasia or adenopathy, indicating that SUVs may not reliably help differentiate between physiologic thymic uptake and thymic neoplasia.

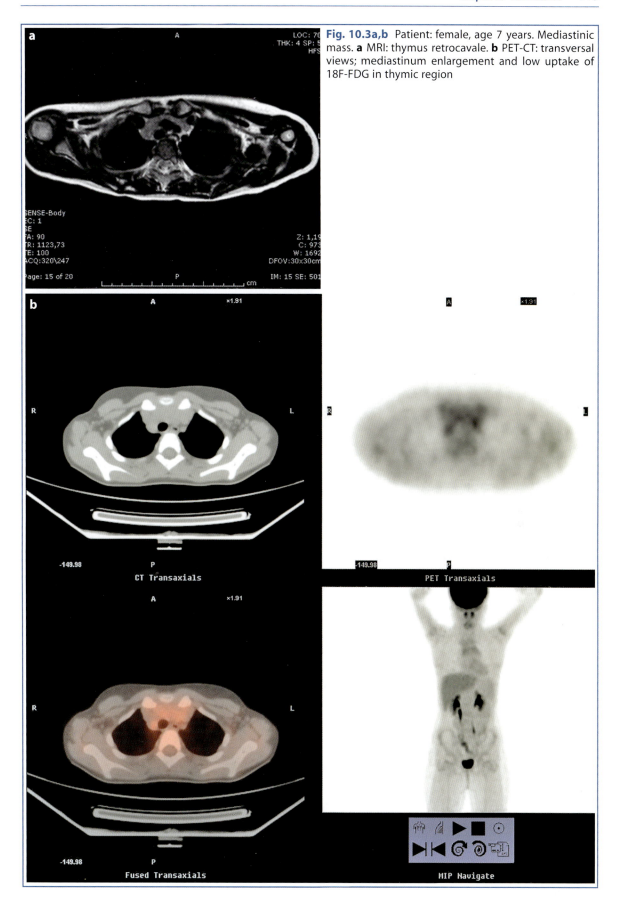

Fig. 10.3a,b Patient: female, age 7 years. Mediastinic mass. **a** MRI: thymus retrocavale. **b** PET-CT: transversal views; mediastinum enlargement and low uptake of 18F-FDG in thymic region

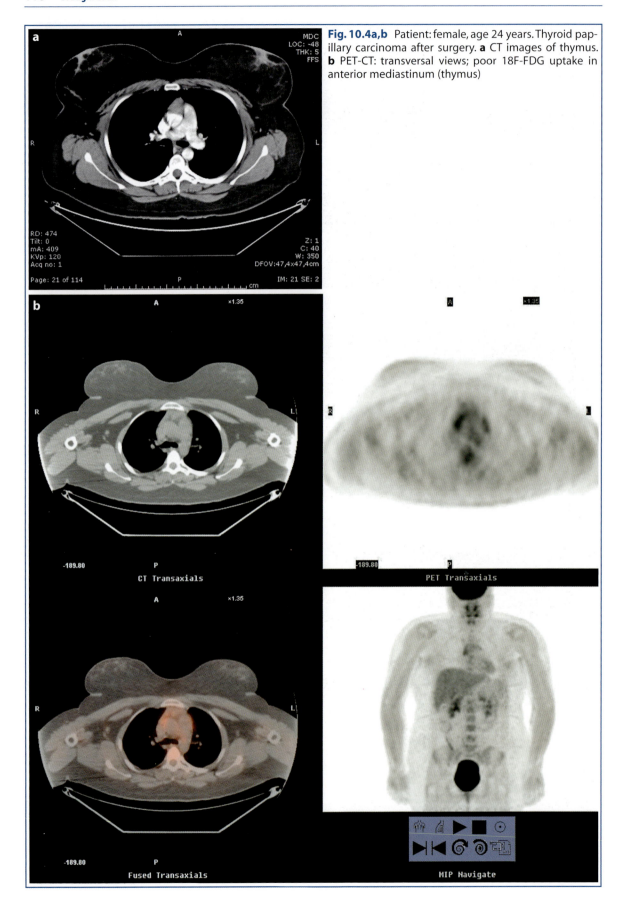

Fig. 10.4a,b Patient: female, age 24 years. Thyroid papillary carcinoma after surgery. **a** CT images of thymus. **b** PET-CT: transversal views; poor 18F-FDG uptake in anterior mediastinum (thymus)

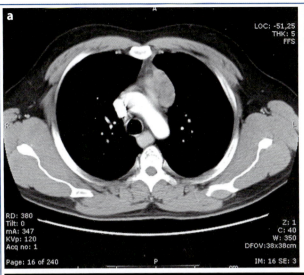

Fig. 10.5a,b Patient: male, age 36 years. Thymoma. **a** CT scan well-defined thymus carcinoma. **b** PET-CT: transversal views; uptake of 18F-FDG in the thymus

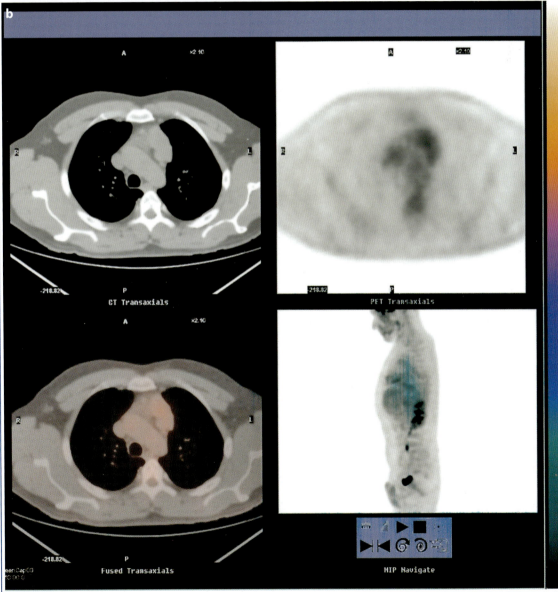

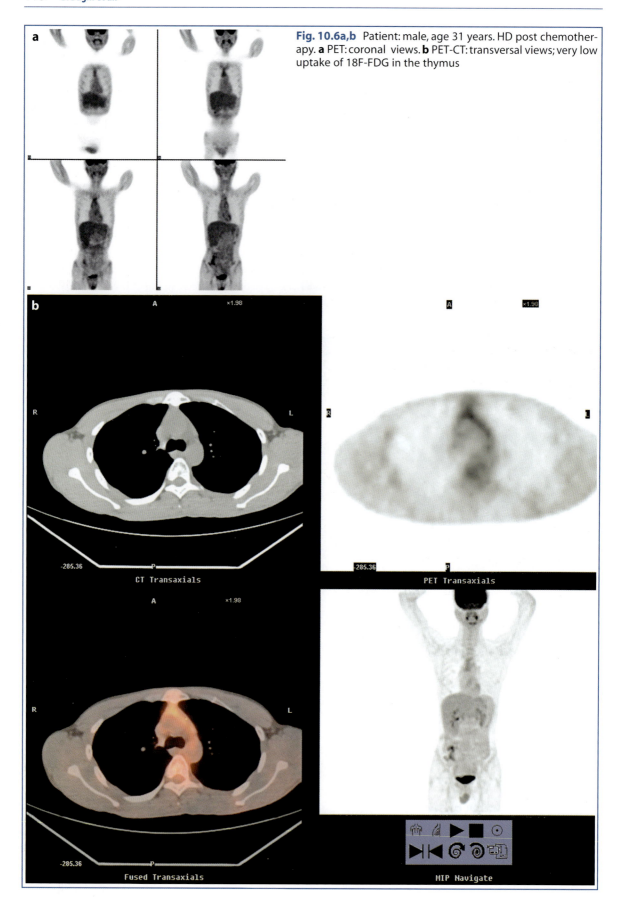

Fig. 10.6a,b Patient: male, age 31 years. HD post chemotherapy. **a** PET: coronal views. **b** PET-CT: transversal views; very low uptake of 18F-FDG in the thymus

The highest SUV value for normal thymus was found be nearly 2.0, whereas the average SUV occurred in the group of adults with lymphoma following chemotherapy reaches until a maximum of 4.0 [19].

SUV and Thymic Neoplasms

SUV may be useful in evaluating the differentiation of thymic carcinoma from other thymic neoplasm, and hyperplasia [20].

Sasaki et al. [21] found a mean SUV of 7.2 for patients with thymic carcinoma. This value was significantly greater than the values found for invasive thymoma (3.8) and noninvasive thymoma (3.0). By using an SUV of 5.0 as a cutoff, the authors achieved reasonable sensitivity (84.6%), specificity (92.3%), and accuracy (88.5%) in differentiating thymic carcinoma from thymoma. They found no statistically significant difference in SUV between invasive and noninvasive thymoma, a finding that is consistent with the histological similarity of the two tumors [21].

Conclusions

As the number of clinical applications of 18F-FDG PET-CT grows, the recognition of physiologic thymic uptake and its differentiation from mediastinal disease will remain important. The correlation with treatment history (e.g., in patients who have undergone chemotherapy) will suggest the possibility of rebound thymic hyperplasia. Morphologic data from CT or MR imaging will continue to play a key role in diagnosis and will aid in differentiating benign thymic uptake from malignancy, but PET-CT may overcome this step with fused images obtained with a hybrid device and 18F-FDG.

Summary

18F-FDG PET is a sensitive method for detecting, staging, and monitoring the effects of therapy of many tumors. PET-CT coregistration is the process of aligning PET and CT images for the purposes of combined image display (fusion) and image analysis. In the evaluation of malignancy with 18F-FDG, a potential pitfall in the assessment of the anterior mediastinum is mistaking normal uptake within the thymus from disease such as adenopathy or local invasion by tumor.

Thymic uptake was classified as "normal" on the basis of morphologic features, size, and contour at 18F-FDG PET. Pediatric patients and, more rarely, adult patients can exhibit normal physiologic thymic uptake of 18F-FDG thymic hyperplasia following chemotherapy, especially in young patients treated for testicular malignancy or malignant lymphoma. 18F-FDG PET provides information regarding the metabolic rate of thymic tissue. Several investigators have examined the relationship between the rate of glucose metabolism and the presence of thymic neoplasia or mediastinal malignancy using standardized uptake value (SUV) to measure 18F-FDG uptake. SUV may be useful in evaluating the differentiation of thymic carcinoma from other thymic neoplasms, and hyperplasia.

References

1. Delbeke D, Coleman RE, Guiberteau MJ et al (2006) Procedure guideline for tumor imaging with 18F-FDG PET/CT. J Nucl Med 47(5):885-895
2. Ayabe Z, Sakakibara N, Matsuura K (1984) 201Tl-chloride imaging of malignant thymus neoplasm. Rinsho Hoshasen 29(2):341-342
3. Srirajaskanthan R, Toubanakis C, Dusmet M, Caplin ME (2008) A review of thymic tumours. Lung Cancer 60(1):4-13
4. Kazuya K, Kiyoshi Y, Masaru T et al (2004) Who histologic classification is a prognostic indicator in thymoma. Ann Thorac Surg 77:1183-1188
5. Sasaki M, Kuwabara Y, Ichiya Y et al (1999) Differential diagnosis of thymic tumors using a combination of 11C-Methionine PET and FDG PET. J Nucl Med 40(10):1595-1601
6. Ferdinand B, Gupta P, Kramer E (2004) Spectrum of Thymic Uptake at 18F-FDG PET. RadioGraphics 24:1611-1616
7. Alibazoglu H, Alibazoglu B, Hollinger EF et al (2001) Normal thymic uptake of 2-deoxy-2[F-18]fluoro-D-glucose. Clin Nucl Med 24(8):597-600
8. Bar-Sever Z, Keidar Z, Ben-Barak A et al (2007) The incremental value of 18F-FDG PET/CT in paediatric malignancies. Eur J Nucl Med Mol Imaging 34(5):630-637
9. Sung YM, Lee KS, Kim BT et al (2006) 18F-FDG PET/CT of thymic epithelial tumors: Usefulness for distinguishing and staging tumor subgroups. J Nucl Med 47(10):1628
10. Del Rocío Estrada-Sánchez G, Altamirano-Ley J, Ochoa-Carrillo FJ (2007) Normal variants and frequent pitfalls with (18)FDG PET/CT. Cir 75(6):491-497
11. Ferdinand B, Gupta P, Kramer EL (2004) Spectrum of thymic uptake at 18F-FDG PET. RadioGraphics 24(6):1611-1616 (review)
12. Patel PM, Alibazoglu H, Ali A et al (1996) Normal thymic uptake of FDG on PET imaging. Clin Nucl Med (10):772-775

13. Liu RS, Yeh SH, Huang MH et al (1995) Use of fluorine-18 fluorodeoxyglucose positron emission tomography in the detection of thymoma: A preliminary report. Eur J Nucl Med 22(12):1402-1407
14. El-Bawab H, Al-Sugair AA, Rafay M et al (2007) Role of flourine-18 fluorodeoxyglucose positron emission tomography in thymic pathology. Eur J Cardiothorac Surg 31(4):731-736
15. Brink I, Reinhardt MJ, Hoegerle S et al (2001) PET: Increased metabolic activity in the thymus gland studied with 18F-FDG. Age dependency and frequency after chemotherapy. J Nucl Med 42(4):591-595
16. Bagga S, Bloch EM (2006) Imaging of an invasive malignant thymoma on PET Scan: CT and histopathologic correlation. Clin Nucl Med 31(10):614-616
17. Bogot NR, Quint LE (2005) Imaging of thymic disorders. Cancer Imaging 5(1):139-149
18. Smith CS, Schöder H, Yeung HW (2007) Thymic extension in the superior mediastinum in patients with thymic hyperplasia: Potential cause of false-positive findings on 18F-FDG PET/CT. AJR Am J Roentgenol 188(6):1716-1721
19. Ferdinand B, Gupta P, Kramer EL (2004) Spectrum of thymic uptake at 18F-FDG PET1. RadioGraphics 24:1611-1616
20. Bar-Sever Z, Keidar Z, Ben-Barak A et al (2007) The incremental value of 18F-FDG PET/CT in paediatric malignancies. Eur J Nucl Med Mol Imaging 34(5):630-637
21. Sung YM, Lee KS, Kim BT et al (2006) 18F-FDG PET/CT of thymic epithelial tumors: Usefulness for distinguishing and staging tumor subgroups. J Nucl Med 47(10):1628-1634

CHAPTER 11
Minimally Invasive and Surgical Diagnosis

Ciro Ruggiero, Corrado Lavini, Younes Mehd, Daniela Paioli, Marco Patelli, Mario De Santis, Antonio Affinita

Introduction

Approximately half of all mediastinal neoplasms are located in the anterior compartment. Masses in the anterior mediastinum include a broad variety of diseases ranging from frankly benign ones to extreme malignancies [1-3].

Thymic disease accounts for a vast proportion of these expansive lesions originating in the anterior mediastinum, ranging from 25% to 30% of cases [4, 5]. Indeed, thymic neoplasms followed by lymphomas, germ-cell tumors, and carcinomas are predominantly located in this area.

Thus, whenever confronted with a neoplasm in the anterior mediastinum, a thymic disease should be suspected.

Indications

Modern imaging techniques are an irreplaceable step in the definition of a mass in the anterior mediastinum of suspected thymic origin.

CT scan and MRI can provide valuable information on the location of the lesion, its characteristics, its relationships with neighboring organs and structures and the presence or absence of local invasion. Radiology often provides hints on the origin of the lesion, allowing to establish if it is benign or malignant, its extension, and whether or not it is possible to radically remove it.

If an expansive lesion of the anterior mediastinum characterized as a thymic neoplasm is definitely resectable at radiological evaluation, surgery should be performed without preoperative diagnosis (which would increase morbidity risks and slow down the therapeutic process [6]).

If, on the other hand, due to the extension of the disease, surgery is contraindicated or questionable, diagnostic investigations should undoubtedly be taken a step further to confirm the possible indication of chemotherapy and/or radiotherapy [1, 2, 7].

Finally, if after radiological investigation doubts remain as to the nature of the lesion, i.e., thymoma or lymphoma, which is treated oncologically, diagnostic biopsy becomes mandatory.

Hence, the histological diagnosis of a suspected thymic neoplasm is indicated in the following cases:
– Nonresectable or possibly nonresectable at radiological evaluation
– Uncertainty in differential diagnosis with respect to lymphoproliferative forms

Thus, a histological diagnosis will be essential to establish operability and correct staging of the disease and to plan, where applicable, chemotherapy and/or radiotherapy.

The diagnostic techniques used in these cases include nonsurgical methods such as traditional endoscopy, possibly EBUS, and interventional radiology techniques such as US/CT-guided transthoracic needle aspiration or US/CT-guided transthoracic needle biopsy (FNAB, CNB) as well as minimally invasive and traditional surgery.

Diagnostic Techniques

1. Endoscopic Techniques

Flexible bronchoscopy is a minimally invasive method which can be used as an effective outpatient procedure. It can be performed under local anesthesia only or under conscious sedation. It allows for visualization of the bronchial tree. Furthermore, it makes it possible to perform endobronchial sampling, biopsy of pulmonary parenchyma, and transbronchial needle aspiration (TBNA) to obtain cytohistologic specimens by needles of several different sizes (19-21 gauge). At the mediastinal level, this method allows to reach lesions adjacent to the trachea, large bronchi, and lymph nodes (stations 2, 4, 7, 10 and 11 according to ATS NSCLC classification) [8].

In case of a suspected thymic neoplasm, bronchoscopy can be proposed if the CT or MRI suggests a direct invasion of lung or bronchi, or in presence of metastatic lymphadenopathies which could be reached by endoscopy.

Flexible bronchoscopy is also suitable as simple preoperative examination in order to exclude other endobronchial alterations in anticipation of thoracic surgery. In this case, along with the white-light (WL) inspection, an additional autofluorescence (AFL) endobronchial examination should be performed if available. It is indeed recommended in heavy-smoking patients or in subjects who have significant risk factors for lung cancer. In literature the Relative Sensitivity of AFL along with WL bronchoscopy varies from 1.3 to 6.3 compared with WL examination alone in detecting preneoplastic lesions or bronchial squamous carcinoma either in situ or early [9, 10].

TBNA

In case of thymoma, surgical resection remains the standard of care for both noninvasive and invasive lesions, as it provides the best prognosis [11-13]. Surgical excision can be used for diagnosis without a preventive biopsy, if no lesion of other nature is suspected, e.g., lymphomas.

However, if lymph node metastases are suspected, it is highly important to verify the neoplastic invasion, since it could exclude surgery.

Thymoma seldom shows lymphogenous metastasis (stage IVb according to Masaoka's clinical staging). In a 2003 study by Kondo et al., only 1.8% of thymomas presented lymph node metastasis, prevailingly in anterior mediastinal lymph nodes and minimally in the other intrathoracic lymph nodes [14].

The thymic carcinoma, on the other hand, which accounts for only less than 10% of thymic neoplasms, showed lymph node metastasis in 26.8% of cases, of which 69.4% were in anterior mediastinal lymph nodes, 34.7% in other intrathoracic lymph nodes, and 30.6% in extrathoracic lymph nodes.

Carcinoid occurs less frequently than carcinoma; it shows 27.5% of lymph node metastasis, out of which 90.9% were in anterior mediastinic lymph nodes; 45.5% in other intrathoracic lymph nodes, and 27.3% in extrathoracic lymph nodes.

Especially in presence of thymic carcinoma, in case of suspected lymph node lesions which could be endoscopically reached by TBNA, bronchoscopy can be suitable for both diagnosis and staging.

TBNA is an operator-dependent technique and it can be performed as a blind procedure in stations 4, 7, and 10, using endobronchial landmarks and prior contrast enhancement CT images of enlarged lymph nodes (Figs. 11.1-11.2). The diagnostic yield, as far

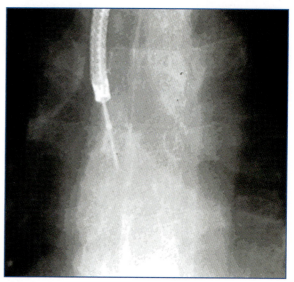

Fig. 11.1 Subcarinal TBNA. Chest X-ray feature

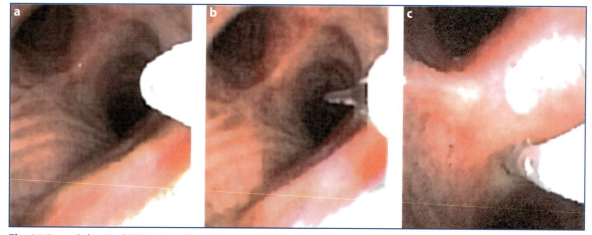

Fig. 11.2a-c Subcarinal TBNA. Step-by-step procedure

as lung carcinoma metastases are concerned, is 78% in two different meta-analyses [15, 16].

There are no studies, in literature, to evaluate the yield of TBNA in thymic neoplasms, due to the scarce occurrence of cases.

There are several specific needles used in flexible bronchoscopy. Instruments used for this procedure share a common architecture and operational concept:
- A distal, retractable, sharp-bevelled, metal needle attached to a flexible catheter that is housed in an outer sheet into which the needle and its catheter can be withdrawn;
- A proximal control device that manipulates the movement of the needle, the stylet, or both, and has a proximal side-port through which suction can be applied [17].

Histology probes are made of an outer 19-gauge needle and a inner 21-gauge needle. The latter acts as a trocar helping the outer needle to penetrate into the incision and preventing it from plugging. The histologic core of tissue, after being captured by the probe, is extracted and placed in a formalin solution before being sent for staining and pathologic analysis. The cytologic sample can be smeared on glass slides, and fixed with air or alcohol. This method will provide for a better preservation of cellular architecture in the sample, in comparison to the flushing, centrifugation, and resuspension technique.

Histologic samples are considered adequate when they show the lymph node histologic architecture. Cytologic samples are considered adequate when they present a moderate number of lymphocytes, although an exact cut-off has not been defined as of today [18].

The presence of a cytopathologist at the moment of procedure ("rapid on-site evaluation", ROSE) could be of some help in determining the adequacy of samples, increasing the yield, and reducing the complication risk and the overall sampling time [19].

With regard to lymph nodes which could not be easily reached by blind procedure due to the lack of endobronchial landmarks (stations 2 and 3), and with regard to small lymph nodes (short axis <1 cm), a new echoendoscope model was recently developed. It makes it possible to visualize lymph nodes and large vessels adjacent to trachea and bronchi, so that real-time, echo-guided sampling can be performed [20, 21].

The ultrasound bronchoscope now available for the so-called EBUS-TBNA (Endobronchial Ultrasound TBNA) features an ultrasound transducer engineered into the tip of the endoscope (distal end outer diameter of the instrument: 6.9 mm). The working channel outlet of the bronchoscope is located immediately before the transducer. When the needle is extracted out of the working channel, it comes into the detection range of the transducer and therefore it can be visualized during aspiration.

The initially developed EBUS technique did not allow any real-time sampling, since it consisted of introducing, through the working channel of the bronchoscope, an ultrasound catheter to locate the target; however, the probe was to be removed afterwards, for the needle to be inserted through the same working channel [22].

Patient characteristics, endosonographer experience, and available expertise for cytologic and histologic review will influence both techniques.

Many studies assessed EBUS as a technique to increase TBNA yield in nonsmall cell lung cancer (NSCLC). Herth et al., with a randomized study comparing EBUS-guided with standard TBNA, concluded that EBUS significantly increased the yield of TBNA in all lymph node stations except for the subcarinal one [23]. A deeper analysis of results indicates, however, that in lymph node stations 4L and 4R yield is similar to conventional TBNA [24].

In case of thymic neoplasms, the EBUS-TBNA can also prove useful when there is a direct invasion of neoplasm in the middle-mediastinum area adjacent to the trachea, to perform a needle aspiration of the neoplastic mass.

EUS

The classic Endoscopic Ultrasound (EUS), performed through a gastroscope, is an effective and safe method of examining the posterior mediastinum through the esophageal wall. Mediastinal lymph nodes may be visualized in the aorto-pulmonary window (station 5) in the subcarina (station 7), the paraesophageal area (station 8), and that adjacent to the inferior pulmonary ligament (station 9).

Two different types of echoendoscopes are available. The radial endoscope provides a 360° ultrasound image; the curvilinear echoendoscope provides a 180° view that is parallel to the shaft of the endoscope, allowing for a real-time visualization of the fine needle aspiration (FNA).

EUS-FNA can usually sample lymph nodes in the posterior mediastinum (stations 5, 6, 8, 9) and subcarina (station 7).

EUS-FNA and TBNA should not necessarily be regarded as competing modalities, but rather as complementary ones towards lymph node station sampling.

EUS-FNA presents a good accuracy (around 90%) and sensitivity (around 90%) in NSCLC [25, 26]. With regard to thymic neoplasms, though, no specific investigation is reported in the literature for assessing the yield of the procedure. There are, however, individual case reports [27].

Cytologic interpretation can be hampered by the presence of blood and benign epithelial cells. EUS-FNA typically yields a small biopsy sample, thereby limiting diagnostic accuracy for some lesions such as lymphomas. Larger caliber cutting needles were designed to overcome many of the problems associated with FNA. In order to obtain larger tissues specimens for histologic examinations, a new technique, the trucut biopsy (TCB) was recently developed [28]. It adopts a special needle, which can be used with linear echoendoscopes. Experience with EUS-TCB is rapidly accumulating [29, 30]. In the literature, there are very few examples of thymic neoplasm diagnosis by EUS-FNA or EUS-TCB [31].

Endobronchial Invasion

Invasive thymomas extend from the anterior mediastinum and they can infiltrate the pericardium, the pleura, the lung, and other mediastinal structures. If CT findings demonstrate a neoplastic mass invading the pulmonary parenchyma, it is seldom possible to detect, upon preoperative bronchoscopic examination, an endobronchial invasion with polypoid growth.

This circumstance is extremely rare in the literature: so far, only 19 such cases have been described, either as a first diagnosis [32-34], or as a case of recurrence [35]. Cough and hemoptysis appear among the symptoms experienced by most patients [36-38]. There is a frequent occurrence of left-upper lobe bronchus invasion.

A possible tumor invasion sequence has been hypothesized by Honda et al. [39] and it can be summarized as follows: the thymoma infiltrates the pleuras and invades a distal bronchus by penetrating through a sufficiently thin section of its wall; then it develops inside the bronchus as polypoid lesion. In most cases, endoscopic biopsy specimens of such polypoid lesions are not thymoma diagnostic due to the necrosis of tissues [40].

In our center's experience, during the past 10 years, we performed 19 bronchoscopic procedures for suspected or established thymic neoplasms. In two cases there was a direct pulmonary invasion in the right-upper lobe. One of them had negative bronchoscopy examination. The other one, examined in 2003, was a 67-year-old woman who presented hemoptoe; at bronchoscopy she showed a necrotic-surface polypoid neoplasm obstructing the right-upper lobe bronchus. She had already undergone mediastinal needle aspiration highly suggestive of thymoma. In order to prevent postobstructive pneumonia and to obtain diagnostic biopsies, the patient underwent rigid bronchoscopy under general anesthesia for laser-assisted endoscopic disobstruction. Endoscopic biopsies indicated the presence of a carcinoma. The patient did not present parathymic syndromes. She was later sent to surgery for complete resection of the mass in the anterior mediastinum along with right-upper pulmonary bilobectomy. The final histologic examination confirmed the presence of a well-differentiated clear-cell thymic carcinoma along with a thymoma type B2 according to WHO histologic classification (cortical). On gross examination, the carcinoma infiltrated the pericardium and pulmonary parenchyma of the right-upper and middle lobe with areas of necrosis and hemorrhage. It also grew into the bronchi of the right-upper lobe for a maximum residual extent of 1.3 cm beyond the part resected by rigid bronchoscopy.

Up to the last follow-up check, in 2006, the patient was alive and disease-free after surgery and adjuvant therapy.

2. Interventional Radiology Techniques

Transthoracic percutaneous biopsy of the anterior mediastinum is widely used for the histological sampling of expansive lesions. It can be fluoroscopy-, US-, or CT-guided, mainly depending upon the location and size of the lesion.

The CT-guided technique is more widespread in that it makes it possible to accurately evaluate the borders and margins of the lesion and in particular its relationships with vascular structures, thus reducing the risk of major complications. The advantage of this technique is that it makes it possible to verify the position of the needle tip and do repeated sampling. This technique can be used to tackle most lesions of the anterior mediastinum.

The US-guided technique is mainly indicated for masses appearing on the surface of the chest wall (i.e., without interposed aerated pulmonary parenchyma).

It is less expensive that the CT-guided technique and enables real-time monitoring of the advancement of the needle, making it possible to precisely select the target and spare, through the use of color Doppler, vascular structures.

This procedure is performed under local anesthesia, using cytology aspiration needles (20-21 G), the sensitivity of which, in relation to epithelial thymic tumors, is reported to attain 61% and 71% [41, 42], or trucut needles (16-18 G), the sensitivity of which, based on several case reports in the literature, is 91.7%, specificity is 100%, global accuracy is 96% [43] (Figs. 11.3, 11.4).

The complications described, though very rare, include pneumothorax and hemorrhage; hence, the patient should be hospitalized and receive standard chest X-ray 24 h after the procedure.

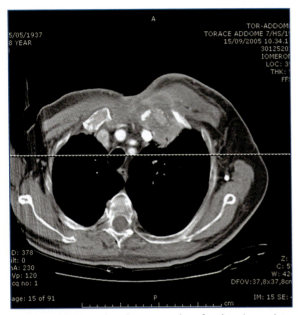

Fig. 11.3 Patient already operated on for thymic carcinoma infiltrating the sternal manubrium. CT findings show a left anterior mediastinal mass infiltrating the chest wall

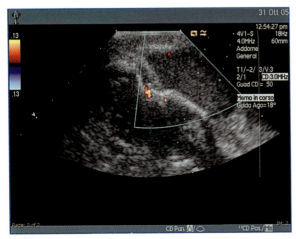

Fig. 11.4 US-guided biopsy of the mass that makes it possible to track the pathway of the biopsy needle. Histology: recurrence of *thymic adenocarcinoma*

No cases have been described of neoplastic seeding along the pathway of the biopsy needle.

3. Surgical Techniques

Mediastinal surgical biopsy, if compared to endoscopic and interventional radiology biopsies, is always superior in terms of quantity and quality of the sample. As a matter of fact, the amount of tissue taken is fundamental in the case of histologically complex thymic neoplasms and where doubts exist as to whether it is a thymic or a lymphoproliferative lesion. The surgical method also makes it possible to perform safe targeted biopsies, allowing, as a result, for the best diagnostic accuracy (as high as 80-100%).

Several authors in the literature have compared the yield of surgical biopsy against that of other, nonsurgical techniques. Fang and coworkers, in a study relating to anterior mediastinal masses, reported, with respect to thymic neoplasms, a diagnostic accuracy of 83.3% with surgical biopsy (mini-mediastinotomy), against 40% with CNB [1].

The decision to do a surgical biopsy on this type of patient should be carefully considered: very often they have superior vena cava syndrome and hence can be demanding in clinical, anesthesiological, and surgical terms as well as in terms of postoperative recovery.

To minimize surgical trauma, a limitedly invasive approach should be selected, to the extent possible. Minimally invasive endoscopic techniques such as videothoracoscopy, videomediastinoscopy, pericardioscopy, and video-assisted minithoracotomy can be the best diagnostic solution and are well tolerated by patients. Amongst nonendoscopic, minimally invasive techniques, mention should be made of anterior mini-mediastinotomy, which minimizes surgical trauma and is optimally tolerated; besides, some authors perform it under local anesthesia.

Only when faced with problems that can make minimally invasive surgery complex, can there be an indication for a traditional surgical approach.

Amongst minimally invasive methods, *videothoracoscopy (VATS)* is the one most commonly used.

It allows for excellent exposure of the anterior mediastinum, is easy, effective, and safe. It is indicated when a thorough exploration of the pleuric cavity is required, such as in the case of anterior mediastinal neoplasms accompanied by pleural effusion [44]. It can also be proposed for pediatric patients [7, 45]. Diagnostic accuracy is very high, attaining 100% of cases [7, 46].

Usually, the operation requires a triangulation with three accesses along the mid- and posterior-axillary line. The exact extension of the disease, the level of infiltration of neighboring structures and where to do targeted biopsies shall be established intraoperatively. Hemostasis at the end of surgery must be highly accurate (Figs. 11.5-11.7).

Videomediastinoscopy (VAM) can be indicated in some cases. Three technical variants of videomediastinoscopy can be used for the diagnosis of thymic neoplasms:
- Cervical VAM
- Anterior VAM
- Retrosternal subxiphoidal VAM.

Cervical VAM can be *prevascular*, which on the anterior plane of the anonymous artery reaches the retrosternal space and the thymic space, or traditionally *retrovascular*, which makes it possible to explore expansive lesions extending from the anterior to the median mediastinum (Figs. 11.8, 11.9).

The presence of a superior vena cava syndrome is not a contraindication for this type of examination, even though a very meticulous dissection is required to avoid excessive traction of the biopsied tissue, followed by a very accurate hemostasis [44, 47]. Intra-op light on the mediastinal compartment is much more limited compared to the VATS access; however, compared to the latter it is less invasive and can be done as an outpatient procedure [48].

Anterior VAM is indicated for anterior mediastinum and retrosternal neoplasms in contact with

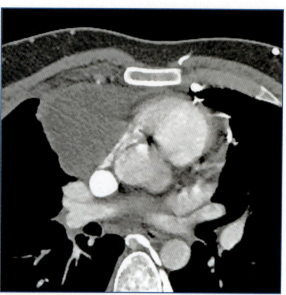

Fig. 11.6 V.P., 30 years old. Detail of chest CT scan. Bulky infiltrating mass in the anterior mediastinum reaching the anterior chest wall and dislocating the large vessels posteriorly and laterally

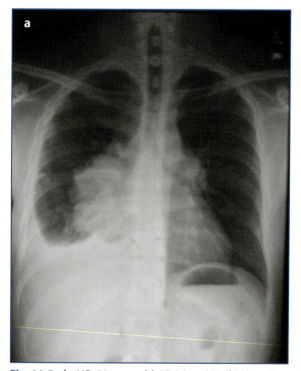
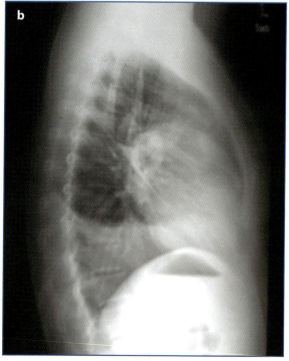

Fig. 11.5a,b V.P., 30 years old. AP (**a**) and LL (**b**) chest X-ray. Right parahilar bulky mass with polycyclic edges. Homolateral consensual pleural effusion

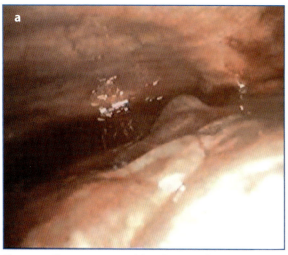 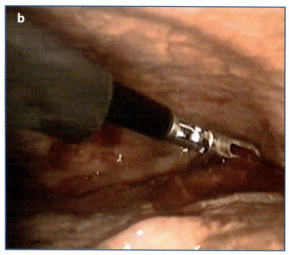

Fig. 11.7a,b V.P., 30 years old. Endoscopic findings at VATS. Bulky, infiltrating neoplasm in the anterior mediastinum. Serum and blood pleural effusion (**a**). Biopsy with oncotom (**b**). Histological diagnosis: *thymic carcinoma*

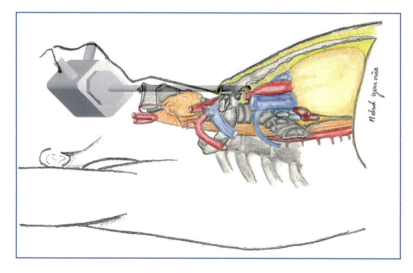

Fig. 11.8 Cervical prevascular VAM

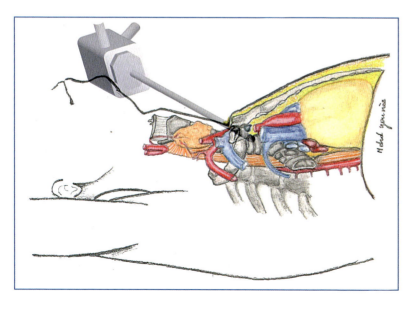

Fig. 11.9 Cervical retrovascular VAM

the anterior chest wall. A minimum intercostal parasternal access is used (2nd, 3rd, 4th intercostal space, as appropriate) (Fig. 11.10).

Intraoperative view of the mediastinum is limited but sufficient to do safe targeted biopsies. It can also be performed under local anesthesia [44, 49, 50].

Some authors have proposed the *retrosternal subxiphoidal VAM*. It requires a subxiphoid incision making it possible to create a tunnel in the retrosternal space to reach, extrapleurally, the anterior mediastinum (Fig. 11.11). It allows for good lighting of the thymic space and gives access to both sides of the mediastinum with a single incision. However, further confirmation is needed on larger patient series [51].

Pericardioscopy (PSC) can sometimes be indicated. Although mainly used for neoplastic pericardial effusions from lung cancer, this method is useful where the anterior mediastinal neoplasm is accompanied by symptomatic pericardial effusion requiring urgent drainage. This investigation, done via a subxiphoid access, makes it possible to evacuate the effusion, locate the neoplasm if it infiltrates the pericardial sac and do targeted biopsies [44, 52].

Anterior mini-mediastinotomy is another minimally invasive technique. It uses the same access as anterior VAM, which is even smaller than in the tradi-

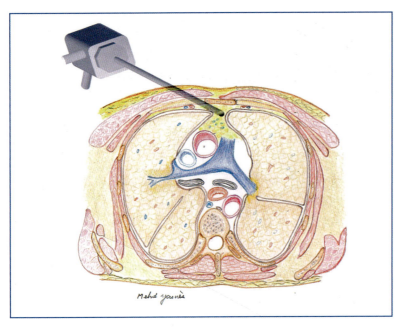

Fig. 11.10 Anterior VAM

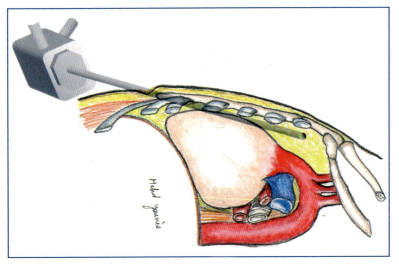

Fig. 11.11 Retrosternal subxiphoidal VAM

tional Chamberlain approach (equally used by several authors, though) [45, 53]. Anterior mini-mediastinotomy is successfully performed also under local anesthesia, without narcosis and orotracheal intubation of these fragile patients, thus reducing risks [1, 47].

VA (video-assisted) minithoracotomy is yet another minimally invasive technique requiring an extremely small thoracotomic incision (4-6 cm). It is an intermediate option between an entirely videoendoscopic access and the traditional "open" access and is thus named *Hybrid VATS*. It can be used where strong adhesions make the biopsy more difficult to perform or when it is necessary to use traditional surgical tools [54].

Usually, traditional "open" techniques such as *minithoracotomy* and *superior partial median sternotomy* (manubriotomy) are only proposed in more complex cases where there are doubts as to the indication of minimally invasive accesses [44] (Table 11.1).

The complications of using surgical diagnostic techniques for neoplasms of the anterior mediastinum range from intraoperative bleeding and nerve damage (i.e., damage to the phrenic nerve and to the recurrent laryngeal nerve) to infection of the surgical wound [7, 47].

Where the mediastinal neoplasm compresses the trachea, the use of narcosis can cause, after removal of the orotracheal tube, an obstruction of the upper airways and major respiratory distress. In this case, it is appropriate to perform a diagnostic examination under local anesthesia like anterior mini-mediastinotomy [44, 47, 55, 56].

There are not many studies on the diagnostic accuracy of surgical techniques in the presence of suspected thymic mediastinal masses. There are, instead, more studies assessing the diagnostic findings of expansive lesions of the entire mediastinum. A prospective study by Gossot and coworkers dealing with VATS and mediastinoscopy has found that the effectiveness of the two methods is almost the same [57]. Furrer and coworkers, instead, comparing cervical mediastinoscopy, anterior mediastinotomy, and VATS, concluded that the diagnostic accuracy of VATS is higher than that of the other two techniques (100% vs. 88%) [46]. Fang and coworkers, presenting one of the few specific studies done on the histological diagnosis of anterior mediastinal masses, concluded by highlighting the diagnostic reliability of minianterior mediastinotomy, which is the same as that of mediastinoscopy and of traditional "open" surgery [1].

Clearly, the opinions of the various authors slightly differ depending on their familiarity with individual procedures and techniques [7].

Conclusions

When a neoplasm is found in the anterior mediastinum, thymic disease should be suspected. It is not, however, always necessary to define histological typization *a priori*. Where the neoplasm is deemed to be resectable at radiologic imaging, exeresis should be done *d'emblée*, which will have diagnostic and therapeutic value.

A histological diagnosis is instead needed where radiological findings leave doubts as to operability, or in case of clear inoperability, or else in the presence of a problem of differential diagnosis between a thymoma and a lymphoma.

Correct clinical methodology provides for the planning of more invasive diagnostic examinations, starting with endoscopic techniques, moving on to interventional radiology, and finally to surgery (Fig. 11.12).

A histological diagnosis is rarely achieved via endoscopy: anterior mediastinal masses only rarely show endobronchial growth and quantitatively appropriate samples might not be obtained with EBUS.

Table 11.1 Biopsy of suspected thymic mediastinal neoplasm. Surgical techniques

Minimally invasive techniques	Traditional "open" techniques
VATS	Minithoracotomy
Pericardioscopy	Partial superior median sternotomy (manubriotomy)
VAM	
Cervical retrovascular	
Cervical prevascular	
Anterior	
Retrosternal subxiphoidal	
Anterior mini-mediastinotomy	
VA Minithoracotomy	

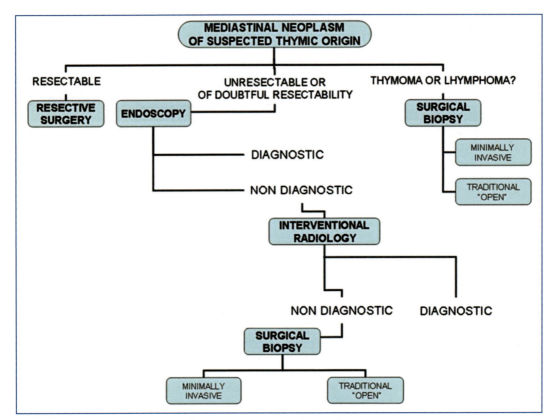

Fig. 11.12 Algorithm for the diagnosis of suspected thymic mediastinal neoplasm

However, fibrobronchoscopy can be useful for diagnosis and staging when CT or MRI findings lead to suspect a direct pulmonary or bronchial invasion and/or metastatic mediastinal lymphadenopathies. Fibrobronchoscopy remains a fundamental preoperative examination in surgical cases to exclude endobronchial lesions.

US/CT-guided interventional radiology techniques such as FNAB and CNB ensure good diagnostic accuracy but are not indicated if there are doubts between an expansive thymic lesion and a lymphoproliferative disease. In the case of lymphomas, indeed, the presence of necrotic intratumoral areas can generate false negatives and, in any case, correct typization, which can be complex in some cases, makes it necessary to take an adequate amount of material, which can only be done via a surgical biopsy.

Surgical techniques are by far the most effective ones from a diagnostic point of view. To achieve an optimal risk-benefit ratio, considering the fragility of most of these patients, priority should be given to minimally invasive techniques, leaving traditional "open" surgery as a second option. Amongst minimally invasive techniques, VATS certainly is the most widespread; the variants of VAM have precise, codified indications; anterior mini-mediastinotomy is well tolerated and can be done under local anesthesia; VA minithoracotomy is easy and resolutive, including in cases difficult to handle with a wholly videoendoscopic access. The traditional "open" approach, with minithoracotomy or manubriotomy, is only indicated for particularly complex situations, as an alternative to minimally invasive access.

References

1. Fang W, Xu M, Chen G et al (2007) Minimally invasive approaches for histological diagnosis of anterior mediastinal masses. Chin Med J 120(8):675-679
2. Restrepo CS, Pandit M, Rojas IC et al (2005) Imaging findings of expansile lesions of the thymus. Curr Probl Diagn Radiol 34(1):22-34
3. Strollo DC, Rosado-de-Christenson ML, Jett JR (1997) Primary mediastinal tumors. Part I. Tumors of the anterior mediastinum. Chest 112:511-522
4. Priola AM, Priola SM, Cardinale L et al (2006) The anterior mediastinum: Diseases. Radiol Med 111:312-342
5. Sousa B, Araùjo A, Amaro T et al (2007) Malignant thymomas – The experience of the Portuguese Oncological Institute, Porto, and literature review. Rev Port Pneumol 13(4):553-585

6. Lara PN Jr (2000) Malignant thymoma: Current status and future directions. Cancer Treat Rev 26:127-131
7. Cirino LM, Milanez de Campo JR, Fernandez A et al (2000) Diagnosis and treatment of mediastinal tumors by thoracoscopy. Chest 117:1787-1792
8. Mountain CF, Dresler CM (1997) Regional lymph node classification for lung cancer staging. Chest 111:1718-1823
9. Haussinger H, Becker H, Stanzel F et al (2005) Autofluorescence bronchoscopy compared with white light bronchoscopy alone for the detection of precancerous lesions: A European randomised multicentric study. Thorax 60:496-503
10. Lam S, Kennedy, Unger M et al (1998) Localization of bronchial intraepithelial neoplastic lesions by fluorescence bronchoscopy. Chest 113:696-672
11. Blumberg D, Port JL, Weksler B et al (1995) Thymoma: A multivariate analysis of factors predicting survival. Ann Thorac Surg 60:908-914
12. Wilkins HB, Sheikh E, Green R et al (1999) Clinical and pathologic predictors of survival in patients with thymoma. Ann Surg 230:562-574
13. Detterbeck FC, Parsone AM (2004) Thymic tumors. Ann Thorac Surg 77:1860-1869
14. Kondo K, Monden Y (2003) Lymphogenous and hematogenous metastasis of thymic epithelial tumors. Ann Thorac Surg 76:1859-1865
15. Detterbeck FC, Jantz MA, Fallace M et al (2007) Invasive mediastinal staging of Lung Cancer: ACCP Evidence-based clinical practice guidelines, 2nd edn. Chest 132:202S-220S
16. Holty JC, Kunschner WG, Gould MK (2005) Accuracy of transbronchial needle aspiration for mediastinal staging of non-small cell lung cancer: A meta-analysis. Thorax 60:949-955
17. Trisolini R, Paioli D, Cancellieri A, Patelli M (2006) Diagnostic bronchoscopic approach to mediastinal diseases. Minerva Pneumol 45:39-51
18. Patelli M, Agli LL, Poletti V et al (2002) The role of fiberscopic transbronchial needle aspiration in the staging of N2 disease due to non small cell lung cancer. Ann Thorac Surg 73:407-411
19. Diette GB, White P, Terry P et al (2000) Utility of rapid on-site cytological evaluation of lung masses and adenopathy. Chest 117:1186-1190
20. Krasnik M, Vilmann P, Larsen SS et al (2003) Preliminary experience with a new method of endoscopic transbronchial real-time ultrasound guided biopsy for diagnosis of mediastinal and hilar lesions. Thorax 58:1083-1086
21. Yasufu K, Nakajima T, Chiyo M et al (2007) Endobronchial ultrasonography: Current status and future directions. J Thorac Oncol 2(10):970-979
22. Herth F, Becker HD (2000) Endobronchial ultrasound of the airways and the mediastinum. Monaldi Arch Chest Dis 55:29-32
23. Herth F, Becker HD, Ernst A (2004) Conventional vs. endobronchial ultrasound-guided transbronchial needle aspiration. A randomized trial. Chest 125:322-325
24. Trisolini R, Agli LL, Patelli M (2004) Conventional versus EBUS-guided transbronchial needle aspiration of the mediastinum. Chest 126:1005-1006
25. Pedersen BH, Vilmann P, Folke K et al (1996) Endoscopic ultrasonography and real time guided fine-needle aspiration biopsy of solid lesions of the mediastinum suspected of malignancy. Chest 110:539
26. Wallance MB, Silvestri GA, Sahai AV et al (2001) Endoscopic ultrasound-guided fine needle aspiration for staging patients with carcinoma of the lung. Ann Thorac Surg 72:1861
27. Larghi A, Noffsinger A, Dye C et al (2005) EUS-guided fine needle tissue acquisition by using negative pressure suction for the evaluation of solid masses: A pilot study. Gastrointes Endosc 62(5):768-774
28. Wiersema MJ, Levy MJ, Harewood GC et al (2002) Initial experience with EUS-guided trucut needle biopsies of perigastric organs. Gastrointest Endosc 56:275
29. Vadarajulu S, Fraig M, Schmulewitz N et al (2004) Comparison of EUS-guided 19-gauge trucut needle biopsy with EUS-guided fine needle aspiration. Endoscopy 36:397
30. Storch I, Jorda M, Thurer R et al (2006) Advantage of EUS Trucut biopsy combined with fine-needle aspiration without immediate on-site cytopathologic examination. Gastrointest Endosc 64:505
31. Larghi A, Rodriguez-Wulff E, Noffsinger A et al (2006) Recurrent malignant thymoma diagnosed by EUS-guided trucut biopsy. Gastrointes Endosc 63(6):859-860
32. Honma K, Mishina M, Watanabe Y (1988) Polypoid endobronchial extension from invasive thymoma. Virchows Arch A Pathol Anat Histopathol 413(5):469-474
33. Asamura H, Morinaga S, Shimosato Y et al (1988) Thymoma displaying endobronchial polypoid growth. Chest 94(3):647-649
34. Abiko M, Sato T, Spiono S et al (1999) A case of invasive thymoma displaying endobronchial extension. Kikansigaku (J Jpn Soci Bronch) 21:289-293
35. Matsuguma H, Furuta M, Tsukiyama I et al (1999) Endobronchial brachytherapy for recurrent thymoma showing endobronchial polypoid growth. Am J Clin Oncol 22(1):84-86
36. Ichimanda M, Okada S, Kai T (1991) A case of invasive thymoma displaying endobronchial and endocaval polypoid growth. Nippon Kyobu Geka Gakkai Zassi 39(6):938-942
37. Kondo K, Uyama T, Sumitomo M et al (1997) Invasive thymoma with endobronchial polypoid growth. Surg Today 27(5):466-468
38. Yokoi K, Miyazawa N, Mori K et al (1990) Invasive thymoma with intracaval growth into the right atrium. Nippon Kyobu Geka Gakkai Zassi 28(3):529-534
39. Honda T, Hayasaka M, Hachiya T et al (1995) Invasive thymoma with hypogammaglobulinemia spreading within the bronchial lumen. Respiration 62(5):294-296

40. Sakuraba M, Sagara Y, Tamura A et al (2005) A case of invasive thymoma with endobronchial growth. Ann Thorac Cardiovasc Surg 11(2):114-116
41. Herman SJ, Holub RV, Weisbrod GL et al (1996) Anterior mediastinal masses: Utility of transthoracic needle biopsy. Radiology 199:489
42. Weisbrod GL (1987) Percutaneous fine-needle aspiration of the mediastinum. Clin Chest Med 8:27
43. Yonemori K, Tsuta K, Tateishi U et al (2006). Diagnostic accuracy of CT-guided percutaneous cutting needle biopsy for thymic tumors. Clin Radiol 61:771-775
44. Porte H, Metois D, Finzi L et al (2000) Superior vena cava syndrome of malignant origin. Which surgical procedure for which diagnosis? Eur J Cardio Thoracic Surg 17(4):384-388
45. Fraga JC, Komlos M, Takamatu E et al (2003) Mediastinal tumors in children. J Pneumol 29(5):253-257
46. Furrer M, Striffeler H, Ris HB (1995) Invasive diagnosis of mediastinal space-occupying lesions: On differential indications between cervical mediastinoscopy, parasternal mediastinotomy and videothoracoscopy. Chirurg 66:1203-1209
47. Dosios T, Theakos N, Chatziantoniou C (2005) Cervical mediastinoscopy and anterior mediastinoscopy in superior vena cava obstruction. Chest 128:1551-1556
48. Mineo TC, Ambrogi V, Nofroni I et al (1999) Mediastinoscopy in superior vena cava obstruction: Analysis of 80 consecutive patients. Ann Thorac Surg 68(1):223-226
49. Rendina EA, Venuta F, De Giacomo T et al (2002) Biopsy of anterior mediastinal masses under local anaesthesia. Ann Thorac Surg 74:1720-1723
50. Santambrogio L, Nosotti M (2006) Anterior videomediastinoscopy. In: Lavini C, Ruggiero C, Morandi U (eds) Video assisted thoracic surgery. Springer-Verlag Italia, Milan, pp 187-190
51. Hutter J, Junger W, Miller K et al (1998) Subxiphoidal videomediastinoscopy for diagnostic access to the anterior mediastinum. Ann Thorac Surg 68(4):1427-1428
52. Porte H, Delebecq T, Finzi L et al (1999) Pericardioscopy for primary management of pericardial effusions in cancer patients. Eur J Cardio Thoracic Surg 16:287-291
53. Kitami A, Suzuki T, Usuda R et al (2004) Diagnostic and therapeutic thoracoscopy for mediastinal disease. Ann Thorac Cardiovasc Surg 10(1):14-18
54. Lavini C, Morandi U (2007) Video-assisted minithoracotomy. A hybrid surgical technique between totally endoscopic and conventional approach. Abstr XIV Nat Congr Ital Soc Thor Endosc, Verona, Oct 11-13, 2007. Min Pneum 46(3 Suppl):6-7
55. Ferrari LB, Bedford LF (1990) General anaesthesia prior to treatment of anterior mediastinal masses in paediatric cancer patients. Anaesthesiology 72:991-995
56. Power CK, Buggy D, Keogh J (1997) Acute superior vena cava syndrome with airway obstruction following elective mediastinoscopy. Anaesthesia 52:989-992
57. Gossot D, Toledo L, Fritsch S et al (1996) Mediastinoscopy vs. thoracoscopy for mediastinal biopsy: Results of a prospective nonrandomized study. Chest 110:1328-133

CHAPTER 12
Surgical Anatomy of the Thymus Gland

Joseph B. Shrager

Introduction

The thymus is an H-shaped, bilobed gland that sits largely in the anterior mediastinum but extends also into the lower neck. In infancy through adolescence the gland it quite large, filling the entire anterior mediastinum and even bulging the pleurae out laterally into each hemithorax. With increasing age, as its role in maturation of the immune system diminishes, the thymus shrinks dramatically. By age 50, the normal thymus is a diminutive, mostly fatty structure.

Since the anterior mediastinum is an anatomical area that both contains and is bordered by a number of vital vascular and nervous structures, the thymus sits in direct relation to a number of important structures. An understanding of these relationships is critical to the performance of safe and effective thymic operative procedures. The location of the gland at a central region of the body which is accessible from a number of directions has given rise to a variety of different operative approaches to the thymus. These include transcervical approaches (TCT), thoracoscopic approaches (VATS), and "open" approaches by median sternotomy or thoracotomy.

We will describe some general aspects of thymic anatomy first, followed by a description of its relationships on all sides – anterior, posterior, inferior, superior, and lateral. Along the way, we will review how each of these points relates to the conduct of thymic operations.

General Anatomical Points

Any discussion of the anatomy of the thymus must differentiate between the main, intracapsular portion of the gland and the ectopic foci of thymic tissue which have been described to be fairly widely dispersed within the mediastinal and cervical fat, well outside of this main portion.

It is the main body of the gland that demonstrates the aforementioned H shape (Fig. 12.1), consisting of elongated left and right lobes that join at their central portions just caudal to the left innominate vein. The cephalad ends of each lobe become thin and are generally well-defined, whereas the caudal ends of each lobe are thicker and less easily definable as they fade into surrounding mediastinal fat as one approaches the diaphragm. It is the H-shaped main body of the gland which must be considered when describing anatomical relations (see following sec-

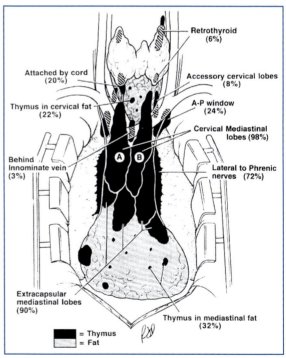

Fig. 12.1 Jaretski's classic depiction of the H-shaped "body" of the thymus, with small extracapsular foci of thymic tissue distributed widely in the mediastinal and cervical adipose tissues. The author would argue that tissues labeled "extracapsular mediastinal lobes" are as likely to be intracapsular and are included in virtually any "extended" thymectomy specimen, regardless of approach. Many of the other smaller ectopic sites are probably only resected by "maximal" thymectomy (reprinted with permission from [1])

tions). This H-shaped gland is contained in a fairly sturdy, thin fibrous capsule which allows the surgeon to place traction upon it and aids in differentiation from the surrounding fat. This feature is particularly important in minimally invasive approaches to thymectomy (VATS and TCT), which rely to some extent on this ability to retract on the gland. During TCT, for example, ties are placed on each of the upper poles of the gland early on in the dissection, and because the capsule is firm enough to allow substantial tension to be placed upon these upper poles, they can be used as "handles" during the dissection as it proceeds into the mediastinum.

The color of the gland is also important in the conduct of surgical procedures. Although it has been described as "salmon pink". I believe that this description overstates the difference in color between the thymus and the surrounding fatty tissue. In fact, the thymus itself is only very subtly different in color from the fat, with a somewhat deeper orangish-yellow and perhaps a very minor hint of pink. It is not only this slight difference in color, but also a clearer difference in texture, that allows the surgeon to differentiate thymic from fatty tissue. The gland itself, by virtue of its capsule, has a smoother, more lobulated appearance while the fat has a less coalesced, less solid appearance. Making this differentiation is particularly challenging during the most caudal portion of a thymic dissection as one approaches the diaphragm, in trying to separate the inferior thymic poles from surrounding normal fat. It is just this difficulty that renders it safest to remove all of this fat rather than try to differentiate it from intracapsular thymus.

"Ectopic" thymic tissue has been described in autopsy [2] and surgical studies [3] to be present at surprisingly high rates in the mediastinal and cervical fat in which the main body of the thymus is embedded (Fig. 12.1). The presence of these ectopic foci stimulated some surgeons to advocate more extensive procedures for thymic resection in myasthenia gravis (MG) which would include all, or at least more, of the tissue at these extrathymic sites. Most surgeons have settled upon the performance of an "extended" thymectomy for MG which includes the body of the gland and all of the mediastinal fat surrounding the thymus between the pleurae – an operation that can be performed via partial or full median sternotomy, TCT, or VATS, depending upon the experience of the surgeon. A few surgeons, however, advocate a "maximal" procedure that includes more aggressive resection of essentially all mediastinal and cervical fat through a combined sternotomy and cervical incision [4]. The absence of clear differences in remission rates following these differing procedures, however, calls into question the physiological significance of the extrathymic, ectopic foci in the pathogenesis of MG [5].

The blood supply to the body of the thymus is derived from small branches which arise from the superior and inferior thyroid arteries, the internal mammary vessels, and less importantly from the pericardiophrenic vessels. These branches can generally be controlled with surgical clips intraoperatively. The venous drainage, on the other hand, is primarily through 1-3 larger branches that drain directly off of the posterior aspect of the gland into the left innominate vein. These are usually of sufficient caliber that formal ligation and division is safest. Other smaller venous branches may accompany the arterial supply and can be clipped.

Anterior and Posterior Relations of the Body of the Gland

The anterior aspect of the intramediastinal portion of the thymus is applied to the endothoracic fascia lining the undersurface of the sternum and the most medial costal cartilages. As they ascend into the neck, the upper poles of the thymus run beneath the manubrium or the clavicular heads and then the strap muscles (sternothyroid and sternohyoid) until they trail off into the thyrothymic ligament at the level of the thyroid isthmus. In performing TCT, the upper poles are identified first, in fact, by blunt dissection beneath these strap muscles (Fig 12.2). When approaching the thymus from the chest, either by sternotomy or VATS, the upper poles are generally dissected last.

Just posterior to the upper poles lie the carotid sheaths containing the vagi, so it is important during dissection in this area to remain directly on the surface of the gland. The posterior aspect of the intramediastinal portion of the gland rests directly on the anterior pericardium. The plane between the gland and the pericardium is usually well defined and easily dissected since it consists of filmy connective tissue. When a tumor, however, breaches this plane and is adherent to the pericardium, it is of little consequence to resect a portion of the pericardium en bloc with the mass. Cephalad to the pericardial reflection, however, the distal ascending aorta/proximal aortic arch and the superior vena cava are in direct contact with the posterior surface of the thymus. Aggressive tumors may traverse the pericardium entirely and invade these structures, or they may invade them directly above the pericardial reflection, rendering complete resection a complicated endeavor which at times may even require cardiopulmonary bypass and complex vascular reconstructions.

The vagus and recurrent laryngeal nerves lie somewhat more posterior than the phrenic nerves but even more medially. Only if one has entered a deeper plane than is generally required to achieve a complete thymectomy are these nerves put at risk. This complication has, however, been described.

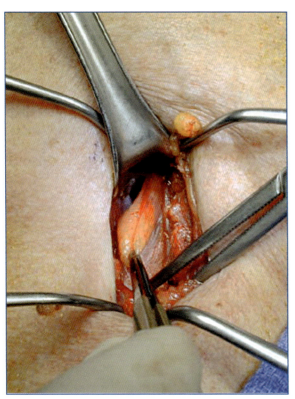

Fig. 12.2 Dissection of the upper pole of the left thymic lobe from beneath the strap muscles during performance of transcervical thymectomy. The view is from the patient's head

The upper portions of the two thymic poles run in the vast majority of cases anterior to the left innominate vein, so the vein usually sits at a posterior relation of the gland at this level, providing venous drainage as described above. If a thymic tumor invades the innominate vein, it may be resected without the need for reconstruction. If the superior vena cava is invaded by a tumor, it too can be resected either incompletely or circumferentially, but a normal lumen must be re-established by either prosthetic or autogenous tissue reconstruction to provide sufficient venous drainage of the upper body.

On occasion, one or even both of the poles of the thymus may run posterior to the innominate vein, and this may complicate the dissection during thymectomy. It is important to note that the phrenic nerves normally run just posterior to the innominate veins and that the most anterior and medial portion of the course of the phrenics is at the level of the vein and above. The phrenics are closest to the thymus, and thus most at risk, then, in this area (Fig. 12.3). When an upper thymic pole runs posterior to the vein, it must be dissected particularly carefully away from the phrenic, which will need to be identified carefully along its course in this region.

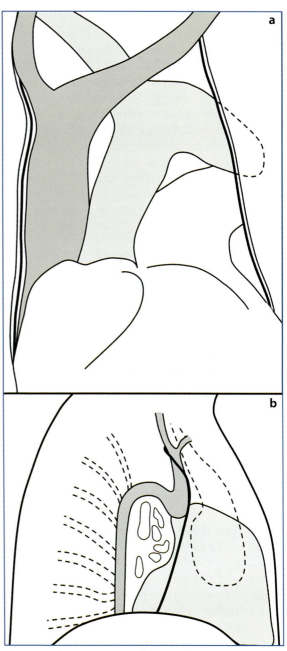

Fig. 12.3a,b **a** Anterior and **b** lateral (right) view of the course of the phrenic nerves as they descend from the neck into the mediastinum. The nerves are represented by the *bold black lines*. Note how the nerves are most anterior and medial, and thus most at risk during thymectomy, at approximately the level of the left innominate vein

A final posterior relation of the thymus in this region around the innominate vein is the thoracic duct. Although injury to the duct is rare during thymectomy, it can occur since the duct enters the posterior aspect of the venous system in the vicinity of the junction of the left internal jugular and innominate veins.

Superior and Inferior Relations of the Gland

At the most cephalad extent of the gland, the upper poles trail off into a thin vascular stalk termed the thyrothymic ligament. This occurs typically just below the thyroid isthmus. It is important to take the proximal end of resection fully into these vessels to assure that no thymic tissue is left in place at this margin when performing a thymectomy.

At its most caudal extent, the gland fades into surrounding mediastinal fat as it approaches the diaphragm (see previous description). A complete thymectomy generally includes resection of the bulk of this fat, all the way down to the diaphragm.

Lateral Relations of the Gland

Laterally in the mediastinum sit some of the most important relations of the gland – the pleurae and the phrenic nerves. The pleurae contact the entire lateral aspect of the gland on each side. Some surgeons believe the mediastinal pleurae must be resected en bloc with the gland to assure complete thymectomy in MG, while others feel that the gland can be separated from the pleurae. Certainly, in cases of thymic tumors, adjacent pleura must be resected with the tumor. Occasionally, a tumor will traverse the pleura to involve the adjacent lung. A portion of lung can easily be resected en bloc with the tumor to provide a complete resection. It is the close relationship between the pleurae and the thymus that results in pleural "drop" metastases being the most common site of recurrence of thymomas. For the same reason, during thymic resections for tumor, the pleural spaces and lungs are carefully examined for the presence of such sites of spread.

At the posterior-most point of the lateral surface over which the thymus and pleurae are apposed lie the phrenic nerves (Fig. 12.3). Most surgeons use the phrenics as the point which defines the posteriormost extent of dissection within the mediastinum during thymectomy, although occasionally functioning thymic tissue can extend even slightly beyond the phrenics. (I question, however, Jaretzki's suggestion that this occurs in approximately 70% of patients.) Thymic tumors may involve the phrenics, causing diaphragm paralysis, diaphragm elevation on imaging studies, and dyspnea. During surgery, it is acceptable to resect one phrenic nerve in cases of unilateral involvement if that will allow a complete resection. This is generally well tolerated in patients without significant underlying pulmonary disease. Bilateral phrenic nerve resection is, obviously, contraindicated. During TCT for MG, paralyzing agents are avoided so that if the dissection inadvertently approaches a phrenic nerve, the surgeon will become aware of this by the resulting diaphragmatic contraction.

Summary

The thymus sits in a central location that puts a number of vital structures at risk during its surgical resection and allows it to be approached from a variety of directions and incisions. Many of the potential complications of thymectomy – phrenic or recurrent nerve injury, bleeding, chylothorax – can be avoided if one has a detailed knowledge of the anatomy of the gland and its relations. Further, the limits of resection for thymic tumors are defined by these critical adjacent structures. The presence of small foci of thymic tissue ectopic to the main body of the gland serves as the pathophysiological basis for the more extensive procedures that have been proposed for thymectomy in MG. Whether the more frequent complications that result from these more extensive operations balance any small improvement in remission rates that may be achieved remains to be seen.

References

1. Jaretzki III A (1997) Thymectomy for myasthenia gravis: Analysis of the controversias regarding technique and results. Neurology 48(Suppl 5):S52-S63
2. Fukai I, Funato Y, Mizuno T et al (1991) Distribution of thymic tissue in the mediastinal adipose tissue. J Thorac Cardiovasc Surg 101:1099-1102
3. Jaretzki A III, Wolff M (1988) "Maximal" thymectomy for myasthenia gravis: surgical anatomy and operative technique. J Thorac Cardiovasc Surg 96:711-716
4. Jaretzki A III, Penn A, Younger D et al (1988) "Maximal" thymectomy for myasthenia gravis: Results. J Thorac Cardiovasc Surg 95:747-757
5. Shrager JB, Deeb ME, Mick R et al (2002) Transcervical thymectomy for myasthenia gravis achieves results comparable to thymectomy by sternotomy. Ann Thorac Surg 74:320-327

CHAPTER 13

Anesthesiological Problems in Thymus Gland Surgery

Vincenzo Lucio Indrizzi, Fabio Gazzotti, Maria Antonietta Fanigliulo, Alberto Tassi

Introduction

In Italy, about 15,000 patients are known to suffer from myasthenia gravis; however, in other cases the condition is not diagnosed or is confused with other pathologies. In Europe, it is thought that about 6 in 100,000 inhabitants are affected, and in the USA the incidence has been estimated at 20 cases for every 100,000 inhabitants. As regards the patient's age at onset, there are two peaks: between 20 and 40 years of age (women most affected) and 60 to 80 years (no difference between the sexes). This data would suggest that myasthenia gravis patients rarely undergo surgery; on the contrary, as thymectomy causes a significant improvement in symptoms in 40-90% of cases and complete remission of the disease in 25% of cases, surgery in patients with myasthenia gravis (especially in large centers with a Chest Surgery Unit) is not uncommon [1].

From an anesthesiological standpoint, the main problems to be tackled in myasthenia patients are: preoperative assessment and adaptation of pharmacological therapy in preparation for surgery, the choice of the type and dose of the agents to be used during surgery, postoperative intensive care (when to extubate, the duration of assisted ventilation required). Although patients with myasthenia gravis should be considered at high anesthesiological and surgical risk, it can be confidently stated that correct planning of the pre-, intra-, and postoperative periods makes it possible to perform the operation in good safety. However, the question is more complicated when the presence of myasthenia is unknown until the time of surgery and suddenly manifests when the patient comes round from the anesthetic with a delay in decurarization and severely compromised ventilatory function.

Preoperative Period

The anesthesiological consultation is of fundamental importance in preparing a myasthenic patient for surgery and although overall it is no different from that performed on any other patient who is to undergo surgery, it also includes a number of particular aspects. In the case of a myasthenic patient scheduled for thymectomy, as with any other type of surgery, it is above all essential to determine the gravity, duration, and evolution of the disease to adapt medical therapy so that the patient reaches the date of the operation in the best possible conditions.

Clinical Classification of Myasthenia Gravis

The most commonly used method for the clinical staging of myasthenia gravis patients is that derived from a study by Osserman [2] in 1971, whereby myasthenia patients are staged into four groups (see Table 13.1).

Table 13.1 Osserman's classification of myasthenia gravis based on symptoms and signs

Group		Description
Group I	Ocular involvement	Mild, nonspecific symptoms: double vision, drooping eyelids, no skeletal muscle symptoms, although the electromyogram may show myasthenic symptoms
Group II	A: generalized nonspecific symptoms	Mild ocular and skeletal symptoms without respiratory muscle involvement. Good response to therapy
	B: moderate generalized symptoms	Ocular and skeletal symptoms are evident but moderate: dysphagia, chewing difficulties and impaired speech. No respiratory muscle involvement. Response to therapy variable
Group III	Severe and acute generalized symptoms	Significant ocular and skeletal symptoms with respiratory muscle involvement. Poor response to therapy
Group IV	Advanced stage of disease	Rapidly worsening generalized symptoms with poor response to therapy

Thorough research into the various signs and symptoms of myasthenia allows the anesthetist to ascertain the degree and gravity of the condition, with important perioperative implications. *Weakness with ready exhaustion of the muscles* is typical of myasthenia patients and may be more or less evident, according to the gravity of the disease and the efficacy of medical treatment. The groups of skeletal muscles involved vary from case to case and may result in very different clinical conditions. The patient often complains of general tiredness and experiences difficult in performing even very simple movements (such as lifting an arm or clenching a fist). This feeling of weakness is exacerbated by physical activity and benefits from rest. In the most severe and advanced cases of myasthenia, the respiratory muscles are involved, with consequent significant ventilation difficulties. Eye muscles involvement is common and leads to the onset of *ptosis* and sight disorders, in particular *double vision*. *Chewing difficulties* should always be sought, as they suggest facial muscle involvement. This may be associated with lack of expressiveness and expression disorders, such as difficulties in smiling. Other particularly important symptoms are difficulties in talking (*dysphonia*) and swallowing (*dysphagia*). Together with respiratory muscles weakness, dysphagia in particular causes reduced cough efficacy, leading to secretion build up in the upper airways and consequent respiratory infections (which in turn may worsen myasthenic symptoms). In the most severe cases, eating difficulties lead to *general physical deterioration,* with altered electrolyte and protein values.

Preoperative assessment of a patient with myasthenia gravis should also take into consideration the possibility of the disease being accompanied by other autoimmune diseases. Rheumatoid arthritis and thyroid disorders are particularly common in this type of patient.

Chemistry Tests and Preoperative Procedures

Chemistry tests and instrumental procedures provide valuable information by specifying the indications provided by evaluation of the clinical signs and symptoms observed in the myasthenic patient, and identifying other concomitant pathologies (see Table 13.2).

In particular, *respiratory function tests* (evaluating vital capacity and pulmonary volume) and *inspiration and expiration tests* (for quantifying respiratory fatigue) make it possible to better identify respiratory muscles involvement and represent important elements for determining the duration of postopera-

Table 13.2 Preoperative blood chemistry tests and instrumental procedures in myasthenic patient

Complete blood count with formula	Electrocardiogram
Blood glucose, uricemia, azotemia and creatininemia	Chest X-ray
Electrolytes	Respiratory function tests
Liver function	Inspiration and expiration tests
Cholinesterase	Neck and chest CT
Creatine phosphokinase	Neck and chest MRI
Proteinemia and electrophoresis	
Full urine sediment examination	
Arterial blood gas analysis	

tive assisted ventilation. The pO_2 and pCO_2 values obtained from arterial blood gas analysis complete the evaluation of the respiratory situation in myasthenic patients.

Medical Therapy in Preparation for Surgery

Myasthenic patients should ideally be operated on during the remission stage of the disease; however, for obvious reasons this is often not possible (such as for emergency cases) and thymectomy is often the treatment of election for the specific pathology [3]. When adequately modulated and managed during the preoperative period, the medical treatment administered for myasthenia gravis can favorably affect both the anesthesiological and postoperative intensive care phases (see Table 13.3).

Anticholinesterase Agents

The medical therapy most commonly used for myasthenic patients is based on an oral administration of *anticholinesterase agents* [4] (see Table 13.4). These inhibit the enzyme anticholinesterase responsible for acetylcholine breakdown and therefore ultimately

Table 13.3 Medical treatment of myasthenia gravis

| Anticholinesterase agents |
| Immunosuppressive agents/immunomodulators |
| Plasmapheresis |
| γ-globulin |

Table 13.4 Anticholinesterase agents

Molecule	Trade name
Pyridostigmine	Mestinon
Neostigmine	Prostigmin
Ambenonium	Mytelase
Edrophonium (used in the diagnosis but not in the treatment of myasthenia)	Tensilon

prolong the action of the mediator on neuromuscular transmission [5]. They cause the onset of muscarinic effects, with consequent side effects such as bradycardia, increased salivation, sudoration and gastric secretion, increased gastrointestinal and uterine motility, and broncospasm.

The most frequently used anticholinesterase agent is undoubtedly pyridostigmine *(Mestinon)*, which is administered orally and has a lasting effect and less severe side effects.

The continuation or suspension of anticholinesterase therapy in view of surgery continues to be controversial. Anticholinesterase agents are known to create problems while under anesthetic as they strengthen vagal responses, make muscle relaxation more problematic, prolong the duration of the narcotic agents, and slowdown metabolism and elimination of ester-based local anesthetic. They can also cause the onset of a cholinergic attack in the immediate postthymectomy period. Their effect of prolonging the activity of acetylcholine at the postsynaptic membrane in a situation in which the removal of the thymus gland has eliminated the main cause of the myasthenia gravis leads to the onset of overdose with muscular fatigue and weakness that can often be difficult to distinguish from those of a true myasthenic attack. For the above reasons, these drugs should be suspended at least 4 days before thymectomy surgery. Suspension can be well tolerated in myasthenic patients with initial and mild forms of the disease; however it can be harmful in the more severe forms, with the possibility of causing a myasthenic attack close to the operation. One frequently adopted approach is to reduce anticholinesterase agents by 20% before the operation.

From a practical standpoint, anticholinesterase medication can be suspended if this is well tolerated by the patient; however in all other cases, it can be suspended on the morning of the operation (the thymectomy should be scheduled as the first operation of the day for this reason) or alternatively not suspended at all (for example, thymectomy scheduled for the early afternoon in patients with severe and acute forms of the disease). One approach is to suspend medication on the morning of surgery to cause muscle weakness and atonia to facilitate orotracheal intubation without use of muscle relaxants. Whatever approach adopted, the anesthetist must adapt his/her intra- and postoperative behavior to suit each individual patient's situation, without hazardous generalizations.

Immunosuppressive Agents

The rationale applied to the use of *immunosuppressive agents* (corticosteroids, azathioprine, cyclophosphamide, cyclosporine, methotrexate and the more recent mycophenolate mofetil, tacrolimus, and rituximab) in treating myasthenia gravis is to restrict synthesis of anticholinergic receptor antibody by the body's immune system. These are used in combination with anticholinesterase drugs when monotherapy is inadequate [4]. To avoid a sudden acute relapse of myasthenia gravis in response to the suspension of the immunosuppressant therapy, administration is not usually interrupted for thymectomy.

Plasmapheresis

The use of *plasmapheresis* removing anticholinergic receptor antibodies from the circulation, as an alternative to high doses of anticholinesterase medication causes a clear improvement in myasthenia symptoms and is performed as preparation for surgical removal of the thymus gland above all in the most serious and acute cases of myasthenia gravis [6]. This technique offers the advantages of improving postoperative respiratory function, thus shortening intensive care stays and assisted ventilation. It is useful to remember that the use of plasmapheresis significantly reduces serum concentrations of pseudocholinesterase, which should be borne in mind when a depolarizing muscle relaxant such as succinylcholine is used for orotracheal intubation.

Human Immunoglobulin

Treatment with *γ-globulin* provides a further therapeutic alternative to anticholinesterase agents. They are administered intravenously at high doses (0.4 gr/Kg/die) and cause a significant reduction in myasthenia symptoms, with an evident improvement in the general clinical situation [7].

Intraoperative Period

During the delicate intraoperative phase, in the case of myasthenic patients, the most important factor is undoubtedly related to the drugs to be used to induce and maintain the general anesthesia. In myasthenia gravis, the transmission of the nerve impulse to the neuromuscular junction is further depressed by the action of the agents most commonly used during general anesthesia. The anesthesiological technique and doses used must consequently be suited to the pathological condition in question, and pre- and postoperative monitoring of the patient's neuromuscular function is essential. These preliminary considerations take on greater importance if we consider that the possibility of early extubation of the patient after the operation is highly conditioned by both the gravity of the disease and the consequences of the general anesthesia.

Pharmacological Interactions in Myasthenia Gravis

Many agents, and not merely those most commonly used for anesthesia, are able to depress the already compromised neuromuscular function in myasthenia gravis patients to a varying extent. The mechanisms of action can be numerous and both pre- and postsynaptic [8]. Certain pharmacological substances are able to cause a clinical worsening in the myasthenia symptoms with high frequencies and dramatic effects. Others are relatively harmful, but may in any case have important and detrimental affects on muscular strength. Others still have effects that can only be considered as potentially hazardous but rarely observable and require great care when used on patients with myasthenia [9]. Use of these kinds of drugs in myasthenia gravis patients must always be justified by real necessity and careful risk-benefit analysis for each individual patient. For each case, the severity of the illness and its symptoms must be considered, with particular attention, above all, on symptoms of respiratory failure.

The active ingredients able to interfere with previously impaired neuromuscular function can be divided into two main groups: nonanesthetic agents and agents used for anesthesia.

Nonanesthetic Agents

The most frequently-used medicines able to depress a previously compromised neuromuscular function in

Table 13.5 Nonanesthetic agents able to depress neuromuscular function

Antiarrhythmics	Procaine amide, quinidine
Antibiotics	Gentamycin, amikacin, tobramycin, streptomycin, kanamycin Tetracycline, doxycycline, lymecycline, minocycline, oxytetracycline Ciprofloxacin, acrosoxacin, cinoxacin, nalidixic acid, norfloxacin, ofloxacin Polymyxin B, colistin Telithromycin
Antimalarials	Chloroquine, hydroxychloroquine
Antirheumatic agents	Penicillamine
Antispasmodics	Flavoxate, oxybutinin, propantheline
Beta-blockers	Propanolol, atenolol, acebutolol, betaxolol, bisoprolol, carvedilol, celiprolol, esmolol, labetalol, metoprolol, nadolol, oxprenolol, pindolol, sotalol, timolol
Antiepileptic agents	Phenytoin
Drugs used in psychiatry	Chlorpromazine, clozapine, flupenthixol, fluphenazine, loxapine, methotrimeprazine, oxypertine, pericyazine, perphenazine, pimozide, risperidone, sulpiride, thioridazine, trifluoroperazine, zuclopenthixol Lithium Phenelzine, isocarboxazid, tranylcypromine

From: http://www.mgauk.org/main/mgdrugs1.htm, modified

patients with myasthenia gravis include cardiac and psychotropic agents and certain antibiotics [9]; however, there is a long list of active ingredients that need to be used with care in myasthenic patients (see Table 13.5).

Cardiac Agents

Many cardiac agents included in the Vaughan-Williams classification (1970) worsen the symptoms of myasthenia gravis, through various different mechanisms. Class I antiarrhythmic drugs, most notably procainamide (IA), depress the action potential due to their local anesthetic effect and should consequently be avoided or used with great care; these include lidocaine (IB), which would appear to be the safest [9]. Beta-blockers (Class II), such as propanolol, must be used with great care as, in combination with anticholinesterase agents, they can cause severe bradycardia [10]. Calcium inhibitors (Class IV), like verapamile, reduce the pre- and postsynaptic conductance of calcium channels and consequently also require great care when used [11]. Diuretic agents can cause potassium deficiency and can influence neuromuscular transmission, which is depressed by furosemide at low doses and facilitated at high doses [12].

Psychotropic Agents

Of the various substances routinely used in epilepsy therapy, trimethiadone is able to cause simil-myasthenic syndromes in patients with myasthenia [13, 14], and is therefore hazardous on account of its interference with neuromuscular transmission. Diphenylhydantoin and carbamazepine may be used with caution when absolutely essential, as they present a relative risk.

Antibiotics

Antibiotics used in the perioperative period can worsen myasthenia symptoms with a mechanism that manifests on both a pre- and post synaptic level. Aminoglycosides, in particular, can strengthen neuromuscular blockade and their effects are poorly antagonized by use of anticholinesterase agents [15]. Fluoroquinolone antibiotics (cyprofloxacin, norfloxacin, trovafloxacin, levofloxacin, etc.) have also been found to heighten muscular weakness in patients with myasthenia gravis, and in some cases, highlighted the presence of the illness when it was still unknown [16, 17]. Cholistin, clindamycin, and lincomycin should also be used with caution and tetracyclines should be administered orally, avoiding intravenous administration.

Anesthetic Agents

Many of the agents used for the various phases of general or local anesthesia can interfere with neuromuscular transmission, and consequently require special caution when administered to myasthenic patients (see Table 13.6).

Curariform Agents

Of the various drugs used to induce and maintain general anesthesia, curariform drugs are those that arouse the greatest concern when administered to patients with myasthenia gravis. Their mechanism of action, which is closely connected to the physiopathology of myasthenia, makes them hazardous

Table 13.6 Anesthetic agents interfering with neuromuscular transmission

Potent neuromuscular transmission depressors	Agents with a mild to no affect on neuromuscular transmission
Depolarizing and nondepolarizing curariform agents	Propofol
Halogenated anesthetics	Barbiturates
Ketamine	Etomidate Droperidol
Benzodiazepine (relative risk)	Opioids
Local anesthetics (relative risk)	Nitrogen protoxide

and great caution is therefore required during use. Moreover, they should only be used when neuromuscular function is monitored closely (muscular response following electrical stimulation of peripheral motor nerves, generally the ulnar nerve).

Muscle relaxants are conventionally classified according to their mechanism of action on the neuromuscular junction, in the case of both depolarizing and nondepolarizing curariform agents.

In the operating theatre, the method of election for monitoring neuromuscular function during surgery and in the postoperative period is defined TOF ("train of four"), in which four consecutive electrical stimuli (2 Hz twitches) are sent for 2 seconds (0.5 second interval), causing a different muscular response according to the efficiency of neuromuscular transmission. Before administering the muscle relaxant, a reference muscle response to four electric stimuli is aroused (T1, T2, T3, T4) and identified as a "control" measurement (Tc): it is characterized by the fact that it is always the same (i.e., T1=T2=T3=T4=Tc). In the presence of nondepolarizing blockade, muscular response to T1 will be inferior to Tc, and T4<T3<T2<T1; the relationship between T4 and T1 is considered as a reference for quantifying the degree of curarization. In the case of a depolarizing blockade (succinylcholine), Tc>T1 but T1=T4.

Depolarizing Curariform Agents

Succinylcholine, a curariform agent with a depolarizing action on the neuromuscular junction, is generally used to create the ideal conditions for orotracheal intubation in the case of general anesthetic. Patients with myasthenia gravis show a certain resistance to depolarizing agents, probably on account of the reduced number of cholinergic receptors typical of the disease and on which these agents perform their specific action [18, 19]. The dose of succinylcholine needed to perform rapid sequence orotracheal intubation is higher (1.5-2 mg/Kg) in myasthenic patients than in normal ones. The effects of succinylcholine in myasthenia gravis patients are therefore very variable: the depletion of plasma cholinesterase due to plasmapheresis or their inhibition by anticholinesterase agents influences the metabolism of the agent, prolonging neuromuscular blockade [20]. The same applies for mivacurium, a short half-life nondepolarizing curariform agent that could be an ideal substitute for succinylcholine [21]. Again, repeated doses of succinylcholine could obtain prolonged muscle relaxation on account of the establishment of type II blockade. On account of these very variable and unpredictable effects, most authors believe the use of depolarizing curariform agents in myasthenia gravis is risky and to be avoided when alternatives exist.

Nondepolarizing Curariform Agents

Patients with myasthenia gravis are very sensitive to the action of nondepolarizing muscle relaxants, which must only be used when truly indispensable and always under close supervision and neuromuscular function monitoring. It is impossible to establish general dosage rules for the use of these agents in patients with myasthenia gravis as the sensitivity of each patient is individual and depends on the degree of illness and the extent to which it affects the various muscle groups. However, the doses must be very low and 1/4 to 1/8 those used in normal patients [9].

Long-action nondepolarizing muscle-relaxants such as pancuronium are generally avoided in cases of myasthenia gravis, although it has been stated in literature that a dose of 0.005-0.01 mg/Kg^{-1} achieves a blockade equal to that which would be achieved in a nonmyasthenic patient [22].

The drugs currently used to obtain muscular resolution during surgery generally have an intermediate duration of action, such as vecuronium, atracurium, cis-atracurium.

Vecuronium is generally used in myasthenic subjects at a dose of between 0.005 and 0.03 mg/Kg^{-1}. This interval depends on the differing individual sensitivity of each single subject and the degree of evolution of the myasthenia [9]. There is evidence that patients with generalized myasthenia are more sensitive to the action of vecuronium than those with primarily ocular involvement [23], whereas serum negativity to anti-Ach antibodies does not seem to make patients more resistant than those with serum positive myasthenia [24].

Atracurium is considered the nondepolarizing curariform muscle relaxant best suited for use in myasthenia patients due to its pharmacokinetics (elimination through the Hoffmann effect) that is thought to make the recovery of neuromuscular function very similar to that observed in normal subjects: the recommended dose would appear to be around 0.1 mg/Kg^{-1} [9, 25]. A number of authors also report that also in the case of atracurium there is a great variability in the amount of agent required to obtain similar results between myasthenic patients and healthy subjects [18, 26].

Myasthenic patients are also more sensitive than healthy subjects to cisatracurium and doses of 0.05 mg/Kg^{-1} cause onset of shorter and more potent neuromuscular blockade [27]. Furthermore, the simultaneous use of sevoflurane to maintain general anesthesia makes it possible to obtain complete neuromuscular blockade with even lower doses equal to 0.025 mg/Kg^{-1} [27].

Short half-life nondepolarizing muscle relaxants (mivacurium, rocuronium) have been used on patients with myasthenia. Findings reported in literature confirm the greater sensitivity of myasthenia patients to the action of mivacurium, which therefore calls for a reduction in dose when using this agent [28]; in any case, its short half-life could facilitate more rapid recovery of muscular resolution in the postoperative period [29]. However, metabolism and breakdown of the agent depend largely on the action of plasma cholinesterase, which calls for great caution in the use of mivacurium in myasthenic patients being treated with anticholinesterase agents, especially when taken on the same day as the operation [18].

Halogenated Anesthetics

The muscle relaxant effect of halogenated anesthetics (halothane, isoflurane, enflurane, sevoflurane, desflurane), potent anesthetics for inhalation, on healthy subjects [30] has been known for a long time; this action is heightened in myasthenic patients. Halogenated anesthetics are highly lipophilic substances and modify the structure of the plasma membrane inside which the postsynaptic cholinergic receptor is located, making it less sensitive to the action of acetylcholine. In those cases in which muscular relaxation is not considered to be fundamental for the performance of the operation, the halogenated ethers commonly used in clinical practice for general anesthesia maintenance are able to achieve satisfactory muscular resolution when used alone. If a muscle relaxant is simultaneously used, the dose should be further reduced. These concepts are valid in both healthy and, above all, myasthenic patients.

The increased potency of neuromuscular blockade in myasthenic patients when using halothane, isoflurane, and enflurane has been extensively documented in studies completed on the subject for many years [30-34].

One of the halogenated ethers currently most frequently used is sevoflurane, a potent neuromuscular transmission inhibitor [35], which was used as a single anesthetic agent able to provide satisfactory neuromuscular relaxation with MAC values of between 0.5-0.7% and 4% and in the absence of other muscular resolution agents in pediatric and adult myasthenic patients undergoing general surgery and transsternal thymectomy [18, 36, 37].

Desflurane is the halogenated ether most recently introduced into anesthesiological practice. It causes a reduction in muscle relaxant requirements in healthy patients and in some cases it has been used alone, without the aid of muscle relaxants in surgery on myasthenic patients [38, 39].

Hypnotic and Neuroleptic Agents

Propofol is currently the most frequently used sedative. It has been extensively used in cases of myasthenia, for both the induction and maintenance of general anesthesia, above all in combination with sevoflurane and especially, with remifentanil in continuous infusion, in what is known as total intravenous anesthesia (TIVA) [40-42]. This agent reduces upper airway reflexes and produces favorable conditions for orotracheal intubation even in the absence of curariform agents [43]. On account of its short half-life, it is eliminated rapidly to favor fast recovery and early postoperative extubation: characteristics that make it particularly well suited to myasthenic patients [42].

Barbiturates would appear to have little effect on neuromuscular transmission. On a presynaptic level, they increase the quantity of acetylcholine freed whereas, postsynaptically, they reduce receptor sensitivity, thus making the final effect null [9]. Etomidate would appear to have a similar action.

Ketamine, on the other hand, could worsen neuromuscular blockade due to its desensitizing effect on the postsynaptic receptors [9].

Benzodiazepines should be used with care and at reduced doses in myasthenic patients, in that its muscle relaxant action takes place in the marrow, thus strengthening the inhibiting action of GABA on muscle tone [9].

Droperidol does not affect neuromuscular transmission at all, whereas a slight effect can be obtained by phenothiazine, by desensitizing the postsynaptic membrane receptors.

Morphine and Other Opioids

Morphine, its derivates and synthetic opioids (especially fentanyl) can be used in myasthenic patients as they do not have any particular affect on neuromuscular transmission; however, the risk of causing respiratory depression calls for caution and close monitoring, especially when used as premedication.

Remifentanil merits a separate comment. This very potent, short half-life agent is used almost exclusively as a continuous infusion. Literature provides extensive evidence of its use in myasthenic patients, in combination with propofol (TIVA) or halogenated ethers (sevoflurane and desflurane) [40, 41, 44, 45]. Its advantages when used on patients with myasthenia gravis could be primarily attributed to its very rapid metabolism when the continuous infusion is interrupted, and for operations not requiring great muscular relaxation, to the possibility of avoiding the use of nondepolarizing muscle relaxants to adapt the patient to mechanical ventilation.

Local Anesthetics

It has been known for some time that, on account of their desensitization of the postsynaptic membrane, local anesthetic agents depress neuromuscular transmission [46]; this occurs if the agent reaches high blood levels. In this sense, ester-based local anesthetics (procaine, tetracaine) are more dangerous, because they are metabolized by plasma cholinesterase, which interacts with the anticholinesterase agents the myasthenic patient is receiving. Amino-amide agents (lidocaine, mepivacaine, bupivacain, levo-bupivacaine) can be used with caution and at reduced doses in patients with myasthenia gravis. In actual fact, combining general anesthesia and local anesthesia techniques has a number of advantages, especially as regards both intra- and postoperative pain control. The use of thoracic epidural anesthetic and thoracic paravertebral blockade, in association with general anesthetic, is widely used and has been amply documented in the literature [18, 39, 44, 47]. The reduction in surgical stress and pain control improve postsurgical outcome and favor a more rapid recovery of respiratory function, especially when employing conservative surgical techniques of different kinds (transsternal or thoracic thymectomy).

Postoperative Period

Postoperative management of the myasthenic patient remains a key issue. The possibility of developing respiratory failure, especially after major surgery and thymectomy, has been amply documented and is the most feared problem during the intensive care of this type of patient [48]. The first significant cases published between 1940 and 1960 reported high surgical mortality of between 10 and 30% [49, 50]. These very unreassuring percentages obviously encouraged a very cautious attitude in the postoperative period and the adoption of precautionary measures that are no longer in use today. Intraoperative tracheotomy was performed in almost all patients and controlled ventilation was continued for at least 1 week after surgery and gradually suspended with the aid of anticholinesterase agents. These measures made it possible to reduce mortality to 1-3% [9].

Thorough preoperative evaluation of myasthenic patients, appropriate monitoring and medical treatment, the use of increasingly safe anesthesia agents and techniques, and the significant progress achieved in postoperative intensive care have now made the need to perform tracheotomy exceedingly rare and, when necessary, it is possible to obtain very rapid extubation times, with good recovery of spontaneous breathing.

Another greatly disputed subject is that relating to the precociousness of extubation of myasthenic patients undergoing surgery. In most cases, extubation is performed early, either in the theatre or in the recovery room from 30 minutes to 2 hours after the end of surgery, provided certain essential conditions are present (patient awake and cooperative, adequate muscular strength, good spirometric and blood gas values, and adequate heating and monitoring) [9]. In other cases, the patients may require controlled ventilation for a longer period of up to 24 hours [9]. In addition to the patient's clinical condition and the evolution of the disease, this variability is also influenced by surgical and anesthesiological techniques used during the operation. For example, transcervical thymectomy would appear to be less prone to postoperative respiratory failure than the transsternal technique, since in the former the integrity of the chest wall is preserved to a greater degree and consequently so are normal pulmonary pressure values, especially vital capacity [1].

It would be very useful to identify the predictive factors able to indicate the possibility of early extubation of the myasthenic patient even before surgery. One attempt in this sense (1974) suggested that in a myasthenic patient with ocular symptoms and positive history of respiratory failure or myasthenic attack and with a vital capacity lower than 2 liters, it was prudent to perform a preventative intraoperative tracheotomy on account of the high possibility of lengthy postoperative respiratory assistance [48]. A later study conducted in 1975 suggested that postoperative respiratory assistance was associated to a pulmonary vital capacity, measured before the operation, of less than 2 liters and simultaneous presence of bulbar symptoms (especially dysphagia), thymoma, and age above 50 [51] (see Table 13.7).

A retrospective analytical study published in 1980 on myasthenic patients undergoing transsternal thymectomy identified four risk factors correlated to the need for postoperative respiratory assistance [52]: duration of myasthenia gravis >6 years, prior episodes of respiratory insufficiency correlated to myasthenia or chronic respiratory disease, daily dose of pyridostigmine higher than 750 mg, and preoperative vital capacity of less than 2.9 liters. Each of these parameters was assigned a score, whose sum produced a maximum rating of 34. If the sum of the various scores was higher than 12, mechanical ventilation was considered necessary; an area of uncertainty was associated to scores of between 10 and 12, and early extubation was performed if the score was below 10 (see Table 13.8). The attempt to validate this score by applying it to different groups of myasthenic patients undergoing thymectomy produced less than convincing results, rather highlighting the predictive importance of certain symptoms correlated to the gravity of the myasthenia, in particular bulbar involvement with talking difficulties and/or dysphagia [53].

To guarantee early extubation after thymectomy, the patient's preoperative respiratory strength and

Table 13.7 Loach's predicting criteria for postoperative respiratory assistance [51]

Vital capacity of less than 2 l in the preoperative period
Presence of thymoma
Presence of bulbar involvement (dysphagia)
Age above 50 years

Table 13.8 Leventhal's score for prediction of the need for postoperative mechanical ventilation in myasthenia gravis [52]

Duration of myasthenia ≥6 years	12
Prior respiratory failure and/or COPD	10
Daily dose of pyridostigmin >750 mg	8
Vital capacity <2.9 liters	6
Maximum rating	34
If <10: rapid extubation	
If between 10 and 12: uncertainty	
If >12: certain mechanical ventilation	

consequently coughing reflex were considered important predictive parameters. The study of the pulmonary volume and of peak inspiration and expiration pressures therefore represents a valuable and essential evaluation in myasthenic patients scheduled for surgery [54, 55].

The above comments suggest that there are still no certain predictive criteria that can be applied in a general way to all myasthenic patients due to have surgery. Evaluation must be performed on a case-by-case basis, considering the many variables that can affect the postoperative course, without hazardous generalizations. However, it can be said that tracheotomy is rarely performed nowadays and only in those patients who will require mechanical ventilation for more than 10 days after the operation [1].

It is also important to use those anesthesiological techniques that, by guaranteeing ever-greater safety to myasthenic patients, also favor rapid extubation, with minimal use of postoperative respiratory assistance.

As discussed at length in the previous paragraphs, both depolarizing and nondepolarizing curariform agents should be avoided where possible in myasthenic patients. Most surgery can be performed without using muscle relaxants and this applies also to thymectomies. Very often, muscle relaxant use is only needed to obtain ideal conditions for orotracheal intubation. The use of agents for general anesthesia induction such as propofol (which provides adequate conditions for easy orotracheal intubation [43]), in combination with local anesthesia of the laryngeal inlet with lidocaine, make it possible to avoid using muscle relaxants for induction. To maintain anesthesia, halogenated ethers (such as sevoflurane and desflurane) are able to grant the surgeon a more than satisfactory condition of muscular relaxation for the whole operation. If the use of nondepolarizing agents (vecuronium, atracurium, cis-atracurium) is considered to be essential, their dosage should be reduced to as little as 1/8 of that usually used. It should, however, be remembered that, in myasthenic patients, intra- and postoperative monitoring of the neuromuscular function (mechanographical and electrographical) is essential, regardless of the anesthetic agents employed.

General anesthesia can be maintained using primarily inhalatory techniques with halogenated anesthetics or totally intravenous anesthetic with a continuous infusion of propofol and remifentanil. When anesthesia maintenance using halogenated anesthetics is chosen, short half-life agents such as sevoflurane and desflurane should be used. As these substances do not have any analgesic properties, simultaneous use of bolus fentanyl or continuous intravenous infusion of remifentanil will be required for postoperative pain relief. In recent years, the use of local anesthetic (thoracic epidural, thoracic paravertebral blockade, subarachnoid anesthesia) with administration of long-lasting anesthetic agents (bupivacaine, levo-bupivacaine, ropivacaine) has become increasingly widespread and makes it possible to maintain a lighter general anesthetic plan but optimal intra and postoperative pain control [44, 47]. Totally intravenous analgesia (TIVA and TIVA-TCI i.e., target control infusion) is based on a simultaneous infusion of propofol and remifentanil, agents with a short half-lives and that do not leave an "anesthetic tail," thus favoring rapid postoperative recovery and early extubation [41]. Comparisons conducted on myasthenic patients undergoing transsternal thymectomy between two general anesthesia techniques, one based on maintenance with a continuous infusion of propofol and the other with sevoflurane by inhalation, without the use of muscle relaxants in either case, showed no difference between the groups in relation to the patients' postoperative recovery with regard to both consciousness and neuromuscular function. In all cases, extubation was performed while still in the theatre, before transferring the patients to intensive care [42].

Despite the safety of the anesthesiological techniques currently used, it must always be remembered that myasthenic patients are nevertheless at high risk and that, despite having performed rapid extubation, it would be imprudent not to transfer the patient to intensive care for 24-48 hours after surgery. In this phase, neuromuscular and respiratory function monitoring (spirometry and blood gas tests) are essential to improving outcome. Pain control is another important factor in this phase and in many cases benefits can be obtained from the local anesthesia techniques that can be implemented (thoracic epidural, thoracic paravertebral block), which should consequently be performed whenever possible in the case of myasthenic patients. Generally speaking, the most frequently used analgesic agents are morphine and opioids in general (such as meperidine, fentanyl, and sufentanil) [1]. It is important to remember that with a mechanism that is not yet completely clear, the effects of morphine are made more potent by anticholinesterase agents: doses should therefore be reduced in myasthenic patients on medical therapy to as little as one third the normal value [1].

The management of anticholinesterase therapy after thymectomy is an important part of the postoperative stage. This phase is characterized by two contrasting conditions: on the one hand there is a variable timeframe (from a few to 48 hours) in which the patient does not need anticholinesterase agents and on the other, and in particular after thymectomy, the sensitivity to anticholinesterase agents is generally increased. In some cases, treatment is reinstated very shortly after reawakening, possible at lower doses and gradually ramped up. In other cases, after considering compatibly with the patient's symptoms, it is recommended later, up to 3-4 days after the operation. If the patient undergoes plasmapheresis before surgery, the reintroduction of anticholinesterase therapy may be further postponed or, in some cases, definitively suspended. It has in fact been observed that 1 year after thymectomy, in 30% of cases there is a complete remission of the myasthenia gravis and 80% undergo a clear improvement in symptoms [1, 56].

References

1. Kaplan JA, Slinger PD (2003) Thoracic anesthesia, 3rd edn. Elsevier Science,pp 281-294
2. Osserman KE, Genkins G (1971) Studies in myasthenia gravis: Review of a twenty-year experience in over 1,200 patients. J Mt Sinai Hosp 38:497-503
3. Hermann C, Lindstrom JM, Kessey JC et al (1985) Myasthenia gravis – Current concepts. West J Med 142:797
4. Romi F, Gilhus NE, Aarli JA (2005) Myasthenia gravis: Clinical, immunological, and therapeutic advance. Acta Neurol Scand 111:134-141
5. Millard CB, Bromfield CA (1995) Anticholinesterases: Medical applications of neurochemical principles. J Neurochem 64:1909-1918
6. Gaidos P, Chevret S, Toyka K (2002) Plasma exchange for myasthenia gravis. Cochrane Database Syst Rev 4:CD002275
7. Gaidos P, Chevret S, Toyka K (2003) Intravenous immunoglobulin for myasthenia gravis. Cochrane Database Syst Rev 2:CD002277
8. Philip E, Levarenne J, Dordain G (1985) Myasthénie et médicaments: Évaluation critique des contre-indications. Press Med 14, 515-516
9. Martin C, Auffray JP (1990) Il periodo perioperatorio del miastenico. Anestesia Rianimazione, 36657 C[10]. EMC, Roma, p 8
10. Viby-Mogensen J (1985) Interaction of other drugs with muscle relaxants. In: Katz RJ (ed) Muscle relaxants. Basic and critical aspects. Gune and Stratton, Orlando, pp 233-256
11. Swash M, Ingram DA (1992) Adverse effect of verapamil in myasthenia gravis. Muscle Nerve 15(3):396-398
12. Scappaticci KA, Ham JA, Sohn J et al (1982) Effects of furosemide on the neuromuscolar junction. Anesthesiology 57:381-388
13. Rall TW, Schleifer LS (1985) Drugs effective in the therapy of the epilepsies. In: Goodman LS, Gilman A (eds) The pharmacological basis of therapeutics. MacMillan Publishing Co., New York, pp 446-472
14. Booker HE, Chun RW, Sanguini M (1970) Myasthenia gravis syndrome associated with trimethadione. JAMA 212(13):2262-2263
15. Orts A, Marti JL, Baltar I et al (1979) Inhibition neuro-musculaire de nouveaux antibiotiques aminoglucosids. Ann Anesthesiol Fr 20:25-30
16. Gunduz A, Turedi S, Kalkan A et al (2006) Levofloxacin induced myasthenia crisis. Emerg Med J 23:662
17. Sieb JP (1998) Fluoroquinolone antibiotics block neuromuscolar transmission. Neurology 50:804-807
18. Abel M, Eisenkraft JB (2002) Anesthetic implications in myasthenia gravis. Mt Sinai J Med 69:31-37
19. Eisenkraft JB, Book VJ, Mann SM et al (1988) Resistance to succinylcholine in myasthenia gravis: A dose-response study. Anesthesiology 69:760-763
20. Baraka A (1992) Suxamethonium block in the myasthenic patient. Correlation with plasma cholinesterase. Anesthesia 47:217-219
21. Seigne RD, Scott RP (1994) Mivacurium chloride and myasthenia gravis. Br J Anaesth 72:468-469
22. Blitt CD, Wright WA, Peat J (1975) Pancuronium and the patient with myasthenia gravis. Anesthesiology 42:624-626
23. Itoh H, Shibata K, Nitta S (2001) Difference in sensitivity to vecuronium between patients with ocular and generalized myasthenia gravis. Br J Anaesth 87(6):885-889
24. Itoh H, Shibata K, Nitta S (2002) Sensitivity to vecuronium in seropositive and seronegative patients with myasthenia gravis. Anesth Analg 95(1):109-113
25. Mann R, Blobner M, Jelen-Esselbom S et al (2000) Preanesthetic train-of-four fade predicts the atracurium requirement of myasthenia gravis patients. Anesthesiology 93(2):346-350
26. Smith CE, Donati F, Bevin DR (1989) Cumulative dose-response curves for atracurium in patients with myasthenia gravis. Can J Anaesth 36:402-406
27. Baraka AS, Siddik S, Kawkabani NI (1999) Cisatracurium in a myasthenic patient undergoing thymectomy. Can J Anesth 46(8):779-782
27. Baraka AS, Taha SK, Kawkabani NI (2000) Neuromuscular interaction of sevoflurane-cisatracurium in a myasthenic patient. Can J Anesth 47(6):562-565

28. Seigne RD, Scott RP (1994) Mivacurium chloride and myasthenia gravis. Br J Anaesth 72:468-469
29. Cordero Escobar I, Benitez Tang SM, Parisi Lopez N (2002) Use of mivacurium chloride during transsternal thymectomy in myasthenic patient. Rev Esp Anestesiol Reanim 49(7):360-364
30. Gissen AJ, Karris JH, Nastuk VL (1966) Effect of halothane on neuromuscular transmission. JAMA 197:770-774
31. Nilsson E, Muller K (1990) Neuromuscolar effects of isoflurane in patients with myasthenia gravis. Acta Anaesth Scand 34:126-131
32. Kadosaki M, Enzan K, Horiguchi T et al (1993) Severity of myasthenia gravis is related to the degree of neuromuscular blocking effect by isoflurane. Masui 42:906-909
33. Eisenkraft JB, Papatestas AE, Sivak M (1984) Neuromuscolar effects of halogenated agents in patients with myasthenia gravis (abstract). Anesthesiology 61:A307
34. Russel SH, Hood JR, Campkin M (1993) Neuromuscolar effects of enflurane in myasthenia gravis (abstract) Br J Anaesth 71:766P
35. Nitahara K, Sugi Y, Higa K et al (2007) Neuromuscolar effects of sevoflurane in myasthenia gravis patients. Br J Anaesth 98(3):337-341
36. Kiran U, Choudhury M, Saxena L et al (2000) Sevoflurane as a sole anaesthetic agent for thymectomy in myasthenia gravis. Acta Anaesth Scand 44:351-353
37. Baraka A, Siddik S, el Rassi T et al (2000) Sevoflurane anesthesia in a myasthenic patient undergoing transternal thymectomy. Middle East J Anesthesiol 15(6):603-609
38. Caldwell JE, Laster MJ, Magorian T et al (1991) The neuromuscolar effects of desflurane alone and combined with pancuronium or succinylcholine in humans. Anesthesiology 74:412-418
39. Hubler M, Litz RJ, Albrecht DM (2000) Combination of balanced and regional anaesthesia for minimally invasive surgery in a patient with myasthenia gravis. Eur J Anaesthesiol 17(5):325-328
40. Ng JM (2006) Total intravenous anesthesia with propofol and remifentanil for video-assisted thoracoscopic thymectomy in patients with myasthenia gravis. Anesth Analg 103(1):256-257
41. Fodale V, Praticò C, Piana F et al (2003) Propofol and remifentanil without muscle relaxants in a patient with myasthenia gravis for emergency surgery. Can J Anaesth 50(10):1083-1084
42. Della Rocca G, Coccia C, Diana L et al (2003) Propofol or sevoflurane anesthesia without muscle relaxant allow the early extubation of myasthenic patient. Can J Anaesth 50(6):547-552
43. De Grood PM, Mitusukuri S, Van Egmond J et al (1987) Comparison of etomidate and propofol for anaesthesia in microlaryngeal surgery. Anaesthesia 42:366-372
44. Bagshaw O (2007) A combination of total intravenous anesthesia and thoracic epidural for thymectomy in juvenile myasthenia gravis. Paediatr Anaesth 17(4):370-374
45. El-Dawlatly AA, Al Kattan K, Hajjar W et al (2005) Anesthetic implications for video assisted thoracoscopic thymectomy in myasthenia gravis. Middle East J Anesthesiol 18(2):339-345
46. Matsuo S, Rao DBS, Chaudry I et al (1978) Interaction of muscle relaxants and local anesthetics at the neuromuscolar junction. Anesth and Analg 57:580-587
47. Lopez-Berlanga JL, Garutti I, Martinez-Campos E et al (2006) Bilateral paravertebral block anesthesia for thymectomy by video-assisted thoracoscopy in patients with myasthenia gravis. Rev Esp Anestesiol Reanim 53(9):571-574
48. Mulder DG, Hermann C, Buckberg GB (1974) Effect of thymectomy in patients with myasthenia gravis. Am J Surg 128:202-206
49. Cohn HE, Solit RW, Schatz NS et al (1974) Surgical treatment in myasthenia gravis: A 27-year experience. J Thorac Cardiovasc Surg 68:876-885
50. Papatestas AE, Alpert LL, Ossermann KE et al (1971) Studies in myasthenia gravis: Effects of thymectomy, results on 185 patients with nonthymomatous and thymomatous myasthenia gravis 1941-1969. Am J Med 50:465-474
51. Loach AB, Young AC, Spalding JMK et al (1975) Postoperative management after thymectomy. Br Med J 1:309-312
52. Leventhal SR, Orkin FK, Hirsh RA (1980) Prediction of the need for post-operative mechanical ventilation in myasthenia gravis. Anesthesiology 53:26-30
53. Gracey DR, Divertie MB, Howard FM et al (1984) Postoperative respiratory care after transsternal thymectomyin myasthenia gravis. A three-years experience in 53 patients. Chest 86:67-71
54. Younger DS, Braun NMT, Jaretzki A et al (1984) Myasthenia gravis: Determinants for independent ventilation after transsternal thymectomy. Neurology 34:336-340
55. Pavlin EG, Holle RH, Schoene RB (1989) Recovery of airway protection compared with ventilation in humans after paralysis with curare. Anesthesiology 70:381-385
56. Oosterhuis HJ (1981) Observations of the natural history of myasthenia gravis and the effect of thymectomy. Ann NY Acad Sci 377:678-690

CHAPTER 14

Conventional Techniques: Cervicotomy

Piero Borasio, Francesco Ardissone

Introduction

Since the pioneering reports by Blalock and associates [1] and Keynes [2], surgical removal of the thymus continues to play a controversial role in the treatment of myasthenia gravis.

Myasthenia gravis (MG) is a rare autoimmune disease of the neuromuscular transmission, with an estimated prevalence of 15/100,000, and an annual incidence of 1.1/100,000 [3]. Typical clinical features of the disease are skeletal muscle weakness, fluctuating in extent and severity over the course of time, and easy muscular fatigability on repeated effort. Approximately half of the patients present with purely ocular muscular involvement in the form of ptosis and/or diplopia. Within 2 to 3 years, most of the patients progress to systemic disease (generalized MG), affecting facial, limb, and axial muscles [4]. Oropharyngeal and respiratory muscle involvement leads to dysarthria, dysphagia, feeding difficulty, and respiratory insufficiency, respectively [5]. However, a minority of patients continue to have only ocular symptoms or they may have a spontaneous remission of the disease [6].

In 85% of MG patients, demonstrable serum antibodies against the acetylcholine receptor (AChR) at the neuromuscular junction are present. AChR antibodies reduce the number of functioning receptors at the postsynaptic terminal of the neuromuscular junction [7]. Besides functional blockade, AChR antibodies cause an accelerated degradation and endocytosis of AChRs, and a complement-mediated destruction of the synaptic folds. Of the 15% of generalized MG patients without detectable serum AChR antibodies, about 50% have antibodies that bind to another synaptic antigen, the muscle-specific receptor tyrosine kinase (MuSK), causing functional blockade of receptors and, possibly, complement-mediated damage of the neuromuscular junction [8]. The remaining seronegative MG patients may have antibodies directed at sites other than the main binding sites.

According to pathologic and immunologic studies [9-12], the thymus is thought to play a primary role in the pathogenesis of MG. A thymoma or a hyperplastic thymus is found in 15% and in 60% of MG patients, respectively. An increased number of AChR-specific T-cells and of B-cells, these latter ones capable of producing AChR antibodies in culture, are found in the hyperplastic thymus. The thymus is the site of T-cell development and education, and it preserves self-tolerance and autoimmunity. Indeed, in animals, complete removal of the thymus in the neonatal period prevents experimental autoimmune MG. In MG patients, removal of residual thymus after incomplete thymectomy achieves complete remission from the disease [13, 14]. However, the starting event in the autoimmune process of MG is not understood nor has the mechanism of the action of thymectomy in MG patients been fully elucidated. Furthermore, there is no other autoimmune disease treated by surgical removal of a gland [15], and the benefit of thymectomy in MG has not been definitely confirmed by randomized, well-controlled trials. Nevertheless, thymectomy is widely practiced in MG patients with and without thymoma.

Indications

Current indications for surgical treatment in MG include the following.
- Thymomatous myasthenia gravis: Thymectomy is formally indicated irrespective of the extent and severity of MG [16-18].
- Nonthymomatous generalized myasthenia gravis: Early-onset AChR antibodies-positive patients with generalized MG and insufficient response to medical therapy should be considered for thymectomy as an option in order to increase the probability of remission or improvement [16-18]. Conflicting information exists about the indication for thymectomy in AChR antibodies-negative patients [19-21].
- Nonthymomatous ocular myasthenia gravis: The debate over the role of thymectomy in the man-

agement of ocular MG has yet to be resolved, given the absence of clear-cut evidence that thymectomy lowers the risk of developing generalized MG or induces full remission in patients with ocular MG. However, it can be offered to young patients with persistent and disabling symptoms who do not respond satisfactorily to medical therapy [15, 22-24].

The Operation

Different surgical approaches and techniques have been recommended for removal of the thymus in MG including transcervical, transsternal, combined transcervical and transsternal, and video-assisted transthoracic thymectomy. All procedures include an extracapsular extraction of the central cervical-mediastinal lobes of the thymus, and differ in the extent of cervical-mediastinal exploration and dissection [25-27].

"Complete thymectomy" is considered the technical goal of surgery. However, since the available evidence does not convincingly demonstrate that more aggressive resections result in better outcomes than lesser resections, controversy continues regarding the best surgical approach and technique to accomplish "adequate excision" of the thymus in order to achieve optimal benefit.

Preoperative Evaluation and Preparation

The referring neurologist plays a central role in the perioperative management of MG patients being considered for thymectomy.

These patients undergo contrast-enhanced computed tomography (CT) scan or magnetic resonance (MR) imaging of the chest in order to check for an associated thymoma. In individuals with suspected thymomas greater than 3 cm in diameter or seemingly invasive, the transsternal approach is to be chosen. Relative contraindications to the transcervical approach include previous cervico-mediastinal surgery and limited neck extension from osteoarthritis.

In view of the potential for postoperative aspiration, ineffective cough, and respiratory failure, patients with more than mild generalized MG or oropharyngeal and respiratory muscle weakness should undergo pulmonary function tests including measurement of maximum expiratory force (MEF). Indeed, MEF is a valuable measure of cough effectiveness and helps to identify patients at an increased risk of postoperative complications [27]. Accordingly, MG symptoms should be medically well controlled before surgery [28]. In patients who cannot be stabilized with anticholinesterase inhibition and/or immunosuppression, plasma exchange or intravenous immunoglobulin is recommended as a short-term treatment in preparation for surgery [18].

Patients take cholinergic inhibitors until the morning of surgery. A general anesthetic is administered with a single-lumen endotracheal tube. Usual anesthetic management consists of a halogenated agent supplemented by intravenous short-acting narcotics as required. Nondepolarizing muscle relaxants are avoided or employed sparingly in order to ensure safe extubation at the end of surgery.

Operative Technique

The anesthetized patient is placed in the supine position with the head at the very end of the operating room table and the arms along the sides. The endotracheal tube is positioned at the patient's right as far laterally as feasible to ensure optimal access to mediastinal exploration and dissection. In order to allow hyperextension of the neck and increase exposure, a bolster or pillow is placed under the shoulders while the occiput is supported by a ring. The neck and anterior chest are prepped as if a sternotomy were needed. Typically, the operating surgeon stands, and later on sits, at the patient's head, wearing a head light.

An 8- to 10-cm curvilinear incision is made, ideally along a skin crease, at the base of the neck, one finger breadth above the sternal notch and the same distance above the clavicle on each side. The incision is deepened through the subcutaneous fascia and platysma down to the deep cervical fascia. Flaps are raised immediately deep to the platysma and superficial to the deep cervical fascia, superiorly to the inferior border of the thyroid cartilage and inferiorly to a point just below the manubriosternal junction in case an upper partial sternal split is needed. The wound edges are retracted by a suitable retractor and the soft tissue at the suprasternal notch is divided with electrocautery down to the external periosteum of the manubrium.

Thereafter, the areolar fascia which joins the strap muscles in the midline is divided and the sternohyoid muscles are retracted laterally to expose the sternothyroid muscles. The thin fascial envelope surrounding these muscles blends imperceptibly with the underlying surgical capsule of the thyroid and thymus glands, so that muscles and glands have to be gradually separated, proceeding from medial to lateral. The superior poles of the thymus are identified and dissected free from their beds up to the thyroid gland. The thyrothymic ligaments are ligated and divided, and, by applying gentle retraction, the anterior surface of thymic lobes is bluntly dissected free down to the thoracic inlet. With sharp and blunt dissection a retrosternal plane is developed to accommodate the placement of a specially designed retractor [29]. Otherwise, a retractor traditionally used for cardiac surgical procedures can be employed [30]. By applying due upward traction on the retractor, the manubrium is lifted and enhanced visualization of the anterior mediastinal area is provided. According to de Perrot and associates [31], a videothoracoscope is a useful adjunct in the full exposure of the distal thymus. Alternatively, an upper partial sternal split is made with or without an additional skin incision, and a specially designed retraction-suspension device, provided with a V-shaped opening (Fig. 14.1), can be used to obtain adequate exposure of the mediastinal portion of the thymus (Fig. 14.2) [32, 33].

At this point, the posterior surface of the superior poles of the thymus is progressively dissected free by blunt and sharp maneuvers to display the central venous drainage into the left innominate vein (Fig. 14.3). These thymic veins are ligated and divided. In the occasional patient in whom part of the thymus is located behind the left innominate vein, careful dissection of this area is needed to avoid retained thymic tissue. With the aid of gentle traction applied upward and forward, the posterior aspect of the thymus is progressively mobilized off the pericardium.

Subsequently, the dissection proceeds laterally sweeping away the thymus and adjacent fat pads from the mediastinal pleura on both sides. The lateral blood supply from the internal mammary artery is ligated or clipped and divided. Utmost care is paid to the visualization and preservation of the phrenic

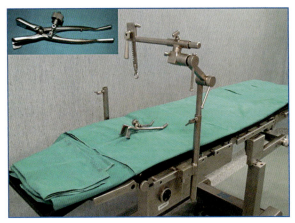

Fig. 14.1 The retraction-suspension device developed by the senior author (P.B.). En cartouche, the self-retaining sternal retractor, provided with a V-shaped opening

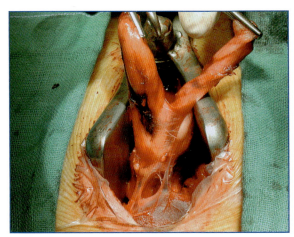

Fig. 14.3 The thymic venous drainage into the left innominate vein is shown

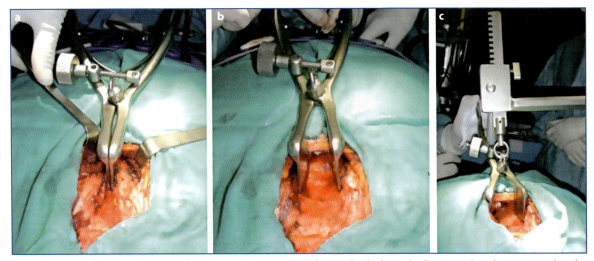

Fig. 14.2a-c **a** The sternal retractor is put into the upper partial sternal split, **b** gradually opened, and **c** connected to the lifting device

nerves. By alternating caudal and lateral dissection, the thymus and surrounding fat are progressively dissected free from their attachments and removed. Then, remnants of fatty tissue in the antero-superior mediastinum are identified and excised as separate specimens.

At the end of the procedure, the space is drained by a small suction catheter which is removed 24 h after surgery. Fortuitous openings of the mediastinal pleura are repaired under a prolonged positive pressure breath. If an upper partial sternal split has been made, the sternum is approximated with interrupted wires. The strap muscles, platysma, and skin are closed with absorbable sutures.

Most patients can be extubated immediately after the operation. An upright chest X-ray is performed in the recovery room.

Results

Several authors [16, 17, 25-27, 34] have raised critical remarks on the literature addressing the role and effectiveness of thymectomy and of the different surgical approaches to thymectomy in the treatment of MG patients. In the absence of randomized controlled trials, these authors have underlined the many confounding differences in the baseline characteristics of patient cohorts, the inconsistency in assessment and statistical analysis of data, and the additional confounders introduced by outcome comparisons between uncontrolled studies.

Bearing in mind these limitations, the transcervical approach appears to offer several advantages. It is a less invasive procedure, which requires a decreased operative time and a minimal postoperative length of stay, reducing costs. Better preservation of lung function contributes to a low postoperative morbidity rate (Table 14.1) and fosters an early return to full activity. Consequently, referring neurologists and patients are provided with a more readily acceptable surgical procedure while earlier referral to surgery and milder clinical manifestations have been shown to allow higher remission rates.

The most accurate measure of the effectiveness of thymectomy in the treatment of MG patients is life table analysis of complete stable remission rates, which has been rarely employed (Table 14.2). In view of the unsettled issue of the pathogenic role of residual thymic tissue after less than "maximal" thymectomy [26], we concur with Shrager and associates [49] in believing that transcervical thymectomy continues to represent "a reasonable choice in the surgical management of MG".

Conclusions

No thymectomy technique appears to achieve unambiguously better results over the other.

Table 14.1 Operative results following thymectomy in MG patients (modified from de Perrot et al. [31])

Surgical approach	Authors [Ref]	Year of publication	Number of patients	Morbidity (%)	Mortality (%)	Mean LoS (days)
Maximal transcervical/ transsternal	Jaretzki et al. [35]	1988	72	7	–	N/A
	Ashour et al. [36]	1995	48	20.8	–	N/A
	Bulkley et al. [37]	1997	202 †	33	–	N/A
Transsternal (standard or extended)	Masaoka et al. [38]	1996	375	N/A	–	N/A
	Detterbeck et al. [39]	1996	100	17	–	6.3
	Budde et al. [40]	2001	113	14	0.9	9.3
	Stern et al. [41]	2001	58	25.9	–	N/A
	Zielinski et al. [42]	2004	118	11.9	–	N/A
	Huang et al. [43]	2005	168	16.6	–	N/A
	Kattach et al. [44]	2006	85	9	–	8
	Park et al. [45]	2006	147	2.7	–	N/A
	Kim et al. [46]	2007	64	6.2	–	N/A
Transcervical (extended)	DeFilippi et al. [47]	1994	53	2	–	3
	Calhoun et al. [48]	1999	100	8	–	1.2
	de Perrot et al. [31]	2003	120	3.3	–	1.9-3.9 ‡
	Shrager et al. [49]	2006	151	7.3	–	1.1

Mean LoS, mean postoperative length of stay; N/A, not available
† Includes 75 extended transsternal thymectomies and 127 maximal transcervical/transsternal thymectomies
‡ Includes 116 patients with an uncomplicated course; 1.9 days after transcervical thymectomy; 3.9 days after conversion to an upper sternotomy

Table 14.2 Complete remission rates following thymectomy in MG patients (modified from de Perrot et al. [31])

Surgical approach	Authors [Ref]	Year of publication	Number of patients	Mean FU (years)	Complete remission Crude (%)	Life table
Maximal transcervical /transsternal	Jaretzki et al. [35]	1988	72	3.4	46	81% (at 7.5 years)
	Ashour et al. [36]	1995	48	1.7	35	N/A
	Busch et al. [50]	1996	65	7.7	19	N/A
	Bulkley et al. [37]	1997	192	5.0	40	N/A
	Klein et al. [51]	1999	51	5.0	40	N/A
Transsternal (standard or extended)	Detterbeck et al. [39]	1996	99	5.3	47	N/A
	Budde et al. [40]	2001	92	4.3	21	N/A
	Stern et al. [41]	2001	53	6.8	53	N/A
	Zielinski et al. [42]	2004	118	6.0	21.7–46.5*	N/A
	Huang et al. [43]	2005	154	8.2	57.8	N/A
	Kattach et al. [44]	2006	85	4.5	17	N/A
	Park et al. [45]	2006	147	7.5	29.2†	37.3 (at 10 years)‡
	Kim et al. [46]	2007	60	4.8	38#	N/A
Transcervical (Extended)	Durelli et al. [32]	1991	400	≥5.0	N/A	30% (at 5 years)
	DeFilippi et al. [47]	1994	53	≥5.0	43	N/A
	Calhoun et al. [48]	1999	78	5.0	35	N/A
	de Perrot et al. [31]	2003	100	4.3	41	91% (at 10 years)
	Shrager et al. [49]	2006	151	4.4	28.8	35% (at 6 years)

Mean FU, mean follow-up; N/A, not available
* 21.7% after standard transsternal thymectomy; 46.5% after extended transsternal thymectomy
† 37.7% nonthymomatous MG; 12.2% thymomatous MG
‡ 45.2% nonthymomatous MG; 27.7% thymomatous MG
# 42% nonthymomatous MG; 33% thymomatous MG

The difference in complete remission rates between limited and aggressive resections has to be balanced against the immediate risks and the long-term consequences of the surgical procedure.

By using the specially designed retraction-suspension device (Fig. 14.1), we can obtain optimal exposure of the mediastinal portion of the thymus.

References

1. Blalock A, Harvey AM, Ford FF, Lilienthal J Jr (1941) The treatment of myasthenia gravis by removal of the thymus gland. JAMA 117:1529-1533
2. Keynes G (1946) The surgery of the thymus gland. Br J Surg 32:201-214
3. Scherer K, Bedlack RS, Simel DL (2005) Does this patient have myasthenia gravis? JAMA 293:1906-1914
4. Grob D, Arsura EL, Brunner NG, Namba T (1987) The course of myasthenia gravis and therapies affecting outcome. Ann N Y Acad Sci 505:472-499
5. Thomas CE, Mayer SA, Gungor Y et al (1997) Myasthenic crisis: Clinical features, mortality, complications, and risk factors for prolonged intubation. Neurology 48:1253-1260
6. Oosterhuis HJ (1981) Observations of the natural history of myasthenia gravis and the effect of thymectomy. Ann N Y Acad Sci 377:678-690
7. Vincent A (2002) Unravelling the pathogenesis of myasthenia gravis. Nat Rev Immunol 2:797-804
8. Hoch W, McConville J, Helms S et al (2001) Auto-antibodies to the receptor tyrosine kinase MuSK in patients with myasthenia gravis without acetylcholine receptor antibodies. Nat Med 7:365-368
9. Wekerle H, Muller-Hermelink HK (1986) The thymus in myasthenia gravis. Curr Top Pathol 75:179-206
10. Younger DS, Worrall BB, Penn AS (1997) Myasthenia gravis: Historical perspective and overview. Neurology 48(Suppl):S1-S17
11. Somnier FE, Skeie GO, Aarli JA, Trojaborg W (1999) EMG evidence of myopathy and the occurrence of titin auto-antibodies in patients with myasthenia gravis. Eur J Neurol 6:555-563
12. Ragheb S, Lisak RP (1998) Immune regulation and myasthenia gravis. Ann N Y Acad Sci 841:210-224
13. Younger DS (2005) Myasthenia gravis. In: Shields TW, LoCicero J III, Ponn RB, Rusch VW (eds) General thoracic surgery, 6th edn. Lippincott Williams & Wilkins, Philadelphia, pp 2617-2623
14. Li J, Lisak RP (2005) Pathophysiology of myasthenia gravis. In: Shields TW, LoCicero J III, Ponn RB, Rusch VW (eds), General thoracic surgery. 6th edn.

Lippincott Williams & Wilkins, Philadelphia, pp 2624-2628
15. Chavis PS, Stickler DE, Walker A (2007) Immunosuppressive or surgical treatment for ocular myasthenia gravis. Arch Neurol 64:1792-1794
16. Gronseth GS, Barohn RJ (2000) Practice parameter: Thymectomy for autoimmune myasthenia gravis (an evidence-based review): Report of the Quality Standards Subcommittee of the American Academy of Neurology. Neurology 55:7-15
17. Gronseth GS, Barohn RJ (2002) Thymectomy for myasthenia gravis. Curr Treat Options Neurol 4:203-209
18. Skeie GO, Apostolski S, Evoli A et al (2006) Guidelines for the treatment of autoimmune neuromuscular transmission disorders. Eur J Neurol 13:691-699
19. Guillermo GR, Tellez-Zenteno JF, Weder-Cisneros N et al (2004) Response of thymectomy: Clinical and pathological characteristics among seronegative and seropositive myasthenia gravis patients. Acta Neurol Scand 109:217-221
20. Evoli A, Tonali PA, Padua L et al (2003) Clinical correlates with anti-MuSK antibodies in generalized seronegative myasthenia gravis. Brain 126(Pt 10):2304-2311
21. Yuan HK, Huang BS, Kung SY, Kao KP (2007) The effectiveness of thymectomy on seronegative generalized myasthenia gravis: Comparing with seropositive cases. Acta Neurol Scand 115:181-184
22. Roberts PF, Venuta F, Rendina E et al (2001) Thymectomy in the treatment of ocular myasthenia gravis. J Thorac Cardiovasc Surg 122:562-568
23. Gilbert ME, De Sousa EA, Savino PJ (2007) Ocular myasthenia gravis treatment: The case against prednisone therapy and thymectomy. Arch Neurol 64:1790-1792
24. Roach ES (2007) Treating ocular myasthenia gravis with inadequate evidence. Arch Neurol 64:1794-1795
25. Jaretzki A III (1997) Thymectomy for myasthenia gravis: Analysis of the controversies regarding technique and results. Neurology 48(Suppl 5):S52-S63
26. Jaretzki A III, Barohn RJ, Ernstoff RM et al (2000) Myasthenia gravis: Recommendations for clinical research standards. Task Force of the Medical Scientific Advisory Board of the Myasthenia Gravis Foundation of America. Ann Thorac Surg 70:327-334
27. Jaretzki A III (2003) Thymectomy for myasthenia gravis: Analysis of controversies – Patient management. Neurologist 9:77-92
28. Krucylak PE, Naunheim KS (1999) Preoperative preparation and anesthetic management of patients with myasthenia gravis. Semin Thorac Cardiovasc Surg 11:47-53
29. Cooper JD, Al-Jilaihawa AN, Pearson FG et al (1988) An improved technique to facilitate transcervical thymectomy for myasthenia gravis. Ann Thorac Surg 45:242-247
30. Komanapalli CB, Person TD, Schipper P, Sukumar MS (2005) An alternative retractor for transcervical thymectomy. J Thorac Cardiovasc Surg 130:221-222
31. de Perrot M, Bril V, McRae K, Keshavjee S (2003) Impact of minimally invasive trans-cervical thymectomy on outcome in patients with myasthenia gravis. Eur J Cardiothorac Surg 24:677-683
32. Durelli L, Maggi G, Casadio C et al (1991) Actuarial analysis of the occurrence of remission following thymectomy for myasthenia gravis in 400 patients. J Neurol Neurosurg Psychiatry 54:406-411
33. Boaron MA (2004) A new retraction-suspension device for limited upper sternotomy. Ann Thorac Surg 77:1107-1108
34. Jaretzki A III, Steinglass KM, Sonett JR (2004) Thymectomy in the management of myasthenia gravis. Semin Neurol 24:49-62
35. Jaretzki A III, Penn AS, Younger DS et al (1988) "Maximal" thymectomy for myasthenia gravis: Results. J Thorac Cardiovasc Surg 95:747-757
36. Ashour MH, Jain SK, Kattan KM et al (1995) Maximal thymectomy for myasthenia gravis. Eur J Cardiothorac Surg 9:461-464
37. Bulkley GB, Bass KN, Stephenson GR et al (1997) Extended cervicomediastinal thymectomy in the integrated management of myasthenia gravis. Ann Surg 226:324-335
38. Masaoka A, Yamakawa Y, Niwa H et al (1996) Extended thymectomy for myasthenia gravis patients: A 20 year review. Ann Thorac Surg 62:853-859
39. Detterbeck FC, Scott WW, Howard JF Jr et al (1996) One hundred consecutive thymectomies for myasthenia gravis. Ann Thorac Surg 62:242-245
40. Budde JM, Morris CD, Gal AA et al (2001) Predictors of outcome in thymectomy for myasthenia gravis. Ann Thorac Surg 72:197-202
41. Stern LE, Nussbaum MS, Quinlan JG, Fischer JE (2001) Long-term evaluation of extended thymectomy with anterior mediastinal dissection for myasthenia gravis. Surgery 130:774-779
42. Zielinski M, Kuzdzal J, Szlubowski A, Soja J (2004) Comparison of late results of basic transsternal and extended transsternal thymectomies in the treatment of myasthenia gravis. Ann Thorac Surg 78:253-258
43. Huang CS, Hsu HS, Huang BS et al (2005) Factors influencing the outcome of transsternal thymectomy for myasthenia gravis. Acta Neurol Scand 112:108-114
44. Kattach H, Anastasiadis K, Cleuziou J et al (2006) Transsternal thymectomy for myasthenia gravis: Surgical outcome. Ann Thorac Surg 81:305-308
45. Park IK, Choi SS, Lee JG et al (2006) Complete stable remission after extended transsternal thymectomy in myasthenia gravis. Eur J Cardiothorac Surg 30:525-528
46. Kim HK, Park MS, Choi YS et al (2007) Neurologic outcomes of thymectomy in myasthenia gravis: Comparative analysis of the effect of thymoma. J Thorac Cardiovasc Surg 134:601-607
47. DeFilippi VJ, Richman DP, Ferguson MK (1994) Transcervical thymectomy for myasthenia gravis. Ann Thorac Surg 57:194-197

48. Calhoun RF, Ritter JH, Guthrie TJ et al (1999) Results of transcervical thymectomy for myasthenia gravis in 100 consecutive patients. Ann Surg 230:555-561
49. Shrager JB, Nathan D, Brinster CJ et al (2006) Outcomes after 151 extended transcervical thymectomies for myasthenia gravis. Ann Thorac Surg 82:1863-1869
50. Busch C, Machens A, Pichlmeier U et al (1996) Long-term outcome and quality of life after thymectomy for myasthenia gravis. Ann Surg 224:225-232
51. Klein M, Heidenreich F, Madjlessi F et al (1999) Early and late results after thymectomy in myasthenia gravis: A retrospective analysis. Thorac Cardiovasc Surg 47:170-173

CHAPTER 15

Conventional Techniques: Median Sternotomy

Alfredo Mussi, Marco Lucchi

Introduction

It is now well known and accepted that the thymus plays a central role in the pathogenesis of autoimmune nonthymomatous and thymomatous myasthenia gravis (MG) [1-5]. While in case of a thymoma oncological reasons make surgery mandatory and the sternotomy route is the golden standard, on the other hand the presence of a radiologically "normal" thymus makes the choices of the thymectomy and of its surgical approach more controversial [6-12]. From retrospective studies it is quite evident that all thymectomies are not equal both in extent of thymic tissue removed and in neurological results [5]. Briefly it can be stated that the more complete the thymectomy the better the results [5]; on the contrary, it is sufficient to leave behind 2 g of residual thymus to reduce the therapeutic value of the thymectomy and produce a lower remission rate [13].

Surgical-anatomic studies proved that thymic tissue can be found out of the thymic lobes both in the neck and mediastinum [13, 14]. It is intuitive that different surgical techniques have advantages and disadvantages in removing all the fat present in the inferior mediastinum or in the neck [5]. The Myasthenia Gravis Foundation of America classified the resectional techniques from T-1a to T-4 (Table 15.1) in order to provide a correct nomenclature able to clarify the resectional technique adopted in different centers [15]. Sternotomy was first described by Milton in 1897 and a standard transsternal thymectomy was used by the pioneers Blalock and Keynes [16, 17].

A standard transsternal thymectomy (T-3a) is limited to the removal of the entire thymic gland but not the mediastinal and cervical fat. The finding of residual thymus in the neck and mediastinum at reoperation suggested that this is an incomplete resection and, as a matter of fact, it was abandoned by most MG centers.

The extended transsternal thymectomy (T-3b), also called "aggressive transsternal thymectomy" and " transsternal radical thymectomy", consists of the en-bloc resection of all the fat and thymic tissue resectable in the neck and mediastinum, from the inferior part of the thyroid lobes to the diaphragm, from phrenic to phrenic nerve [6, 18]. Removing neck tissue without a neck dissection and from below, this technique can leave some thymic tissue in the neck. It is less radical than a transcervical and transsternal thymectomy (T-4) [5, 7], but because of a lower invasiveness and morbidity has been used and appreciated by most surgeons in the MG centers.

Technique

The patient is in a supine position with the arms secured at the patient's sides. An oro-tracheal intubation is sufficient in all thymectomies and a selective bronchial intubation should be reserved only in case of invasive thymomas.

The skin incision is median and vertical, starting just below the sternal notch and extending at the tip of the xyphoid process. The skin incision may be reduced for cosmetic reasons at the preference of the surgeon.

The pectoral fascia is divided and the periosteum is scored with the electrocautery. At the jugulum the interclavicular ligament must be divided

Table 15.1 The MGFA Thymectomy Classification

T-1	Transcervical thymectomy (a) Basic (b) Extended
T-2	Videoscopic thymectomy (a) Classic VATS (b) VATET
T-3	Transsternal thymectomy (a) Standard (b) Extended
T-4	Transcervical & transsternal thymectomy

and, before dividing the sternum with the saw, the anesthetist should stop ventilation to avoid damage to the lung.

The sternum may be divided by using either an electric or air-powered saw. This vertical and strictly median osteotomy may be performed either from above downwards (our preference), or from below upwards. Once the sternum is split, periosteal bleeding should be controlled with cautery. Bone wax can be avoided for a thymectomy because anticoagulation is not necessary during the procedure and bleeding will stop with the closure of the sternum.

A small retractor (Finochietto-like or others) will allow the progressive opening of the sternum. Usually a mild retraction will be sufficient to perform an extended thymectomy in a comfortable way.

The resection starts from the fat of the inferior mediastinum. The anterior mediastinal fat is removed beginning from the diaphragm going upward. Then, the gland with the fat is elevated toward the brachiocephalic trunk, and the draining veins and the thymic branches of internal mammary artery are ligated. Finally, the cervical horns of each lobe and all the fat tissue around are resected by a blunt dissection. Surgeons generally try to avoid opening the mediastinal pleura; however, it can happen. Some surgeons [8] open the mediastinal pleura to recognize the phrenic nerves and remove all the fat without injuring them.

At the end of the procedure one mediastinal drainage (24 F or less) is placed through incision at the epigastrium; mediastinal pleura can be closed, and rarely the pleural spaces must be drained. Sternotomy closure can be performed by means of stainless steel wires or, better, by means of absorbable polyglycolic acid sutures. A subcuticular suture is used for skin closure.

Conclusions

Even though thymectomy has been used in the management of nonthymomatous autoimmune myasthe-

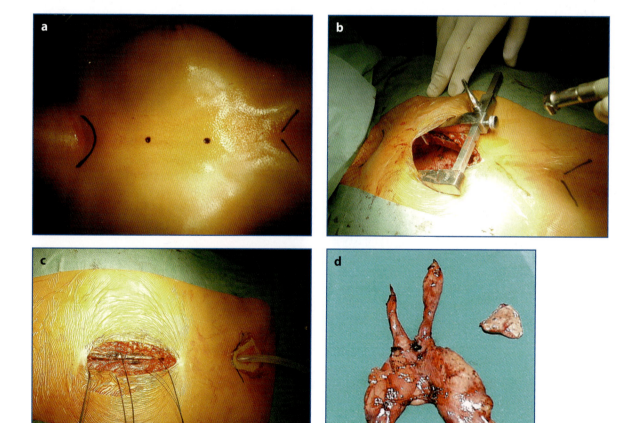

Fig. 15.1a-d **a** Skin sparing incision for a vertical median sternotomy. **b** Operative view. **c** Sternotomy closure by means of absorbable sutures. **d** The surgical specimen

nia gravis in the last decades, there is no randomized controlled trial confirming its role [4, 5]. However, large retrospective studies prompted most neurologists to believe that the procedure is part of the multimodality treatment of the disease [4]. Furthermore, also surgeons have debated about the entity of the thymectomy and which route is to be preferred, without being able to draw any definitive statement. As concerns the neurological results, life table analysis, using the Kaplan-Meier method, should be used for the analysis of complete remissions following thymectomy [5]. Unfortunately, uncorrected crude data analysis for comparative analysis of thymectomy results has been commonly used and the conclusions of such studies should not be accepted. Selection bias of patients who are candidates for thymectomy and the absence of standardized methods for assessing patient status made the different techniques of thymectomy not comparable. Only when all the MG centers follow the MGFA recommendations [15] will comparison among institutional experiences be possible.

The skin scar of a vertical median sternotomy is a major concern to some patients, especially young women. Various skin incisions have been proposed for a thymectomy through a median sternotomy. The transverse submammary skin incision [18] and small median skin incisions (7-8 cm) (Fig. 15.1) [19] appear to offer the best cosmetic advantages despite the potential complications originating from a large skin flap. Exposure can be obtained by means of retractors and instruments and technology used for mini-invasive surgery.

Up to now every VATS [10] or robotic technique [20] should be considered in the investigative phase. These techniques are feasible and safe but we must wait for a longer follow-up before discussing the goal of a thymectomy, which is the MG complete remission rate. The only exception can be for the VATET technique, which seems to reproduce the maximal thymectomy through a cervicotomy plus a bilateral VATS approach instead of a cervicosternotomy, and whose results were recently published [21].

As thoracic surgeons, therefore, we must do our best to perform the least invasive operation possible, with attention to cosmetic appearance, while respecting criteria for a radical resection.

With regard to completeness of surgery, our opinion is that every surgeon should use the approach with which he feels most comfortable, but we believe that radical "extended" thymectomy is actually necessary and it can better be performed through a median sternotomy.

References

1. Papatestas AE, Genkins G, Kornfeld P et al (1987) Effects of thymectomy in myasthenia gravis. Ann Surg 206:79-88
2. Perlo VP, Poskanzer DC, Schwab RS et al (1966) Myasthenia gravis: Evaluation of treatment in 1355 patients. Neurology 16:431-439
3. Blossom GB, Ernstoff RM, Howells GA et al (1993) Thymectomy for myasthenia gravis. Arch Surg 128:855-862
4. Gronseth GS, Barohn RJ (2000) Practice parameter: Thymectomy for autoimmune myasthenia gravis (an evidence-based review). Report of the quality standards subcommittee of the American Academy of Neurology. Neurology 55:7-15
5. Jaretzki A 3rd (2003) Thymectomy for myasthenia gravis: Analysis of controversies-patient management. Neurologist 9(2):77-92
6. Masaoka A, Yamakawa Y, Niwa H et al (1996) Extended thymectomy for myasthenia gravis patients: A 20-year review. Ann Thorac Surg 62:853-859
7. Jaretzki A, Penn AS, Younger DS et al (1988) "Maximal thymectomy" for myasthenia gravis. J Thorac Cardiovasc Surg 95:747-757
8. Detterbeck FC, Scott WW, Howard JF et al (1996) One hundred consecutive thymectomies for myasthenia gravis. Ann Thorac Surg 62:242-245
9. Hatton PD, Diehl JT, Daly BD et al (1989) Transternal radical thymectomy for myasthenia gravis: A 15-year review. Ann Thorac Surg 47:838-840
10. Mack MJ, Landreneau RD, Yim AP et al (1996) Results of video-assisted thymectomy in patients with myasthenia gravis. J Thorac Cardiovasc Surg 112:1352-1360
11. Bril V, Kojic S, Ilse W, Cooper JD (1998) Long-term clinical outcome after transcervical thymectomy for myasthenia gravis. Ann Thorac Surg 65:1520-1522
12. Jaretzki A (1997) Thymectomy for myasthenia gravis: An analysis of the controversies regarding technique and results. Neurology 48(Suppl 5):52-63
13. Jaretzki A, Wolff M (1988) "Maximal" thymectomy for myasthenia gravis: Surgical anatomy and operative technique. J Thorac Cardiovasc Surg 96:711-716
14. Masaoka A, Nagaoka Y, Kotake Y (1975) Distribution of thymic tissue in the anterior mediastinum: Current procedures in thymectomy. J Thorac Cardiovasc Surg 70:747-754
15. Jaretzki A, Barohn RJ, Ernstoff RM et al (2000) Myasthenia gravis: Recommendations for clinical research standards. Task Force of the Medical Scientific Advisory Board of the Myasthenia Gravis Foundation of America. Ann Thorac Surg 70:327-334
16. Blalock A, Mason MF, Morgan HJ, Riven SS (1939) Myasthenia gravis and tumors of the thymic region: Report of a case in which the tumor was removed. Ann Surg 110:544-561
17. Keynes G (1949) The results of thymectomy in myasthenia gravis. Br Med J 2:611-616

18. Granone P, Margaritora S, Cesario A, Galetta D (1999) Thymectomy in myasthenia gravis via video-assisted infra-mammary cosmetic incision. Eur J Cardiothorac Surg 15:861-863
19. Mussi A, Lucchi M, Murri L et al (2001) Extended thymectomy in myasthenia gravis: A team-work of neurologist, thoracic surgeon and anaesthesist may improve the outcome. Eur J Cardiothorac Surg 19(5):570-575
20. Rea F, Marulli G, Bortolotti L et al (2006) Experience with the "da Vinci" robotic system for thymectomy in patients with myasthenia gravis: Report of 33 cases. Ann Thorac Surg 81(2):455-459
21. Mantegazza R, Baggi F, Bernasconi P et al (2003) Video-assisted thoracoscopic extended thymectomy and extended transsternal thymectomy (T-3b) in non-thymomatous myasthenia gravis patients: Remission after 6 years of follow-up. J Neurol Sci 212(1-2):31-36

CHAPTER 16
Conventional Techniques: Transthoracic Approach

Uliano Morandi, Christian Casali

Introduction

Thymomas are the most frequent neoplasms of the anterior mediastinal compartment, accounting for approximately 20% of all mediastinal tumors in adults. They are, however, a rare neoplasm, with an incidence of approximately 0.15 cases in 100,000 habitants per year in the USA [1]. Thymomas are neoplasms of epithelial origin which, despite being considered tumors with an often indolent growth pattern, have a well-documented capability to invade adjacent structures and develop metastases in the pleura as well as, though more rarely, distant metastases. Although several histological classifications have been proposed over the last few years, today there is a wide consensus on the use of the classification proposed by the World Health Organization (WHO) in 1999, as reviewed and confirmed in 2003, which breaks down thymic neoplasms into 6 groups based on the presence of cellular atypias and based on the relationship between epithelial and lymphatic cells (Table 16.1) [2]. By now, a unanimous consensus has been reached on the staging system proposed by Masaoka in 1981 and reviewed in 1994 (Table 16.2) [3], which classifies neoplasms based on the presence or absence of a macroscopic or microscopic invasion of the capsule, of adjacent structures, and the presence of metastases. A significant correlation was recently demonstrated between the current histopathological classification and the staging system: the majority of sub-types A and AB are stages I and II and there is a trend towards an increase in the percentage of III and IV in types B1, B2, and B3 [4]. C forms are almost exclusively stage III and IV [4]. Quite peculiar and of fundamental importance for the purposes of diagnosis and therapy is the possible association with several autoimmune diseases in 28% of patients with thymoma. Amongst these, myasthenia gravis (MG) is the most frequent one, accounting for 30-60% of patients with thymoma, while only 10-15% of patients with MG can develop a thymic neoplasm [5]. Generally, thymomas accompanied by MG are at an earlier stage compared to those unrelated to MG and most frequently they are WHO type B [4]. Erythroid aplasia, systemic lupus erythematosus and hypogammaglobulinemia occur more rarely.

Table 16.1 Histological classification of epithelial neoplasms of the thymus (World Health Organization 2003)

WHO Type	Traditional nomenclature
Type A	Medullary, spindle-shaped cells
Type AB	Mixed
Type B1	Organoid, predominately cortical, lymphocyte predominant
Type B2	Cortical
Type B3	Well-differentiated thymic carcinoma, epithelial predominant
Type C	Thymic carcinoma

Table 16.2 Staging of epithelial neoplasms of the thymus [3]

Masaoka stage	Diagnostic criteria
I	Macroscopically and microscopically capsulated
II	(A) Microscopic invasion of the capsule; (B) macroscopic invasion of the surrounding adipose tissue or adherent to but not infiltrating the mediastinal pleura and the pericardium
III	Macroscopic invasion of adjacent organs. (A) Without invasion of large vessels; (B) with invasion of large vessels
IV	(A) Pleural or pericardial metastases; (B) hematogenous or lymphatic metastases

Surgical Indications

The treatment of thymomas depends on the stage of disease and the copresence of accompanying autoimmune diseases, in particular MG. Each patient with MG, erythroid aplasia, or hypogammaglobulinemia should receive contrast enhancement chest CT scan so as to exclude the presence of an asymptomatic mass in the mediastinum. All of the patients with a mediastinal mass should instead receive a neurological assessment so as to exclude the presence of latent MG.

Surgical exeresis is the treatment recommended for stage I and II thymomas. Clinically operable masses in the anterior mediastinum do not require preoperative histological diagnosis and are an indication for surgical exeresis. While surgery is sufficient for capsulated (stage I) forms, starting from stage II the proportion of local recurrences following radical exeresis increases significantly. Despite the lack of evidence in prospective randomized studies, many authors believe that adjuvant radiotherapy is indicated for stage II [6, 7].

The approach to locally-advanced (stage III) thymomas or thymomas with isolated metastasis involving the parietal pleura alone (stage IVa) has changed significantly over the last few years in that several authors have reported good outcomes using an integrated therapeutic approach where surgical exeresis is only considered after chemotherapy or as part of protocols combining neoadjuvant chemotherapy and postoperative radiotherapy [8-10]. Where CT scan reveals infiltration of a mediastinal mass, it is preferable to do a minimally-invasive biopsy and delay the surgical exeresis until after neoadjuvant chemotherapy.

The table enclosed shows, as an algorithm, the role of surgical treatment in relation to the stage of disease (Fig. 16.1).

Transthoracic Approach: Indications and Surgical Technique

Median sternotomy is the ideal surgical approach for the majority of thymic neoplasms, in particular those accompanied by MG, in that it gives an excellent view of most thymomas and allows to perform radical thymectomy with removal of the mediastinal adipose tissue. The various types of thoracotomy are indicated in selected cases of large thymic neoplasms involving one hemithorax, in the rare cases of thymoma developing in the anterior cardiophrenic recess (Fig. 16.2), or in the cases of thymoma with focal pleural metastases in respect of which exeresis is opted for. Only thymomas not accompanied by MG are an indication for the thoracotomic approach. Indeed, the main limitation of this approach is the difficulty in performing radical thymectomy and hence where it is not possible to remove the thymic tissue in its entirety, several authors opt for thoracotomy combined with one-stage sternotomy (hemi-clamshell) or with delayed sternotomy [11]. With large mediastinal neoplasms involving both hemithoraces, Patterson and coworkers proposed to perform anterior bilateral thoracotomy in the fourth space with transverse incision of the sternum ("clamshell" incision) [12]. Thus, many surgeons continue to prefer posterolateral thoracotomy in that it ensures an excellent surgical field. In our experience, muscle-sparing lateral thoracotomy does, however, allow to approach most thymic neoplasms requiring a thoracotomic approach.

Irrespective of the stage of disease, the objective of the surgical treatment of a thymic neoplasm must be the oncologically radical removal of the neoplasm (i.e., microscopically negative resection margins) [13]. For capsulated forms, complete removal of the neoplasm is sufficient, providing, however, that the entire capsule be removed, considering that in a small

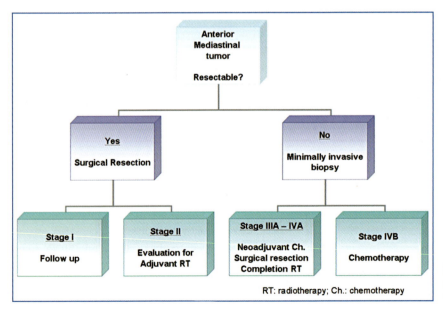

Fig. 16.1 Algorithm of decision-making in the treatment of neoplasms of the thymus

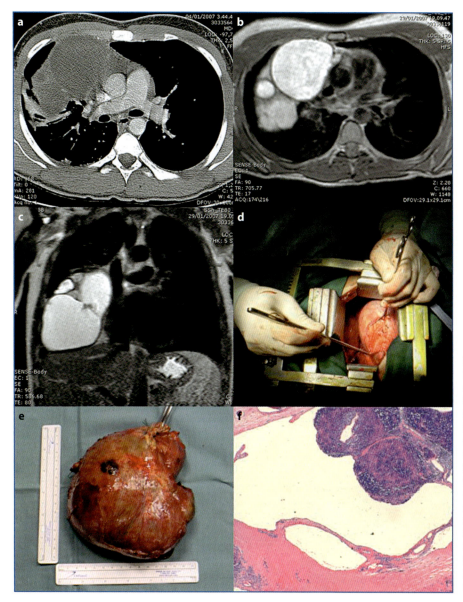

Fig. 16.2a-f 18-year-old patient with multilobulated cystic neoplasm starting from the anterior mediastinum and extending to involve the right pericardium-phrenic recess (**a**, **b**), with cleavage plane versus the vascular structures of the mediastinum (**c**). Radical removal of the cystic neoplasm via lateral thoracotomy (**d**, **e**). Histological findings confirm the presence of a 15-cm giant cystic thymoma Type AB WHO 2004 without capsular invasion (Masaoka Stage I) (**f**)

percentage of capsulated neoplasms the capsule is microscopically invaded [14]. For resectable infiltrating forms, removal of the neoplasm must always be combined with the removal, possibly en bloc, of infiltrated structures.

Also in the absence of MG, many authors agree to combine the removal of thymoma with thymectomy [13]. Besides the possible neoplastic recurrence in the thymic residue, if any, there have been reports of onset of MG immediately postoperatively or later in time after surgery for thymoma [15]. In our experience we have not found any occurrence of MG after the thoracotomic exeresis of thymomas.

From a technical point of view, the first stage consists of assessing the extension of the lesion and its relationships with adjacent structures, which, if removable, must be removed en bloc with the neoplasm. Furthermore, the visceral and parietal pleural surfaces must be explored to identify any metastatic areas. It has been proven that thymic neoplasms tend to develop focal metastases in the parietal pleura (droplet metastases), most frequently in the posterobasal pleura and in the diaphragm, at times unrevealed at preoperative CT scan. The larger the neoplastic component projecting into the pleural cavity or adhering to the mediastinal pleura, the more frequent this metastatization pattern is.

Infiltration of resectable structures such as the pericardium and the mediastinal and pulmonary pleura is no contraindication for surgical exeresis as long as the structures involved are radically removed with the thymic neoplasm. Lobectomies and wedge resections are classified in relation to the extent of lung involvement. Likewise, the presence of isolated pleural metastases is no contraindication for surgical treatment. These foci of neoplastic tissue must be radically removed via localized extrapleural resection. In case of widespread pleural metastatization or of lung involvement requiring pneumonectomy, the role of surgical exeresis is still a matter of debate. Wright and coworkers recently reported a 5-year survival rate of 75% after pleuropneumonectomy for stage IVa thymoma with multiple pleural metastases [16]. Monolateral infiltration of the phrenic nerve is a relative contraindication for surgical exeresis. The phrenic nerve can be sacrificed as long as the patient has a good respiratory reserve. Symptomatic postsurgical diaphragm relaxation requires plastic surgery of the hemidiaphragm via placation at a later stage. In patients with reduced respiratory reserve and those with MG, resection – including monolateral resection – of the phrenic nerve is not indicated. Bilateral infiltration of both phrenic nerves, infiltration of the aorta, of the pulmonary artery, of the recurrent nerve and of the trachea are an absolute contraindication for surgical exeresis. Partial infiltration of the wall of the superior vena cava and/or of one of the two brachiocephalic veins is no contraindication for the exeresis. As illustrated in Chap. 18, en bloc resection of the thymoma and of the vessel involved followed by prosthetic reconstruction or mere vascular suture in cases of tangential involvement, has led, in select cases, to satisfactory outcomes. The radicality of the surgical approach to large thymomas should, however, warrant utmost care in that recent evidence seems to confirm a higher rate of local recurrences after the resection of masses over 8 cm in diameter [17].

Unfortunately, imaging diagnostics (CT scan, MRI) cannot be relied upon in all cases to characterize the invasiveness of a lesion, most especially as regards invasion of the mediastinal pleura (Fig. 16.3), of the adjacent lung and of vascular structures: hence, resectability can only be evaluated intraoperatively. In these cases, the path to be taken remains a matter of debate. The role of debulking is controversial [18-19] and recent phase II studies have demonstrated a benefit in terms of survival after chemotherapy and radiotherapy alone in nonresectable locally advanced disease [20]. Despite the lack of guidelines in this respect, in case of nonresectable disease we believe it is useful to perform a debulking procedure, providing residual disease does not exceed 10% and is bounded by metal clips in

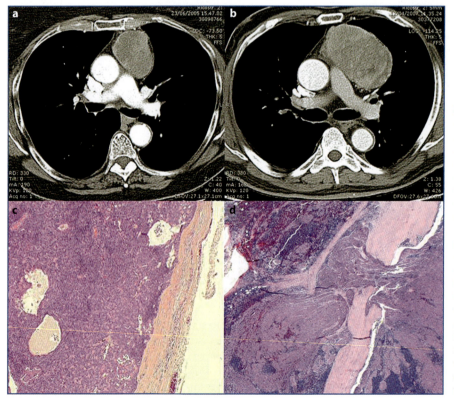

Fig. 16.3a-d a,c Neoplasm of the anterior mediastinum with clear margins and adipose plane between the lesion and mediastinal vascular structures. Histological findings of the specimen show a capsulated thymoma (Masaoka Stage I). **b, d** Neoplasm of the anterior mediastinum with regular margins extending to the left hemithorax with a broad area of contact at the level of the mediastinal pleura. Histological findings of the specimen show an invasive thymoma at the level of the capsule and of the mediastinal adipose tissue (Masaoka Stage II)

view of subsequent radiotherapy. Diagnostic biopsy followed by surgical assessment after induction therapy should instead be done, we believe, where debulking is not an option.

Outcomes of Surgical Treatment

The mortality rate following exeresis of a thymoma not accompanied by MG ranges between 3% and 7%, depending on case histories [21-31]. In locally-advanced disease, the mortality rate is significantly higher compared to initial stages. Adequate preoperative preparation of patients with MG, using plasmapheresis and gammaglobuline infusion, has reduced the proportion of postoperative myasthenic crises and in the latest case reports the postoperative mortality rate of patients with MG does not significantly differ from non-MG patients. Accompanying MG has long been seen as an adverse prognostic factor for long-term survival. Recent experiences have instead proven that accompanying MG has no significant impact on long-term prognosis, possibly due to the generally earlier stage of thymic neoplasms with accompanying MG [17, 32].

Although a range of clinical and pathological characteristics are analyzed, the two main prognostic factors for thymic neoplasms are stage and resection type. It has by now been broadly demonstrated that the Masaoka classification is an adequate staging system with a good prognostic stratification between stages (Table 16.3) Capsulated neoplasms (stage I) show excellent long-term survival rates, close to 100%, after radical exeresis. Invasion of the capsule or of adjacent structures (stages II and III) increases the percentage of recurrences after radical surgery by 5% and 25%, respectively [29].

In practice, all surgical case reports in literature show better survival rates after complete resection. The broader surgical case histories currently available [29], demonstrate that debulking is better than surgical biopsy alone. As mentioned earlier, we believe that debulking should only be performed in selected cases of locally-advanced disease found to be nonresectable intraoperatively.

Over the last few years, several studies have investigated the prognostic impact of the WHO histological classification. Some authors have demonstrated that types A and AB have a better prognoses than B and that the latter is significantly better than C. Others have highlighted that the prognosis for B3 is in between that of C and other, less aggressive forms. A recent review [4] of all the main studies on this topic concluded that the WHO classification appears to only be effective in distinguishing type C from less aggressive ones, while doubts still remain as to the prognostic stratification within the other subtypes (A, AB, B1, B2 e B3)

Conclusions

Within the framework of exeresis of thymic neoplasms, the thoracotomic approach should be reserved for selected cases of thymic neoplasm extensively involving one hemithorax and lying in the pericardium-phrenic angle and for operable focal pleural metastases. Where radical thymectomy with removal of mediastinal adipose tissue is not an op-

Table 16.3 Outcomes of surgical treatment of thymomas

Author	N° pts.	Thoracotomies (%)	R+ (%)	Overall survival at 5-10 yrs (%)			
				Masaoka stage			
				I	II	III	IV
Chalabreisse 2002 [22]	90	NA	33	NA	NA	NA	NA
Okumura 2002 [23]	311	NA	6	89'	91'	20'	0'
Nakagawa 2003 [24]	130	NA	5	100-100	100-100	81-76	47-47
Sperling 2003 [25]	65	21	35	88-80	71-71	61-45	48-16
Strobel 2004 [26]	545	NA	NA	100	90	75	47
Park 2004 [27]	150	NA	13	100	88	63	22
Rea 2004 [28]	132	42	18	93-84	93-82	60-51	36-0
Kondo 2005 [29]	1320	NA	8	100	98	88	70
Kim 2005 [30]	108	NA	18	100-95	91-81	74-46	NA
Rena 2005 [31]	197	NA	16	100	100	85	NA
Wright 2005 [17]	179	NA	11	0*	5*	70*	25*

NA, not available; *, recurrence rate; ', survival at 20 years

tion, the thoracotomic approach can be combined with sternotomy in a one-stage procedure (hemi-clamshell) or with delayed sternotomy.

References

1. Engels EA, Pfeuffer RM (2003) Malignant thymoma in the United States: Demographic patterns in incidence and associations with subsequent malignancies. Int J Cancer 105:546-551
2. Muller-Hermelink H, Engel P, Harris N et al (2004) Tumors of the thymus. In: Travis W, Brambilla E, Muller-Hermelink (eds) Tumors of the lung, thymus and heart. Pathology and genetics. IARC Press, Lyon
3. Masaoka A, Yamakawa Y, Niwa H et al (1994) Thymectomy and malignancy. Eur J Cardiothoracic Surg 8:251-253
4. Detterbeck FC (2006) Clinical value of the WHO classification system of thymoma. Ann Thorac Surg 81(6):2328-2334
5. Thomas CR, Wright CD, Loehrer PJ (1999) Thymoma: State of the art. J Clin Oncol 17:2280-2289
6. Ogawa K, Uno T, Toita T et al (2002) Postoperative radiotherapy for patients with completely resected thymoma. Cancer 94:1405-1413
7. Mangi AA, Wright CD, Allan JS et al (2002) Adjuvant radiation therapy for stage II thymoma. Ann Thorac Surg 74:1033-1037
8. Venuta F, Rendina EA, Longo F et al (2003) Long-term outcome after multimodality treatment for stage III thymic tumors. Ann Thorac Surg 76:1866-1872
9. Lucchi M, Ambrogi MC, Duranti L et al (2005) Advanced stage thymomas and thymic carcinomas: Results of multimodality treatments. Ann Thorac Surg 79:1840-1804
10. Kim ES, Putnam JB, Komaki R et al (2004) Phase II study of multidisciplinary approach with induction chemotherapy followed by surgical resection, radiation therapy and consolidation chemotherapy for unresectable malignant thymomas: Final report. Lung Cancer 44:369-379
11. Gotte JM, Bilfinger TV (2007) Resection of giant right-sided thymoma using a lateral thoracotomy approach followed by median sternotomy for completion thymectomy. Thoracic Cardiovasc Surg 55(5):336-338
12. Patterson GA (1992) Thymomas. Semin Thorac Cardiovasc Surg 4:39-44
13. Port JL, Ginsberg RJ (2001) Surgery for thymoma. Chest Surg Clin North Am 11:421-437
14. Kornstein MJ, Curran WJ Jr, Turrisi AT 3rd et al (1988) Cortical versus medullary thymoma: A useful morphologic distinction? Hum Pathol 19(11):1335-1339
15. Shields TW (2005) Thymic tumors. In: Shields TW (ed) General thoracic surgery. Lippincott Williams & Wilkins, Philadelphia, pp 2581-2617
16. Wright CD (2006) Pleuropneumonectomy for the treatment of Masaoka Stage IVa thymoma. Ann Thorac Surg 82:1234-1239
17. Wright CD, Wain JV, Wong DR et al (2005) Predictors of recurrence in thymic tumors: Importance of invasion. WHO histology and size. J Thoracic Cardiovasc Surg 130:1413-1421
18. Kohman LJ (1997) Controversies in the management of malignant thymoma. Chest 112:296S-300S
19. Liu HC, Chen YJ, Chen CY et al (2006) Debulking surgery for advanced thymoma. Eur J Surg Oncol 32:1000-1005
20. Loehrer PJ, Chen M, Kim K et al (1979) Cisplatin, doxorubicin and cyclophosphamide plus thoracic radiation therapy for limited-stage unresectable thymomas: An intergroup trial. J Clin Oncol 15:3093-3099
21. Maggi G, Casadio C, Cavallo A et al (1991) Thymoma: Results of 241 operated cases. Ann Thorac Surg 52(1):175-176
22. Chalabreisse L, Roy P, Cordier J-F et al (2002) Correlation of the WHO schema for the classification of thymic epithelial neoplasms with prognosis. Am J Surg Pathol 26:1605-1611
23. Okumura M, Ohta M, Tateyama H et al (2002) The World Health Organization histologic classification system reflects the oncologic behavior of thymoma: A clinical study of 273 patients. Cancer 94:624-632
24. Nakagawa K, Asamura H, Matsuno Y et al (2003) Thymoma: A clinicopathologic study based on the new World Health Organization classification. J Thorac Cardiovasc Surg 126:1134-1140
25. Sperling B, Marschall J, Kennedy R et al (2003) Thymoma: A review of the clinical and pathological findings in 65 cases. Can J Surg 46(1):37-42
26. Ströbel P, Bauer A, Puppe B et al (2004) Tumor recurrence and survival in patients treated for thymomas and thymic squamous cell carcinomas: A retrospective analysis. J Clin Oncol 22:1501-1509
27. Park MS, Chung KY, Kim KD et al (2004) Prognosis of thymic epithelial tumors according to the new World Health Organization histologic classification. Ann Thorac Surg 78:992-998
28. Rea F, Marulli G, Girardi R et al (2004) Long-term survival and prognostic factors in thymic epithelial tumors. Eur J Cardiothorac Surg 26:412-418
29. Kondo K, Yoshizawa K, Tsuyuguchi M et al (2004) WHO histologic classification is a prognostic indicator in thymoma. Ann Thorac Surg 77:1183-1188
30. Kim DJ, Yang WI, Choi SS et al (2005) Prognostic and clinical relevance of the World Health Organization schema for the classification of thymic epithelial tumors: A clinicopathologic study of 108 patients and literature review. Chest 127:755-761
31. Rena O, Papalia E, Maggi G et al (2005) World Health Organization histologic classification. An independent prognostic factor in resected thymomas. Lung Cancer 50:59-66
32. Regnard JF, Magdeleinat P, Dromer C et al (1996) Prognostic factors and long-term results after thymoma resection: A series of 307 patients. J Thorac Cardiovasc Surg 112:376-384

CHAPTER 17
Open Videoassisted Techniques: Transcervical Approach

Marc de Perrot, Shaf Keshavjee

Introduction

Blalock's initial experience in the early 1940s and subsequently published series of surgically treated patients led to the widespread acceptance of thymectomy in the treatment of MG despite the absence of a prospective randomized trial comparing surgery with medical treatment alone [1]. Controversies remain, however, with regard to the timing and extent of surgery to be performed.

The transcervical approach was first described in the late 19th century for thymic enlargement in children and consisted in an enucleation of the thymus from within its capsule. Although initially reported in an adult patient with MG by Sauerbruch in 1912, the transcervical approach was modified to completely remove the thymus with its capsule and reintroduced in the 1960s for patients with MG. Through this approach, Kark and his colleagues reported fewer postoperative complications when compared to the transsternal approach [2]. Consequently, their patients were operated on earlier in the course of the disease and were shown to have more rapid rate of improvement.

In order to improve exposure and to facilitate removal of the thymic gland and extracapsular thymic tissue through the neck, Cooper and colleagues described the use of a special right-angle manubrial retractor to elevate the sternum (Cooper retractor, Pilling Company, Fort Washington, PA) [3]. Using the same retractor, we observed that the routine use of a videothoracoscope introduced through the cervicotomy further improves visualization of the mediastinum and permits teaching of the technique under direct supervision [4]. Currently, the combination of early surgical referral, optimization of medical status when necessary by plasmapheresis, video-assisted transcervical thymectomy, and careful perioperative management have led to optimized care for patients with myasthenia gravis in our institution.

Preoperative Care

All patients with a diagnosis of MG are referred to surgery unless they are over 50 years of age and/or experience only ocular symptomatology, in which case the decision to proceed with surgery is decided on a case-by-case basis.

All patients have computed tomography (CT) scan of the thorax before surgery in order to exclude a thymoma. If a thymoma is detected a transsternal approach is always chosen. Relative contraindications to a transcervical approach include prior cervico-mediastinal surgery and/or radiation, and cervical spine pathology limiting extension of the neck. Age, gender, obesity, and exposure to steroids were not considered contraindications to the transcervical approach.

Patients undergoing thymectomy should have their medical condition optimized prior to surgery with anticholinesterase medications along with the use of plasmapheresis in selected cases. Corticosteroids are generally avoided preoperatively in order to minimize the perioperative complications associated with steroid use.

There is no role for urgent thymectomy in patients with myasthenic crisis as immediate clinical improvement postoperatively should not be expected. Rather, a period of 3-12 months is most often observed before clinical improvement can be seen following thymectomy. Furthermore, surgery in the setting of myasthenic crisis predisposes the patient to a significantly increased risk of postoperative respiratory failure.

Perioperative Management

Anesthetic assessment is performed at an ambulatory preadmission clinic visit. Patients are admitted on the day of surgery. They either take their morning dose of pyridostigmine as usually scheduled or take it immediately prior to surgery. If surgery is delayed or scheduled for the afternoon, another dose of pyridostigmine is given before surgery. No other premedication is administered. Anesthesia is induced with propofol and fentanyl, and is maintained with isoflurane and nitrous oxide. Propofol is used in addition to inhaled anesthetics for maintenance of anesthesia in many patients. In general, for transcervical thymectomy, no muscle relaxants are required. A short acting agent such as atracurium or rocuronium is used at reduced doses in less than 20% of cases in our experience. Patients are routinely extubated at the end of surgery in the operating room or occasionally in the recovery room.

Video-assisted Transcervical Approach

Surgery is performed in the supine position. Patients are intubated with a single lumen endotracheal tube. The neck is extended and an inflatable pillow is placed beneath the patient transversely, at the level of the scapulae, to permit further hyperextension of the neck. The neck and full chest are prepped in case a sternotomy is required. A curvilinear incision is made in the skin at the base of the neck, one finger breadth above the sternal notch, and extended on each side to the medial border of the sternocleidomastoid muscle (Fig. 17.1). The incision is extended through the platysma muscle and flaps are developed superiorly to the level of the inferior aspect of the thyroid cartilage and inferiorly to the sternal notch. The interclavicular ligament is divided. The strap muscles are then split vertically in the midline and elevated bilaterally in order to expose the superior poles of the thymus gland, which lie opposed to the posterior surface of the sternothyroid muscles. It is imperative that this be done using careful sharp dissection with meticulous attention to control small blood vessels with electrocautery. A bloodless field makes it significantly easier to delineate the upper poles of the thymus gland from fatty tissue in the neck. Each superior pole of the gland is mobilized near the inferior thyroid vein. The upper pole is divided between ties at the point where the thymic tissue terminates. A heavy silk suture, cut long, is placed on each upper pole and used as a "traction" suture to facilitate retraction of the gland. The thymus gland is then followed inferiorly to the thoracic inlet using a combination of blunt and sharp dissection. The retrosternal space is cleared with blunt finger dissection. This dissection is immediately substernal and extends at least 5-8 cm to accommodate the placement of the Cooper retractor without tension on the thymus gland. If the dissection is not deep enough, the thymus will be pulled into the mediastinum by the retractor as it is inserted. The Upper Hand retractor (Poly-Tract, Pilling Company, Fort Washington, PA) is then set up with the Cooper Thymectomy retractor blade (Pilling Company), which is then placed beneath the sternum to elevate it and open the thoracic inlet (Fig. 17.2). The inflatable pillow that was placed at the start of the procedure is deflated at this point to further improve the thoracic inlet exposure. Care is taken to make sure that the patient's

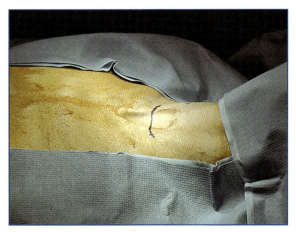

Fig. 17.1 The patient is in supine position and intubated with a single lumen tube. A small curvilinear incision is made at the base of the neck, one finger breadth above the sternal notch, extending to the medial border of the sternocleidomastoid muscle

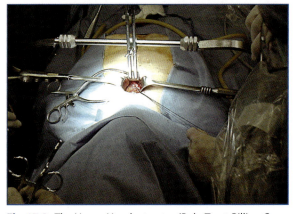

Fig. 17.2 The Upper Hand retractor (Poly-Tract, Pilling Company, Fort Washington, PA) is set up on each side of the patient and the Cooper Thymectomy retractor blade (Pilling Company) is then placed beneath the sternum to elevate it and open the thoracic inlet. The inflatable pillow is deflated at this point to further improve the thoracic inlet exposure

head is not elevated off the operating table pillow by the sternal retraction.

The 5-mm 30° videothoracoscope is then placed at the right lateral aspect of the neck incision to provide light for direct operating and a video magnified view of the operating field on a monitor for the surgeon and assistants (Fig. 17.3). Pressure is maintained laterally with the thoracoscope in order to keep the telescope out of the line of sight of the operating surgeon as much as possible. The dissection of the gland is carried down into the thorax using primarily blunt dissection. The thymic veins draining into the innominate vein are identified posteriorly and divided between stainless steel clips. Two clips are placed on the innominate vein side. The arterial vessels entering the gland laterally from the internal mammary arteries are also clipped with stainless steel clips. The ventilatory tidal volume and rate are frequently reduced in order to facilitate exposure in the mediastinum. The dissection is carried down along the pleura to the inferior poles of the gland alternatively on both sides. A dissecting "peanut" on a curved Swedish-Debakey dissector is used to sweep each inferior pole up. The dissector is placed on the pericardium, distal to the inferior pole of the thymus gland, and in a sweeping motion the gland is extracted from the inferior mediastinum. After this maneuver, the "socket" in which the inferior pole of the gland resided is clearly visible, as is the underlying pericardium. This technique can be done under direct vision with the light of the thoracoscope as an aid; or surgeons comfortable with thoracoscopic operating can operate using the thoracoscopic images on the monitor to perform the operation. The assistance of the videothoracoscope routinely provides good visualization of the lower mediastinum, down to the diaphragm if necessary. On occasion, when it is impossible to complete the operation through the transcervical route using direct vision only, the videothoracoscope can enable successful completion of a thymectomy without having to convert to a sternotomy.

Once the gland is excised (Fig. 17.4), if there is any further mediastinal fatty tissue present that is suspicious for being thymic tissue, this is excised or biopsied for frozen section analysis to ensure that no residual thymic tissue is left behind. A #7 Jackson-Pratt (JP) drain (Zimmer, Dover, OH) is inserted through a lateral stab wound in the neck, placed down into the mediastinum, and the manubrial retractor is removed. The strap muscles are approximated with a single figure of eight vicryl suture (Davis & Geck, Danbury, CT) and the platysma is closed with a running 3-0 vicryl suture.

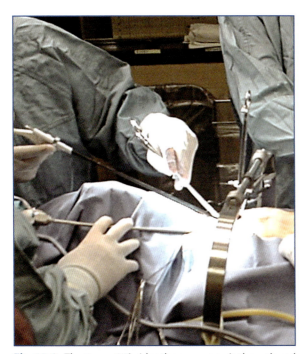

Fig. 17.3 The 5-mm 30° videothoracoscope is then placed at the right lateral aspect of the neck incision to provide light for direct operating and a video magnified view of the operating field on a monitor for the surgeon and assistants. The assistance of the videothoracoscope routinely provides good visualization of the lower mediastinum down to the diaphragm if necessary

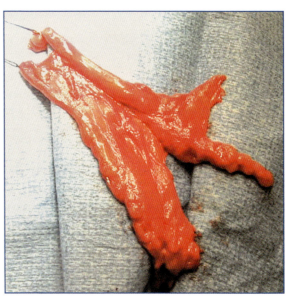

Fig. 17.4 Excised thymus with heavy silk sutures placed on each upper pole and used as "traction" suture to facilitate retraction of the gland during dissection of the lower poles

The skin is closed with a running 4-0 vicryl subcuticular suture. If it is felt that a total thymectomy cannot be safely completed through the transcervical route, the operation is converted to a partial upper sternotomy. This is carried out by the addition of a vertical incision extending down from the cervical incision to just below the manubrium. The incision in the sternal bone is then "J'd" out into the third or fourth intercostal space with the oscillating saw, to create a partial upper sternotomy, which provides sufficient exposure to easily complete the operation.

Postoperative Care

Analgesia is given orally using acetaminophen with or without codeine. Morphine is rarely required. Oral pyridostigmine at the patient's usual dose is reintroduced 4-6 h after surgery. If patients are on steroid therapy before surgery, an intravenous dose is given preoperatively and oral steroids are continued the next morning. The vast majority of our patients are ready to be discharged the next day after removal of the JP drain. Their preoperative medications are not altered until 1 month after surgery when they are seen by the surgeon and the neurologist. Some patients may get transiently worse postoperatively and the medication regimen may have to be altered to include prednisone or azathioprine. An occasional patient may deteriorate considerably. These patients should be expediently treated with plasmapheresis to prevent deterioration to the point of requiring ventilatory support.

Comments

In our experience, over 180 patients underwent transcervical thymectomy between January 1991 and December 2007. Approximately 70% of patients are female with an age ranging between 12 and 79 years (median 35 years). Postoperative complications are rare and the vast majority of our patients are discharged on the first postoperative day. This experience is very similar to other groups performing transcervical thymectomy (Table 17.1).

Long-term follow-up after transcervical thymectomy demonstrate excellent results with a cumulative complete remission rate of up 91% at 10 years after transcervical thymectomy [4]. Preoperative disease severity and the need for preoperative immunosuppression have been shown to be associated with delayed postoperative improvement in myasthenia gravis symptoms [4, 5].

Conclusions

In conclusion, considerable improvement has been made since the time when only selected patients with severe MG unresponsive to medical therapy underwent thymectomy. Currently, transcervical thymectomy requires hospitalization for less than 24 h in the vast majority of cases and is associated with very little morbidity. Patients therefore tend to be referred earlier in the course of their disease when they are in a more stable clinical condition. In the long term, this approach achieved excellent results comparable to other surgical techniques.

References

1. Drachman DB (1994) Myasthenia gravis. N Engl J Med 330:1797-1810
2. Kark AE, Kirschner PA (1971) Total thymectomy by the transcervical approach. Br J Surg 58:321-326
3. Cooper JD, Al-Jilaihawa AN, Pearson FG et al (1988) An improved technique to facilitate transcervical

Table 17.1 Results of extended transcervical thymectomy

Author (Ref)	Year of publication	No. patients	Surgical approach	Morbidity (%)	Mean FU (years)	Complete remission	
						Crude	Life table
Shrager et al. [5]	2006	164	Transcervical	7	4.4	40%	45% (at 6 years)
de Perrot et al. [4]	2003	120	Video-assisted transcervical	3	4.3	41%	91% (at 10 years)
Calhoun et al. [6]	1999	100	Transcervical	8	5	46%	N/A
Bril et al. [7]	1998	52	Transcervical	N/A	8.4	44%	N/A
De Filippi et al. [8]	1998	53	Transcervical	2	5	43%	N/A

thymectomy for myasthenia gravis. Ann Thorac Surg 45:242-247
4. de Perrot M, Bril V, McRae K, Keshavjee S (2003) Impact of minimally invasive transcervical thymectomy on outcome in patients with myasthenia gravis. Eur J Cardio-thoracic Surg 24:677-683
5. Shrager JB, Nathan D, Brinster CJ et al (2006) Outcomes after 151 extended transcervical thymectomies for myasthenia gravis. Ann Thorac Surg 82:1863-1869
6. Calhoun RF, Ritter JH, Guthrie TJ et al (1999) Results of transcervical thymectomy for myasthenia gravis in 100 consecutive patients. Ann Surg 230:555-561
7. Bril V, Kojic J, Ilse WK, Cooper JD (1998) Long-term clinical outcome after transcervical thymectomy for myasthenia gravis. Ann Thorac Surg 65:1520-1522
8. DeFilippi VJ, Richman DP, Ferguson MK (1994) Transcervical thymectomy for myasthenia gravis. Ann Thorac Surg 57:194-197

CHAPTER 18
Open Videoassisted Techniques: Subxiphoid Approach with Bilateral Thoracoscopy

Chung-Ping Hsu, Cheng-Yen Chuang

Introduction

For more than 50 years, sternal splitting thymectomy has been the gold standard ever since Blalock first introduced thymectomy for treatment of myasthenia in 1939 [1]. Jaretzki [2] and Masaoka [3] have demonstrated varied distribution of ectopic thymic tissues in the mediastinum and the neck. They both recommend a more extensive resection of tissue beyond the thymic gland itself, using a transcervical-transsternal approach. Minimally invasive thymectomy was introduced by Yim et al. using a right thoracoscopic approach in the early 1990s [4]. Some concern regarding this minimally invasive approach was raised mainly due to questioning the limited exposure, limited working space, and completeness of extended thymectomy which could endanger the therapeutic results [2]. Though controversy surrounds the selection of operation for patients with myasthenia gravis, we developed a novel technique to perform extended thymectomy using video-assisted thoracoscopy by a subxiphoid bilateral approach in early 2001.

Indications

Ideal candidates for our approach include patients with the following conditions:
- Non-thymomatous myasthenia gravis
- Thymoma less than 2 cm in size in upper half of thymus or less than 3 cm in size in the lower half of thymus
- Thymic cysts.

Contraindications

Patients who are not suitable for our approach include:
- Patients with extensive intrapleural adhesions
- Patients with previous history of median sternotomy
- Patients with previous history of mediastinal irradiation
- Patients with cardiomegaly.

Patients and Methods

Patient Profiles and Measurements

Between 2001 and 2007, a cohort of 50 patients receiving thoracoscopic thymectomy using the mentioned technique were enrolled in this study (Table 18.1). The patients included 12 males and 38 females with a mean age of 36.8 years (21-80 years). The severity of clinical symptoms were MGFA class I, II, III, and IV in 7, 23, 19, and 1 cases, respectively. The resected thymus weights, thoracic drainage periods, complications and outcomes were compared. Follow-up information was obtained by reviewing hospital records or telephone

Table 18.1 Demographic data and surgical results of 50 myasthenic patients receiving thymectomy by subxiphoid bilateral approach

Sex (male/female)	12/38
Age (years, mean)	21-80 (36.8±14.4)
Body mass index	23.4
MGFA class (I/IIB/IIIA/IIIB/IV)	7/23/7/12/1
Thymic weights (grams, mean)	
Overall	25-130 (65.8±26.5)
Non-thymoma	25-130 (61.7±26.2)
Pathology	
Thymoma	9 (18%)
Masaoka stage I	5
Masaoka stage II	4
Non-thymoma	41 (82%)
Thymic hyperplasia	30
Normal thymus	3
Involutional change	6
Others	2
Operation time (minutes, mean)	80-200 (136.2±25.3)
Thoracic drainage (days, mean)	2-10 (3.6±1.3)

contact at intervals of 3 months in the first postoperative year, and then annually. End result interpretation included complete remission (CR) (no medication required), improved (taking mestinon equal to or less than 120 mg/day, but no prednisolone required), stationary (taking mestinon more than 120 mg/day, or any dose of prednisolone), worse (requiring more medication than before surgery). The follow-up period was 4-72 months (mean of 21.7 months).

Preference Card

- Thoracoscope with a side arm working channel (0 degree, 5-mm working channel, 13-in, Karl Storz, Tuttlingen, Germany) (Fig. 18.1).
- Kent retractor set and its accessories (Takasago Medical Industry Co., Tokyo, Japan)
- Instruments which can be introduced from the subxiphoid incision:
  - Ring forceps of various lengths
  - Long slight tissue forceps
  - Long suction catheter (15-in long)
- Instruments specific for thoracoscopic use:
  - Thoracoscopic trocars (12 mm)
  - Endoscopic hook cautery, grasper, clip applier (5 mm)
  - Endoscopic LigaSure LS1500 (5-mm Sealer/Divider, Valley Lab, TycoHealthcare LP, Boulder, CO, USA.)
  - Sternal saw and standard thymectomy tray ready to use.

Patient Setup and Preparation

Under general anesthesia with split lung ventilation, the patient was put in a supine position with 90° abduction of bilateral upper extremities (Fig. 18.2). A rolling pad was put underneath the patient's shoulders to facilitate neck extension. Kent retractor set was fixed to the side bar of the operation table on the patient's head side. The basic settings are shown in Fig. 18.2. Except for patients with MGFA class I myasthenia gravis, 2 to 3 courses of plasmaphoresis were performed before surgery. Intravenous methylprednisolone (1000 mg in 24 h) was administered in the perioperative period.

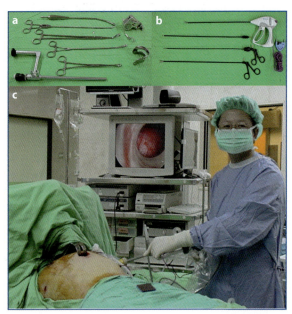

Fig. 18.1a-c Preference card and patient setup. **a** Thoracoscope with a side arm working channel, Kent retractor accessories, and instruments which can be introduced from the subxiphoid incision such as: long suction catheter, slight tissue forceps, and ring forceps of various lengths. **b** Endoscopic instruments such as: LigaSure, hook cautery, and graspers. **c** After finishing the right-side procedure, the operator stands on the patient's left side controlling the thoracoscope with the assistance of Kent retractor to elevate the sternum

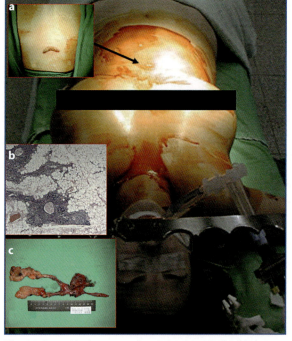

Fig. 18.2a-c Under general anesthesia with double lumen endobronchial tube, the patient was put in supine position with 90° abduction of both upper extremities. **a** A 5-cm-long curved incision was made just below the xiphoid process. **b** Pathology revealed involutional change of the thymus. **c** Extended resection of the thymus showing both upper horns and bilateral pericardial fat pads (60 gm in weight)

Procedure in Details

The majority of the dissection was accomplished by an endoscopic hook cautery or Ligasure cautery introduced through the thoracoscope (controlled by operator) with the help of long, curved-tip ring forceps and/or suction catheter introduced from the subxiphoid incision (controlled by assistant) for traction and dissection of the thymic tissues. The surgical procedure has been revised several times since the initial experience in 2001 [5-7].

The operation started with a 4- to 6-cm long semi-curved incision created just above the tip of xiphoid process (Fig. 18.2a). The anterior rectal sheath was detached from its insertion to the xiphoid process and the bilateral lowest rib cartilages. After excision of the xiphoid process, the retrosternal space was created by finger dissection for introduction of the Kent retractor to lift the sternum, facilitating thoracoscopic and instrumental manipulation. Additional thoracic port sites (1 cm each) were created at the bilateral anterior axillary line in the 5th or 6th intercostal space to introduce the thoracoscope. After thorough evaluation of the pleural cavity, pleural reflection at the lowest sternocostal junction was opened from the subxiphoid incision with guidance from the thoracoscope. The mediastinal dissection was started by freeing the fat pad in the pericardiophrenic sinus cephalically along the anterior border of the phrenic nerve. As part of this avascular plan of dissection, the thymic lobe was also separated from the underlying ascending aorta. With meticulous dissection, the conjunction of the brachiocephalic vein and superior vena cava was identified. The gland was pulled medially by long, curved-tip ring forceps introduced from the subxiphoid incision. Another long suction was introduced from the same incision to push aside the pleural reflection at the pleural apex. This maneuver provides ample space facilitating dissection and delivery of the upper horn of the thymic gland. The upper horn of the thymic gland was delivered from the neck using a combination of blunt dissection and traction. After pulling down the upper horn, the course of the brachiocephalic vein was traced to expose all the thymic veins. Usually, two to three thymic veins were encountered and divided between endoscopic clips or using cautery.

On the left side, the thoracoscopic port site can be created at the same level just opposite to the right side, or can be made one intercostal space higher than the right side to keep an adequate distance from the heart border. The entire procedure is similar to that on the right side. Adequate hemostasis should be obtained either by cautery or metallic clips during delivery of the left upper thymic horn so as to prevent thoracic duct injury.

Finally, the totally freed thymic gland and its accompanying mediastinal fatty tissues (Fig. 18.2b) could be brought out from the subxiphoid incision for pathological examination (Fig. 18.2c). A 16-Fr pig-tail catheter was put into each side of the pleural cavity through the thoracoscopic port site and secured to the chest wall. The rectal sheath was reattached, and the subxiphoid incision was closed by subcuticle sutures. Postoperative chest film was taken to make sure no residual pneumothoraces existed (Fig. 18.3). Typically, the pig-tail catheters were removed on the 3rd to 4th postoperative day, and patients were discharged on the same day.

Results

The resected thymus showed thymoma in 9 cases, which included Masaoka class I in 5 and class II in 4. For the remaining 41 non-thymomatous group, the pathology comprised of thymic hyperplasia in 30, normal thymus in 3, involutional change in 6, thymic cyst in 1, and thymolipoma in 1. The mean operation time, weights of resected specimens, and days of chest tube drainage were 80-200 (136.2±25.3) min, 25-130 (65.8±26.5) grams, and 2-10 (3.6±1.3) days, respectively (see Table 18.2).

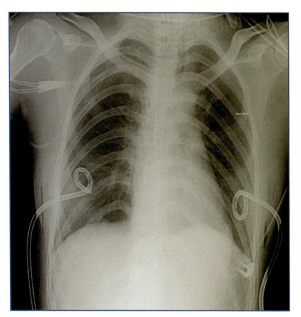

Fig. 18.3 Postoperative chest film shows well-expanded lung with pig-tail catheter in each side of pleural cavity through the thoracoscopic port sites

Table 18.2 Complications and outcomes of patients receiving thymectomy by subxiphoid bilateral approach

Complications	
Prolonged intubation (>24 h)	3
Intraoperative arrhythmia	2
Chylothorax	1
Brachiocephalic vein injury	1
Outcomes*	
Complete remission	19
Improved	28
Stationary	2

* One patient who had been converted to upper partial sternotomy was excluded from outcomes analysis

Complications included prolonged tracheal intubation (>24 h) in 3, intraoperative arrhythmia in 2, chylothorax in 1 and brachiocephalic vein injury in 1. After exclusion of 1 patient who was given an upper partial sternotomy due to bleeding, CR, improvement and stationary status were observed in 19 (38.8%), 28 (57.1%), and 2 (4.1%) patients, respectively. As shown in Fig. 18.4, the cumulative CR rate was 57.2% at 5 years using Kaplan-Meier analysis.

Discussion

Once the gold standard surgical approach, the transsternal thymectomy has been mercilessly challenged by lesser traumatic surgical intervention using thoracoscope. Though the transcervical-transsternal approach provides the only possible way to perform so-called maximal thymectomy, accumulative experience has documented equal medium-term results regardless of different surgical approaches supposing adequate mediastinum adipose tissue has been resected together with the thymus [8-10]. The reported CR rates of the recently developed minimally invasive procedures are between 30% and 50%. This may be due to shorter follow-up periods in the thoracoscopy group. However, studies contributing this relatively lower CR were influenced by the existence of ectopic thymic tissue in mediastinal fat [2, 11, 12]. Özdemira et al. reported that ectopic mediastinal thymic tissue can be found in 27.8% of resected specimens. Multivariate analysis revealed the presence of mediastinal ectopic thymic tissue to be an independent predictor of poorer outcomes (odds ratio, 7.75). They concluded that complete removal of the thymic tissue is essential for a favorable clinical outcome [13].

Nevertheless, minimally invasive procedures have gradually replaced the role of transsternal thymectomy due to their faster recovery. Among these, the transcervical approach has the benefit of a smaller incision, but the inadequate exposure of the more caudal thymic and mediastinal fat tissue. Video-assisted thoracic surgery (VATS) procedures through the right side [4] or left side [8] of the chest wall provides an excellent view of the operative side, but limited exposure to the contralateral side due to

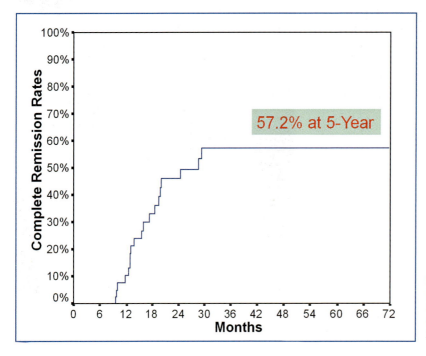

Fig. 18.4 Cumulative CR rates (57.2% at 5 years) of the patients after video-assisted thoracoscopic extended thymectomy by the subxiphoid bilateral approach

limited degrees of freedom of conventional endoscopic instruments which subsequently endangers complete removal of the contralateral-side mediastinal fat. Using mediastinoscope, Kido et al. first introduced the feasibility of using the retrosternal route to perform a resection of anterior mediastinal tumors [14]. Unlike thoracoscopy, this procedure avoids opening the chest and can be performed in patients with pleural adhesions or pulmonary insufficiency in whom split lung ventilation is impossible. Adapting the same idea, Takeo et al. designed another setup for sternal lifting from both ends of the sternum; however, their technique is basically identical to the bilateral thoracoscopic approach [15]. Uchiyama et al. subsequently reported a larger series using infrasternal mediastinoscopy for resection of thymus and anterior mediastinal mass [16, 17]. With or without additional cervical incision, the whole procedure is accomplished exclusively through the working channel of the mediastinoscope. Because the pleural is not routinely opened, maximal excision of the mediastinal and pericardial fat becomes questionable.

Using the same idea of sternal lifting, we designed a novel thoracoscopic setup to overcome the disadvantages of the previously described minimally invasive procedures for thymectomy [5]. Initial experiences using the subxiphoid incision as the main working route were abandoned and replaced by bilateral thoracic ports at the 5th or 6th intercostal space in the anterior axillary line due to interference between the endoscopic instruments [6, 7]. By changing position of the thoracoscope (0° thoracoscope with side arm working channel, Karl Storz, Tuttlingen, Germany), and the main working route, a panoramic view of the operative fields is possible. Moreover, instrumental manipulations are much easier. Unlike other methods, our setup provides a unique advantage of simultaneous bilateral access to the pleural cavities, which greatly improves the possibility of extended thymectomy.

As experience accumulates, worldwide reports have demonstrated video-assisted thoracoscopic approaches can be used for whatever means feasible and safe for resection of thymus. However, one major concern of these procedures is their efficacy in treating myasthenia gravis. Though short- and medium-term follow-up results are promising [10, 18-20], long-term remission rates are inferior to maximal thymectomy performed by a combined transcervical-transsternal approach [21, 22]. Rückert et al. compared the results of three different surgical approaches to carry out thymectomy [10]. They reported that though the thoracoscopic approach required the longest operation time, postoperative morbidity rate was the lowest. There were no differences regarding remission rates; however, they believe the thoracoscopic group has the best cosmetic results and the best chance for a further increase of CR rate due to having the shortest follow-up in this group.

Worldwide reports concerning different types of thymectomy for myasthenia indicate that the remission rate is closely related to the extent of thymectomy [23]. In a long-term follow-up study (154 patients, mean follow-up duration of 98.9 months) from one of our branch hospitals, Huang et al. reported that CR was achieved in 57.8%, and marked clinical improvement in another 30.5% after transsternal thymectomy. Favorable prognosis was observed especially in young patients (<35 years old), and in patients with short disease interval before surgery (<24 months) [24]. Except for a longer operation time, another prospective design study from Taiwan also confirmed the benefits of thoracoscopic thymectomy using a bilateral thoracic approach [25]. In the current study, we found an overall CR rate of 38.8%, an overall improvement rate of 57.1%, or a cumulative CR rate of 57.2% at 5 years. Though the CR rate was lower than the trans-sternal thymectomy group in our hospital (52.9% CR rates and 32.9% improvement rates in 85 patients, unpublished data), the improvement rate was higher. This can be attributed to a relatively shorter follow-up period (mean, 21.7 months) in the thoracoscopic group of patients.

As with any newly adapted technique, longer operation times are almost inevitable in the learning period. As experience grew, however, all operations performed in the recent 3 years (28 cases) were accomplished within 150 min. This is comparable with traditional transsternal approach regarding operation time. But, less pain, rapid recovery, shorter pleural drainage period, shorter hospital stay, and better cosmetic satisfaction of the patient were observed when compared with our historical experience by transsternal thymectomy.

Our approach completely eliminates the possibility of sternal osteomyelitis. Wound healing was excellent, and invisible after surgery due to its location. Three patients in this series required prolonged tracheal intubation for more than 24 h postoperatively. Except for one patient who had respiratory failure before surgery, the other two were extubated within 48 h. Intraoperative arrhythmias, including one bradycardia and one ventricular tachycardia, were encountered. This was caused by putting too much pressure on the heart surface by instruments during tissue dissections. Both of these episodes recovered after releasing heart compression. One patient developed left-side chylothorax probably due to injury of the thoracic duct at its junction with subclavian vein. The chylous leak healed spontaneously 10 days after discontinue of oral intake and total parenteral nutrition support.

Though concomitant thymoma is not an absolute contraindication for thoracoscopic thymectomy, our experience suggests that larger thymomas (larger than 2 cm in diameter) require a longer operation time for resection with additional risk of opening the capsule. The only conversion occurred in one patient who had a Masoaka stage IIb thymoma. Uncontrolled bleeding occurred on separation of the tumor from its underlying brachiocephalic vein. Immediate upper partial sternotomy was performed, and the torn vein was secured. The tumor measured $3 \times 1.5 \times 1.5$ cm^3 in size, and the pathology revealed a WHO type B2 thymoma. This complication suggests that a thymoma of 2 cm across or larger may not be a good candidate for thoracoscopic resection, especially when the tumor is located in the upper half of the thymus. In addition, a sternal saw and standard thymectomy tray ready to be used should be available. Nevertheless, the majority of the thymomas were completely removed without additional incisions. None of these patients had tumor recurrence or metastasis, and two of them have had CR thus far.

In summary, our experience has demonstrated minimally invasive procedures using subxiphoid and bilateral thoracoscopic approaches can safely accomplish promising outcomes in myasthenic patients as with standard transsternal thymectomy. Moreover, our approach has the advantages of (1) feasibility of extended thymectomy; (2) direct retrieval of the specimen from the subxiphoid wound; (3) providing excellent cosmesis with a concealed wound; and (4) less pain, shorter pleural drainage period, and subsequently shorter hospital stay.

References

1. Blalock A, Masson MF, Morgan HJ, Riven SS (1939) Myasthenia gravis and tumors of the thymic region: Report of a case in which the tumor was removed. Ann Surg 110:544-561
2. Jaretzki A III, Wolff MM (1988) "Maximal" thymectomy for myasthenia gravis. J Thorac Cardiovasc Surg 96:711-716
3. Masoaka A, Nagaoka Y, Kotake Y (1975) Distribution of thymic tissue at the anterior mediastinum – Current procedures in thymectomy. J Thorac Cardiovasc Surg 70:745-754
4. Yim AP, Kay RLC, Ho JKS (1995) Video-assisted thoracoscopic thymectomy for myasthenia gravis. Chest 108:1440-1443
5. Hsu CP (2002) Subxiphoid approach for thoracoscopic thymectomy. Surg Endosc 16:1105
6. Hsu CP, Chuang CY, Hsu NY, Shia SE (2002) Subxiphoid approach for video-assisted thoracoscopic extended thymectomy in treating myasthenia gravis. Interactive Cardiovasc Thorac Surgery 1:4-8
7. Hsu CP, Chuang CY, Hsu NY, Chen CY (2004) Comparison between the right side and subxiphoid bilateral approaches in performing video-assisted thoracoscopic extended thymectomy for myasthenia gravis. Surg Endosc 18:821-824
8. Mack MJ, Landreneau RJ, Yim AP et al (1996) Results of VATS thymectomy in patients with myasthenia gravis. J Thorac Cardiovasc Surg 112:1352-1360
9. Savcenko M, Wendt GK, Prince SL, Mack M (2002) Video-assisted thymectomy for myasthenia gravis: An update of a single institution experience. Eur J Cardio Thorac Surg 22:978-983
10. Rückert JC, Sobel HK, Göhring S et al (2003) Matched-pair comparison of three different approaches for thymectomy in myasthenia gravis. Surg Endosc 17:711-715
11. Ashour M (1995) Prevalence of ectopic thymic tissue in myasthenia gravis and its clinical significance. J Thorac Cardiovasc Surg 109:632-635
12. Fukai I, Funato Y, Mizumo T et al (1991) Distribution of thymic tissue in the mediastinal adipose tissue. J Thorac Cardiovasc Surg 101:1099-1102
13. Özdemira N, Karab M, Dikmenb E et al (2003) Predictors of clinical outcome following extended thymectomy in myasthenia gravis Euro J Cardio Thorac Surg 23:233-237
14. Kido T, Hazama K, Inoue Y et al (1999) Resection of anterior mediastinal masses through an infrasternal approach. Ann Thorac Surg 67:263-265
15. Takeo S, Sakada T, Yano T (2001) Video-assisted extended thymectomy in patients with thymoma by lifting the sternum. Ann Thorac Surg 71:1721-1723
16. Uchiyama A, Shimizu S, Murai H et al (2001) Infrasternal mediastinoscopic thymectomy in myasthenia gravis: Surgical results in 23 patients. Ann Thorac Surg 72:1902-1905
17. Uchiyama A, Shimizu S, Murai H et al (2004) Infrasternal mediastinoscopic surgery for anterior mediastinal masses. Surg Endosc 18:843-846
18. Wright GM, Barnett S, Clarke CP (2002). Video-assisted thoracoscopic thymectomy for myasthenia gravis. Int Med J 32:367-371
19. Wolfe GI, Gross B (2004) Treatment review and update for myasthenia gravis. J Clinic Neuromuscular Dis 6:54-68
20. Manlulu A, Lee TW, Wan I et al (2005) Video-assisted thoracic surgery thymectomy for nonthymomatous myasthenia gravis. Chest 128:3454-3460
21. Jaretzki A III, Aarli JA, Kaminski HJ et al (2003) Thymectomy for myasthenia gravis: Evaluation requires controlled prospective studies. Ann Thorac Surg 76:1-3

22. Mantegazza R, Baggi F, Bernasconi P et al (2003) Video-assisted thoracoscopic extended thymectomy and extended thymectomy (T-3b) in non-thymomatous myasthenia gravis patients: Remission after 6 years of follow-up. J Neurol Sci 212:31-36
23. Jaretzki A III (2003) Thymectomy for myasthenia gravis: Analysis of controversies – Patient management. Neurologist 9:77-92
24. Huang CS, Hsu HS, Huang BS et al (2005) Factors influencing the outcome of transsternal thymectomy for myasthenia gravis. Acta Neurol Scand 112:108-114
25. Chang PC, Chou SH, Kao EL et al (2005) Bilateral video-assisted thoracoscopic thymectomy vs. extended transsternal thymectomy in myasthenia gravis: A prospective study. Eur Surg Res 37:199-203

CHAPTER 19

Open Videoassisted Techniques: Transcervical-Subxiphoid-Videothoracoscopic Maximal Thymectomy

Marcin Zieliński, Łukasz Hauer, Jarosław Kużdżał, Witold Sośnicki, Maria Harazda, Juliusz Pankowski, Tomasz Nabiałek, Artur Szlubowski

Introduction

There is a general agreement that thymectomy has a beneficial effect on the results of treatment of myasthenia, although any prospective randomized studies have never been performed to compare the results of operative and conservative treatment of the disease.

There are several techniques of thymectomy utilizing the transsternal, transcervical, videothoracoscopic (VTS), subxiphoid, and combined transcervical-VTS approaches [1-10]. The problem of which technique of thymectomy should be preferred is still a matter of debate. In this report we present the technique of transcervical-subxiphoid-VTS "maximal" thymectomy, developed by the authors of this study [11, 12].

Surgical Technique

The operative technique of this procedure is as follows: a patient is positioned supine on the operating table with a roll placed beneath the thoracic spine to elevate the chest and to hyperextend the patient's neck. Under general anesthesia an endobronchial tube is inserted to conduct selective lung ventilation during the latter part of the procedure. To shorten the operative time and to facilitate performance of the procedure, an operation may be performed by two teams – one called the "cervical team" working from above and the second one called "the subxiphoid team" working from below the sternum with control of the videothoracoscope (VTS). The position of all four members of both surgical teams and the scrub nurse is shown on Fig. 19.1. Alterna-

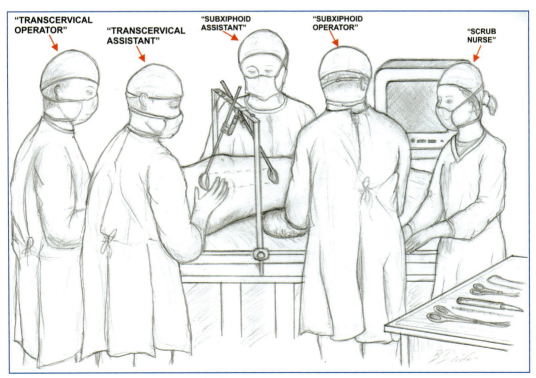

Fig. 19.1 The position of all four members of both teams

tively, the whole operation is performed by one surgical team performing "the cervical" and "the subxiphoid" parts of the operation sequentially.

All operative steps are described without specifying if one or two teams are involved. The cervical part of the operation: a transverse 5- to 8-cm incision is made in the neck above the sternal notch. The platysma and superficial cervical fascia are divided; the anterior jugular veins are divided and suture-ligated. The strap muscles are split along their median raphe and retracted laterally. The whole thyroid gland is visualized and all foci of the adipose tissue are removed downwards from the level of the upper poles of the thyroid gland. The parathyroid glands and both laryngeal recurrent nerves are visualized and carefully preserved (Figs. 19.2, 19.3). The fatty tissue containing the superior poles of the thymus is separated from the lower poles of the thyroid gland with 1-4 inferior thyroid veins ligated and divided (Fig. 19.4). Alternatively, such devices as a harmonic knife, LigaSure, or vascular clips can be used to secure the vessels throughout the procedure. The thymus with the surrounding fat is then separated from the sternohyoid and sternothyroid muscles, the trachea, the internal surface of the sternum, the carotid arteries, the innominate artery, the aorta, and the right innominate vein. At this point a sternal retractor connected to the firm frame with a traction mechanism is inserted under the manubrium of the sternum to el-

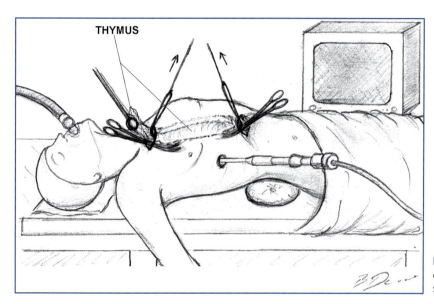

Fig. 19.2 Scheme of transcervical-subxiphoid-videothoracoscopic maximal thymectomy

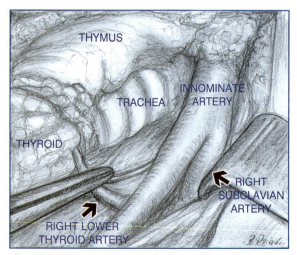

Fig. 19.3 Dissection of the right laryngeal recurrent nerve. Reproduced from [12] with permission from the European Association of Cardio-thoracic Surgery. Copyright 2005

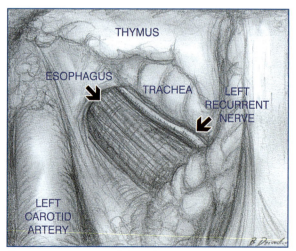

Fig. 19.4 Dissection of the left laryngeal recurrent nerve. Reproduced from [12] with permission from the European Association of Cardio-thoracic Surgery. Copyright 2005

evate it several centimeters to provide access to the anterior mediastinum. The lower thyroid veins (1-4) and the thymic veins (1-4) are dissected, clipped, and divided close to the left innominate vein (Fig. 19.5). The fatty tissue from the area called "the aorta-caval groove" is removed. The boundaries of this space are the division of the innominate artery and the aorta (medially), the trachea (posteriorly), the right innominate vein and the right mediastinal pleura (laterally), and the right main bronchus, the azygos vein, and the superior vena cava (inferiorly) (Fig. 19.6). The dissection proceeds caudally, below the left innominate vein, and the specimen is separated from the pericardium at a distance of several centimeters. The most difficult, but very important part of this operation is the dissection of the adipose tissue from the aorta-pulmonary window. Further dissection of two other branches of the left innominate vein, namely the left internal thoracic vein and the accessory hemiazygos vein is mandatory. These two veins are subsequently divided and their ends are secured with clips or sutures (preferably) (Fig. 19.7). The division of these veins provides much better access to the aorta-pulmonary window above the left innominate vein, which is retracted towards the aorta. The next step is the visualization of the left phrenic nerve, which runs very close to the left internal thoracic vein and the left vagus nerve, which runs laterally to the left common carotid artery. With blunt dissection using a peanut sponge, the fatty tissue containing the aorta-pulmonary window is dissected from these nerves, the aorta, and the left mediastinal pleura. At the bottom of the aorta-pulmonary window the left pulmonary artery is visualized (Fig. 19.8). In difficult cases the dissection

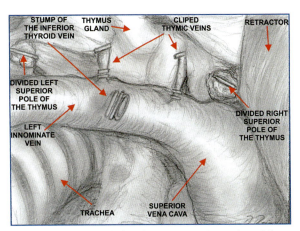

Fig. 19.6 Division of the thymic veins. Reproduced from [12] with permission from the European Association of Cardio-thoracic Surgery. Copyright 2005

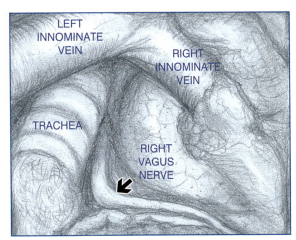

Fig. 19.7 View of the aorta-caval groove after removal of its adipose, lymphatic, and thymic contents. Reproduced from [12] with permission from the European Association of Cardio-thoracic Surgery. Copyright 2005

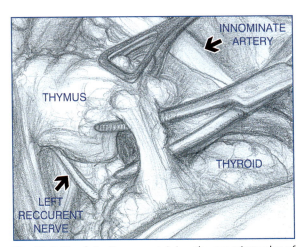

Fig. 19.5 The fatty tissue containing the superior poles of the thymus is separated from the lower poles of the thyroid gland with 1-4 inferior thyroid veins ligated and divided. Reproduced from [12] with permission from the European Association of Cardio-thoracic Surgery. Copyright 2005

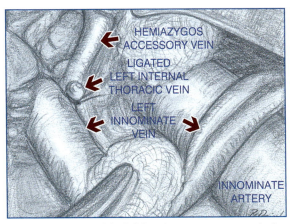

Fig. 19.8 Division of the left hemiazygos accessory vein. Reproduced from [12] with permission from the European Association of Cardio-thoracic Surgery. Copyright 2005

of the aorta-pulmonary window is completed at a later stage of the operation with a videothoracoscopic camera inserted inside the chest.

The subxiphoid part of the operation: a transverse 4- to 6-cm incision is made above the xiphoid process. The subcutaneous tissue is cut and the medial parts of the rectus muscles are cut near the insertions to the costal arches. The xiphoid process is divided transversely and left without removal. The selective left lung ventilation is started resulting in the collapse of the right lung. The anterior mediastinum is opened from below the sternum. A second sternal retractor connected to the traction frame (the same as one which is used for traction of the manubrium) is placed under the sternum, which is elevated to facilitate access to the anterior mediastinum from below. A thoracoscopic port for a 5-mm, 30° oblique thoracoscope is inserted into the right pleural cavity in the 6th intercostal space in the anterior axillary line. The right mediastinal pleura is cut near the sternal surface up to the level of the right internal thoracic vein, which is left intact. The prepericardial fat and right and left epiphrenic fat pads are dissected from the pericardium and diaphragm with blunt dissection using a peanut sponge and a sharp dissection using scissors. Dissection of the prepericardial fat containing the thymus gland proceeds upwards under the control of the VTS camera with en bloc fashion, without any attempt to dissect the thymus gland separately (Fig. 19.9). The right phrenic nerve is a margin of dissection. At this moment the thymus is attached to the pericardium only with its left-lower pole. Ventilation of the right lung is resumed and the ventilation of the left lung is disconnected. A thoracoscopic port for a 5-mm, 30° oblique thoracoscope is inserted into the left pleural cavity, as on the right side. The operating table is rotated on the right side with elevation of the left side, which lowers the mediastinum, improving access to the left pleural cavity. Under the control of the VTS camera the left mediastinal pleura is divided along the sternum and the left prepericardial fat is dissected from the pericardium above the level of the left internal thoracic vein previously divided. The left-lower pole of the thymus is separated from the pericardium and the specimen is removed. Dissection of the aorta-pulmonary window is completed, if necessary, at this stage of the operation. Hemostasis is checked, the VTS ports are removed and the chest tubes are inserted into both pleural cavities through the incisions made for insertion of the ports. Ventilation of both lungs is resumed. The cervical and subxiphoid incisions are closed in the standard manner. Generally, a patient is extubated immediately after the operation.

Methods

Generally, patients with type I-III of myasthenia according to Osserman-Genkins Classification were operated on. During this period of time, patients with thymoma and the patients undergoing repeated thymectomy (rethymectomy) were operated on using the technique of extended transsternal thymectomy, similar to the technique described by Bulkley [3]. In case the myasthenia is severe and the clinical state of the patients is not stable, the preliminary treatment modalities, such as steroids (in dose of 1 mg/kg/day of prednisone), immunosuppressive drugs (azathioprine), intravenous immunoglobulins, or plasmapheresis are used until the patient's clinical state becomes optimal. Operating time and intraoperative and postoperative complications were recorded.

To estimate late results of treatment of myasthenia, questionnaires with questions regarding the clinical state and antimyasthenic drugs intake were sent to all patients at 1-year intervals. Based on the answers to the questionnaires, the complete remission rates (lack of myasthenic symptoms with no need for any myasthenic drugs, including corticosteroids and other immunosuppressive drugs), the improvement rates, the no-improvement rates, deterioration rate, and the late mortality rates (the death from MG or other causes) were calculated.

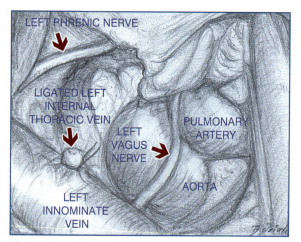

Fig. 19.9 View of the aorta-pulmonary window after removal of its adipose, lymphatic, and thymic contents. Reproduced from [12] with permission from the European Association of Cardio-thoracic Surgery. Copyright 2005

Results

259 patients were operated on in the period from July 1st, 2000 to July 30th, 2007. The mean operative time

for one team approach was 201.5 min (120-330 min) and for two-team approach it was 141 (95-210 min). There was no mortality and the morbidity rate was 12%. The complications are listed in Table 19.1.

The rates of complete remission after 1-, 2-, 3-, 4-, and 5-years of follow-up were 25%, 36.8%, 43.2%, 47.8%, and 51.2%, respectively (Figs. 19.10, 19.11).

Table 19.1 Complications in 259 patients with myasthenia gravis operated on with transcervical-subxiphoid-VATS "maximal" thymectomy

Type of complication	N (%)
Superior vena cava or left innominate vein laceration (managed with clips or sutures without sternotomy)	3 (1.2%)
Postoperative bleeding necessitating revision	5 (1.9%)
Temporary laryngeal recurrent nerve paresis	3 (1.2%)
Permanent laryngeal recurrent nerve paresis	0
Pleural hematoma necessitating VTS	1 (0.4%)
Pleural hematoma necessitating needle aspiration	1 (0.4%)
Respiratory insufficiency – ventilator	11 (4.2%)
Pneumonia without respiratory insufficiency	1 (0.4%)
Minor wound complications	4 (1.5%)
Subarachnoid hemorrhage	1 (0.4%)
Pneumothorax	1 (0.4%)
Overall	31 (12%)

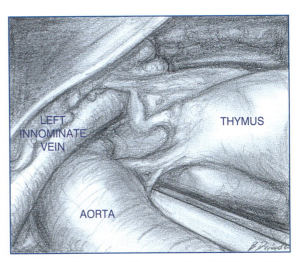

Fig. 19.10 Dissection of the prepericardial fat containing the thymus gland. Reproduced from [12] with permission from the European Association of Cardio-thoracic Surgery. Copyright 2005

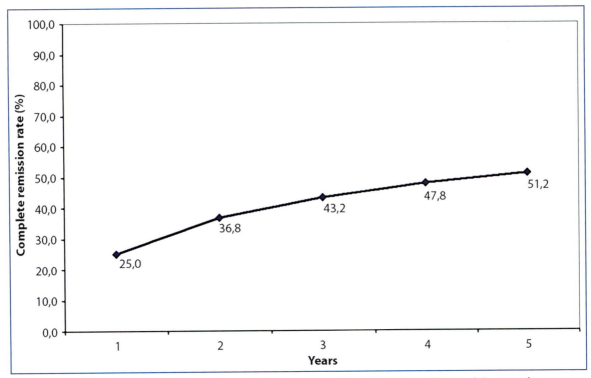

Fig. 19.11 The complete remission rates of myasthenic symptoms after 1-, 2-, 3-, 4-, and 5-years follow-up after transcervical-subxiphoid-VATS "maximal" thymectomy

Discussion

The "maximal" transcervical-subxiphoid-VATS thymectomy is a relatively safe procedure, with no mortality and 12% morbidity, including only 4.2% of patients needing ventilator support. This technique avoids sternotomy, which considerably reduces postoperative pain. Although there were only few complications connected with a sternotomy wound in previous experience in our department, with only two sternal dehiscences in 680 thymectomies (including thymomas and rethymectomies), there is always a potential for such complications [13]. Moreover, after sternotomy the patients' postoperative discomfort is more pronounced and the cosmetic result after sternotomy is less favorable. Results of complete remission rates of patients operated on with a "maximal" transcervical-subxiphoid-VATS thymectomy are comparable to the results achieved with use of the extended transsternal approach (46.6% after 4-years follow-up) [14].

Conclusions

The transcervical-subxiphoid-VTS "maximal" thymectomy is a highly extensive procedure, performed partly in the open fashion, avoiding use of sternotomy. Two-team approach helps to shorten the operative time.

Acknowledgement

The authors would like to thank Mr. Bodgan Dziadzio, the renown artist, for preparing the drawings.

References

1. Masaoka A, Yamakawa Y, Niwa H et al (1996) Extended thymectomy for myasthenia gravis patients: A 20-year review. Ann Thorac Surg 62:853-859
2. Jaretzki A III (1997) Thymectomy for myasthenia gravis: Analysis of the controversies regarding technique and results. Neurology 48(Suppl 5):S52-S63
3. Bulkley GB, Bass KN, Stephenson GR et al (1997) Extended cervicomediastinal thymectomy in the integrated management of myasthenia gravis. Ann Surg 226:324-335
4. Cooper J, Al-Jalaihawa A, Pearson F et al (1988) An improved technique to facilitate transcervical thymectomy for myasthenia gravis. Ann Thorac Surg 45:242-247
5. Mineo T, Pompeo E, Lerut T et al (2000) Thoracoscopic thymectomy in autoimmune myasthenia: Results of left-sided approach. Ann Thorac Surg 69:1537-1541
6. Yim A, Kay R, Izaat M, Ng S (1999) Video-assisted thoracoscopic thymectomy for myasthenia gravis. Semin Thorac Ann Cardiovasc Surg 11:65-73
7. Tomulescu V, Ion V, Kosa A et al (2006) Thoracoscopic thymectomy mid-term results. Ann Thorac Surg 82:1003-1007
8. Uchiyama A, Shimizu S, Murai H et al (2001) Infrasternal mediastinoscopic thymectomy in myasthenia gravis: Surgical results in 23 patients. Ann Thorac Surg 72:1902-1905
9. Novellino L, Longoni M, Spinelli L et al (1994) "Extended" thymectomy, without sternotomy performed by cervicotomy and thoracoscopic technique in the treatment of myasthenia gravis. Int Surg 79:378-381
10. Takeo S, Sakada T, Yano T (2001) Video-assisted extended thymectomy in patients with thymoma by lifting the sternum. Ann Thorac Surg 71:1721-1723
11. Zieliński M, Kużdżał J, Szlubowski A, Soja J (2004) Transcervical-subxiphoid-videothoracoscopic "maximal" thymectomy – Operative technique and early results. Ann Thorac Surg 78:404-410
12. Zieliński M, Kużdżał J, Nabialek T (2004) Transcervical-subxiphoid-VATS "maximal" thymectomy for myasthenia gravis. Multimed Man Cardiothorac Surg doi:10.1510/mmcts.2004.000836. MMCTS Online http://mmcts.ctsnetjournals.org
13. Zieliński M, Kużdżał J, Staniec B et al (2004) Safety for preoperative use of steroids for transsternal thymectomy in myasthenia gravis. Eur J Cardiothorac Surg 26:407-411
14. Zieliński M, Kużdżał J, Szlubowski A, Soja J (2004) Comparison of late results of basic transsternal and extended transsternal thymectomies in the treatment of myasthenia gravis. Ann Thorac Surg 78:253-258

CHAPTER 20

Open Videoassisted Techniques: Thoracoscopic Extended Thymectomy with Bilateral Approach and Anterior Chest Wall Lifting

Hiroyuki Shiono, Mitsunori Ohta, Meinoshin Okumura

Rationale

A thymectomy is now generally accepted as a major option of treatment for myasthenia gravis (MG) patients, both with and without thymomas. In recent years, developments in endoscopic surgical procedures have achieved the benefit of less invasiveness, though that has led to discussion regarding the most suitable surgical approach. The rationale for choosing a thymectomy for nonthymomatous MG is based on its function to remove the germinal centers (GCs) in the thymi, where acetylcholine receptor (AChR)-specific B cells clonally proliferate, and differentiate into antibody producing cells with a high affinity, as demonstrated by the author when working with Willcox [1, 2]. In addition, we found that a decrease in antibody titer 1 year after a thymectomy had a significant inverted correlation with the number of GC B cells in thymic lymphocytes in those patients [3]. Further, the author and Willcox reported that lymphocytes in remnant thymi adjacent to tumors spontaneously produce anti-AChR antibodies in MG patients with a thymoma [4]. Importantly, thymic glands are widely scattered in gross adipose tissue even outside of the mediastinal thymus [5, 6]. Therefore, the final goal of surgery is a total thymectomy, which means removal of as much thymic tissues as widely as possible in the mediastinum. Masaoka and Monden examined the prognoses of patients thymectomized in Osaka University Hospital and defined an extended thymectomy procedure for MG treatment by proposing a benchmark of the feasible area [7]. Since then, that procedure under a median sternotomy has been performed for MG at Osaka University. When introducing an endoscopic approach for a thymectomy used to treat MG patients in 2002, we confirmed that the same amount of clearance of the thymus including adipose tissue could be achieved under a thoracoscopic surgery approach. One of the authors reported the first experiences of video-assisted thoracoscopic surgery (VATS) with a novel chest wall lifting method for some benign mediastinal tumors [8], after which we added some modifications to apply it for an extended thymectomy for MG.

Indication and Preoperative Management

Patients with generalized symptoms and positive for the anti-AChR antibody are encouraged to undergo a VATS thymectomy. Those with a thymoma who have anti-AChR antibodies, even without myasthenic symptoms, also require an extended thymectomy including the tumor using a VATS procedure, unless image findings clearly show tumor invasion. At the present time, we do not plan an operation for the patients with anti-muscle-specific kinase (MuSK) autoantibodies. We usually plan the operation as soon as possible after diagnosis without introducing steroids. However, patients with severe bulbar symptoms are treated with low-dose steroids before the operation.

Techniques for Video-assisted Thoracoscopic Extended Thymectomy

Anesthesia Management

General anesthesia with an endotracheal double-lumen tube is necessary for selective unilateral pulmonary ventilation. Muscle relaxants are not allowed, because some MG patients are hypersensitive to them. Further, intravenous glucocorticoids are administered to patients treated with steroids before the operation.

Operative Position

The patient is placed in a supine position, and after a small pillow is inserted behind the back, both arms are placed just beside the chest (Fig. 20.1). This position is important to provide a wide area at the side chest walls for instrument and scope excursion. Outward rotation of the arms often disturbs free excursion during the diaphragm procedures. This back pillow forces the neck to become slightly extended, allowing easy access to the cervical procedures, and is also effective in emergency sternotomy cases. The operating table is rotated for easy access to the anterior mediastinum, thus both sides of the hips should be firmly guarded. Draping to gather fatty breasts medially can be useful for wide exposure of side chest wall. We successfully operated on a woman with breast implants without causing an injury by using such a draping maneuver.

Operative Approach

Our standard procedure comprises (1) a bilateral intrathoracic approach, (2) lifting of the anterior chest wall to attain a wide view and an easy access in the anterior mediastinum, and (3) a direct open approach through a neck incision to counter the disadvantage of VATS by providing a better access to the upper poles of the thymus [9]. Basically three trocars are positioned in the bilateral pleural cavities. Recently, we prefer a mini-thoracotomy in place of the two cranial trocars with wound edge protectors (Lap-Protector, Hakko, Japan) (Fig. 20.2). The original custom-made costal hooks can now be purchased from

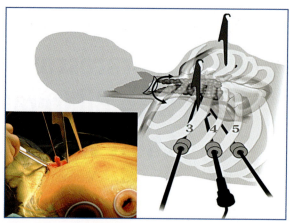

Fig. 20.2 An open direct approach for the dissection of the upper poles of the thymus, which provides a clearance of 3.2% more for cervical fat tissues [9]. The photo shows the upper poles isolated through a neck incision, which cannot be achieved from the pleural cavity

Sonne Medical Instruments (Tokyo, Japan) after a slight modification (Fig. 20.1). Both hooks are connected with a laparoscopic lifting device (VarioLift, Aesculap, Tokyo, Japan) and the chest wall can usually be lifted about 3 cm with a power of 10 kg. An assistant surgeon holding an endoscope stands alongside the operator. Direct dissection of the upper poles is performed after a bilateral VATS procedure. We always make sure to isolate the thymic tissues from the backside of the sternum during the last stage of the operation, in order to keep the effect of lifting at maximum.

The most difficult manipulation during thymectomy is safe dissection of the thymic veins and exposure of the left brachiocephalic vein (LBV). Thus, preoperative identification of these veins using multidetector-low CT scanning is useful, as we reported previously [10] (Fig. 20.3).

Surgical Technique

In cases that undergo bilateral VATS, fewer switches are required for unilateral ventilation. We prefer to start with exploration of the right cavity. A 10-mm trocar is introduced through the fifth intercostal space at the anterior axillary line for a 30° oblique camera. After confirming that lung collapse is adequate and there are no anesthesia complications, a vertical skin incision of about 3 mm is made 2 cm lateral of the sternum at the upper edge of the third rib. These scars become indistinct late after the surgery. We make sure not to injure the internal thoracic artery and intercostal vessels when inserting the costal hooks, which catch

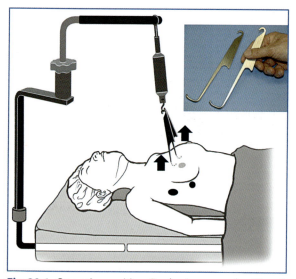

Fig. 20.1 Operative position. Our basic approach utilizes 3 trocars, though recently we prefer to use a mini-thoracotomy and 1 trocar positioned through the bilateral side chest wall. The anterior chest wall is lifted about 3 cm upward using the costal hooks connected to a lifting device

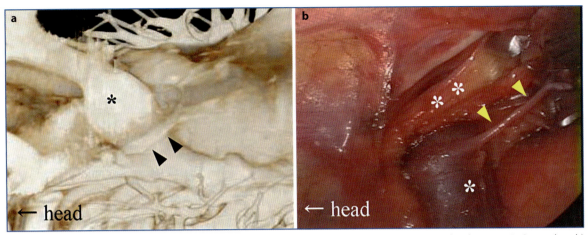

Fig. 20.3a,b **a** Three-dimensional image based on multidetector-low CT imaging showing the thymic vein (*arrowheads*) is shown in a position identical to that found during VATS in the right pleural cavity (**b**). Preoperative information regarding actual numbers and branching patterns is helpful for safer manipulation during this most delicate stage [10]. *Left brachiocephalic vein. ** The thymus (used with permission of Springer-Verlag, Heidelberg)

the third ribs. After switching the collapse of the right lung to the left, the left costal hook is inserted in the same manner by visualization through the left fifth intercostal space. Two more trocars are then placed through the third and fourth intercostal spaces, and dissection of the left lobe can be started after a full lift of the anterior chest wall.

The left mediastinal pleura is incised just anterior to the phrenic nerve: the lateral boundary of an extended thymectomy. The thoracoscopic view can easily identify the nerves, even if the thick fat tissues are extended beyond it, in which case an ultrasound energy source is useful for bloodless division. By careful dissection of cephalad thymic tissues in the left cavity, the most upper part of the LBV can usually be identified. During exposure of the LBV when medially extended, the thymic veins can be identified and then divided using a recently introduced ultrasound energy device (Fig. 20.4). When the LBV cannot be easily found, we try to expose it in the right pleural cavity. Blunt dissection can be safely performed on the pericardium and the diaphragm, so that isolation of the thymus extends to the right side. However, identification of the contralateral phrenic nerve is difficult at this moment. Leaving the upper portion extending to the neck, we finally dissect along the backside of the sternum.

The collapsed side is then switched and two more trocars are added to the right cavity. The pleura anterior of the phrenic nerve are incised and the thymic tissues are separated from the underlying pericardium extending onto the aorta. The bridging vein from the internal thoracic vein to the superior vena cava (SVC) can be preserved, unless it severely disturbs access to the upper portion. The SVC is a good landmark for identification of the LBV in the right cavity. Exposure of the LBV is carefully extended to the left side and some remaining thymic veins may be identified. When the mediastinal pleura is dissected behind the sternum, the thymus and fat tissue, except for the upper poles, become free from the mediastinum. The connective tissues around the upper poles should be dissected before neck manipulation.

Next, we add a 2-cm low collar incision, which is usually caught up in a wrinkle later. After the neck muscles are divided, the fibrous cords between the thyroid and thymus are exposed. We dissect it using

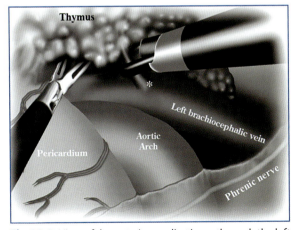

Fig. 20.4 View of the anterior mediastinum through the left pleural cavity. The thymus is mobilized upward and the left brachiocephalic vein is exposed. The thymic veins (*) are cut using an ultrasound energy device. The phrenic nerve is easily visible with a thoracoscope

electric cauterization, and mobilize the upper poles by inserting a finger in front of the trachea and behind the manubrium. Both lateral sides of the poles are carefully dissected with an electric cautery to ensure that the recurrent laryngeal nerves are not injured (Fig. 20.2). A combination of thoracoscopic views makes this stage more comfortable to perform. Finally, all thymic tissue can be removed from the cavity. After removal of the costal hooks, both cavities are explored to ensure hemostasis and complete resection. A silicon chest tube is then placed from one cavity to another through the anterior mediastinal bed, which is usually removed the next day.

Postoperative Management

The patient is extubated immediately after the operation when respiration is fully recovered. Cholinesterase inhibitors are resumed at a half dose and steroids are only introduced when the symptoms are not well reduced by their administration. Immunosuppressants are resumed at the same dose after the operation.

Results

A total of 42 patients have undergone a bilateral VATS extended thymectomy with our anterior chest wall lifting method as a standard procedure since 2002 at Osaka University Hospital, of which 28 were nonthymomatous MG cases, and the remaining 14 patients had thymomas. In 2 female MG patients without tumors, conversion to a sternotomy was necessary, because of bleeding at the confluence of the thymic vein with the LBV. VATS could not be performed in another patient, because unilateral ventilation caused intolerable hypoxia during the thoracoscopic exploration. In that case, it seemed likely that severe obesity disturbed ventilation while in the supine position. As for patients with a thymoma, 2 needed a sternotomy, because of tumor invasion to the pericardium. In another with lung invasion by a thymoma, a partial lung resection was done using endoscopic staplers and VATS was completed.

The median diameter of tumors resected from our patients was 3.5 cm (range, 1.5 to 9.5 cm). No deaths within 90 days of surgery occurred and no transfusion was needed, including converted cases. Further, there was no significant morbidity, except for a pulmonary embolism that occurred in a female patient, who recovered well with oxygenation and anticoagulation therapy. A neck incision was not performed in 3 patients, because of either a tracheotomy scar, a short neck caused by severe obesity, or patient choice. One male patient suffered from hoarseness caused by the recurrent laryngeal nerve paralysis, which may have originated during the neck procedure. The average time period for the operation was 237 min for nonthymomatous patients and 273 min for those with a thymoma, while, the average blood loss in those groups was 135 and 252 g, respectively, including converted cases. Five patients without and 1 with a thymoma required reintubation in the operating or recovery room because of deterioration of MG.

The postintervention symptoms in 38 of the patients who underwent a thymectomy and completed by VATS were evaluated using MG-ADL score. The median length of follow-up was 38 months (range, 3 to 69 months). Status was classified into 5 groups, i.e., remission, improvement, no change, more medication and/or worse symptoms, and death caused by MG, then remission rate (RR) and palliation rate (PR) were calculated as described previously [11] (Fig. 20.5). Three patients without a tumor and 2 with tumors attained remission for at least 1 year, and were classified as Complete Stable Remission (CSR) as defined by the MGFA (Myasthenia Gravis Foundation of America) Postintervention Status classification [12].

Controversy remains regarding which approach is most suitable for a thymectomy used to treat MG [12]. What makes it complicated seems that there are no objective or integrated parameters for MG symptoms, and that other treatment modalities are usually combined. The MGFA proposed some valued clinical classifications and advocates life-table analysis as the best method for follow-up of MG patients [12]. However, we still doubt the application of their

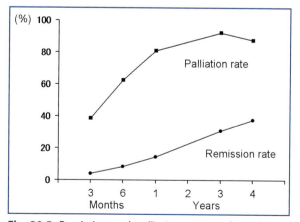

Fig. 20.5 Remission and palliation curves of nonthymomatous MG patients who underwent a thoracoscopic extended thymectomy

recommendation, because relapsed patients after remission cannot be evaluated. Another reason is that improved status is not taken into account in long clinical courses of MG. Particularly in Japan, both medical staff and patients tend to be against treatment with steroids, thus a longer period of time may be required to attain remission. We have adopted the evaluation described by Masaoka for comparison between endoscopic and transsternal approaches in larger series.

Unfortunately, the Thymectomy Classification by the MGFA grouped together various surgical procedures only according to the primary approach. Further, Jaretzki states that removal of the thymo-fatty tissue on the pericardium is not certain in "T-2: Videoscopic Thymectomy" [12]. However, skillful use of a thoracoscope allows better operative views and manipulation as compared to open surgery, i.e., along the phrenic nerve and near the diaphragm. Considering the final goal of the operation, which is total removal of as much thymic gland as possible, the most objective parameter for evaluation of surgical approaches is the amount of removed tissue by the procedure. We previously reported results of a prospective study that indicated the necessity of an additional open approach in the neck, which would lead to the removal of additional fat tissue including the glands below the thyroid [9]. Also, it is important to note that the average weight of the removed tissue in the present series was slightly higher than that in our previous series of patients who underwent a transsternal extended thymectomy, though the difference were not statistically significant (data not shown). Therefore, we consider that our endoscopic approach should be substantially classified into the same category as "T-3(b), Transsternal Extended Thymectomy" in MGFA classification [12].

We believe that use of our thoracoscopic thymectomy method can achieve a proper balance between invasiveness and radicality, leading to improved acceptance and benefits for MG patients.

Acknowledgement

We thank Mrs. Yuko Tonohira in Cornell University, N.Y., for preparing the medical illustration.

References

1. Sims GP, Shiono H, Willcox N et al (2001) Somatic hypermutation and selection of B cells in thymic germinal centers responding to acetylcholine receptor in myasthenia gravis. J Immunol 167:1935-1944
2. Shiono H, Roxanis I, Zhang W et al (2003) Scenarios for autoimmunization of T and B cells in myasthenia gravis. Ann N Y Acad Sci 998:237-256
3. Okumura M, Ohta M, Takeuchi Y et al (2003) The immunologic role of thymectomy in the treatment of myasthenia gravis: implication of thymus-associated B-lymphocyte subset in reduction of the anti-acetylcholine receptor antibody titer. J Thorac Cardiovasc Surg 126:1922-1928
4. Shiono H, Wong YL, Matthews I et al (2003) Spontaneous production of anti-IFN-alpha and anti-IL-12 autoantibodies by thymoma cells from myasthenia gravis patients suggests autoimmunization in the tumor. Int Immunol 15:903-913
5. Fukai I, Funato Y, Mizuno T et al (1991) Distribution of thymic tissue in the mediastinal adipose tissue. J Thorac Cardiovasc Surg 101:1099-1102
6. Scelsi R, Ferro MT, Scelsi L et al (1996) Detection and morphology of thymic remnants after video-assisted thoracoscopic extended thymectomy (VATET) in patients with myasthenia gravis. Int Surg 81:14-17
7. Masaoka A, Monden Y (1981) Comparison of the results of transsternal simple, transcervical simple, and extended thymectomy. Ann N Y Acad Sci 377:755-765
8. Ohta M, Hirabayasi H, Okumura M et al (2003) Thoracoscopic thymectomy using anterior chest wall lifting method. Ann Thorac Surg 76:1310-1311
9. Shigemura N, Shiono H, Inoue M et al (2006) Inclusion of the transcervical approach in video-assisted thoracoscopic extended thymectomy (VATET) for myasthenia gravis: a prospective trial. Surg Endosc 20:1614-1618
10. Shiono H, Inoue A, Tomiyama N et al (2006) Safer video-assisted thoracoscopic thymectomy after location of thymic veins with multidetector computed tomography. Surg Endosc 20:1419-1422
11. Masaoka A, Yamakawa Y, Niwa H et al (1996) Extended thymectomy for myasthenia gravis patients: A 20-year review. Ann Thorac Surg 62:853-859
12. Jaretzki A 3rd, Barohn RJ, Ernstoff RM et al (2000) Myasthenia gravis: Recommendations for clinical research standards. Task Force of the Medical Scientific Advisory Board of the Myasthenia Gravis Foundation of America. Neurology 55:16-23

CHAPTER 21

Totally Endoscopic Techniques: Left-Sided Thoracoscopic Thymectomy

Klaus Gellert, Sven Köther

Introduction

Standard surgical procedures of thymectomy available – as a positive impact on the course of the condition in patients with myasthenia gravis – comprise transsternal, transcervical, extended transsternal, and thoracoscopic thymectomy. All four options have been shown to have a positive impact on the outcome of the disease. Of importance of these approaches is the complete excision of thymic tissue. Up until the present time, however, the question as to what constitutes the optimal approach to thymectomy is still a matter of controversial debate. The development of minimal invasive surgery with its well-known advantages also led to the introduction of thoracoscopic thymectomy, a procedure that can be performed from either the right or the left side. Results of thoracoscopic thymectomy have proved to be comparable with those of other thymectomy procedures.

The open thymectomy contains a substantial operational expenditure with appropriate width of complications for the patient whereby particularly the pain symptomatology after the sternotomy as well as the possible instability of the thorax are most important.

In the present time the underlying problem of acceptance of operation is due to patient concerns about the esthetic or cosmetic effect of all the different procedures, since the region of decolletage of young wives, for instance, is changed by a large scar resulting from a sternotomy.

Advantages of thoracoscopic thymectomy include small operation trauma; an outstanding intraoperative overview, which means that the danger of injury to organs and structures unrelated to the procedure can be limited; and slight postsurgical pain and therefore more rapid mobilization of the patients. Furthermore, thoracoscopic thymectomy has an excellent cosmetic result with very small scars.

Under these aspects we preferred and standardized the thoracoscopic thymectomy especially with a left-sided approach, and excluded patients with large thymoma or suspicion of malignancy. In these cases the open procedure with sternotomy was performed. In analyzing results obtained with this thoracoscopic technique the comparison to those obtained with conventional thymectomy as reported in literature shows lower postoperative morbidity, good early clinical and surgical results, and an excellent cosmetic effect. That led to an increased acceptance of this method by patients and neurologists alike.

Left sided Thoracoscopic Thymectomy

Indication

For thoracoscopic thymectomy the indication should be for all patients with myasthenia gravis in stage I-II B of the Ossermann/Genkins classification [1], as well as patients with nonmalignant hyperplasia of the thymus gland or with encapsulated, noninvasively grown thymomas with a maximum diameter of about 3 cm. For patients with suspicion of malignancy or with bigger thymomas the indication for open procedure exists. Thoracoscopic thymectomy should be performed when myasthenia gravis is in a stable condition and not as an "emergency operation". Therefore, the patient's medications should be adjusted against myasthenia preoperatively. In serious or unstable stages of myasthenia gravis plasmapheresis and/or immunoadsorption represent a better alternative in the acute phase. Additionally immunoglobulins can be used. For these reasons it is desirable to determine the value of ACh antibodies and to prepare a CT or MR from the frontal mediastinal space.

Perioperative Procedure

In preparing for an operation a premedication on the previous evening of promethacin (1 mg/kg body mass) for anxiolysis is recommended. A second dose of promethacin should be given 45 min before the operation. During the operation pyridostigmine can be administered by a stomach tube.

Enlarged monitoring with a central venous catheter, invasive blood pressure measurement, and relaxometry with TOF-Watch (M. adductor pollicis longus) are necessary for thoracoscopic thymectomy. Because of the one-lung ventilation, an intraoperative bronchoscopy may become necessary. For example, in case of intubation problems a bronchoscopic intubation could be performed. Due to the problems of weaning of respiration, which can be expected postoperatively in case of a tracheotomy, this procedure should be obsolete as a prophylactic procedure.

Because of possible complication patients should always be supervised in an intensive care unit after the operation.

Surgical Technique

Thoracoscopic thymectomy is performed under insufflation anesthesia with single-lung ventilation, using a double-luminal endobronchial tube. The patient is placed in a right-lateral position at 30° to the horizontal. For arrangement of thoracoscopic trocars and sufficient space conditions during operation, the left arm is placed over the head. Three thoracoscopic trocars are inserted into the pleural cavity in the 3rd to 5th intercostal spaces (Fig. 21.1). To achieve good cosmetic results, particularly for females, the incisions should be placed in a triangular position around the mamma, so that the scars are hidden after healing (Fig. 21.2). For the best view over the precardial and mediastinal operation area a camera

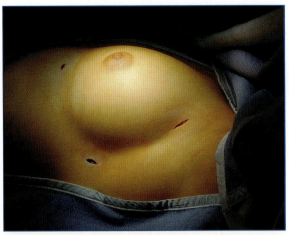

Fig. 21.2 Placement of incisions for good cosmetic result

with a 30° optic proved well. For best handling the camera instrument should be taken over by an assistant. Dissection is begun at the lower-left pole of the thymus gland close to the phrenic nerve, including the perithymal fat tissue (Fig 21.3). The nerve represents thereby a guidance structure. The entire thymic tissue together with pericardial fat is dissected cranially using both blunt and sharp technique. For preparation an ultrasonic scissor could be recommended.

In the next step of extirpation of the thymus gland, the retrosternal working space is prepared to the right pleura. The thymus gland is then lifted from the pericard and then the brachiocephalic vein is exposed (Fig 21.4). There in most cases exist very intensive junctions and adhesions to the region of

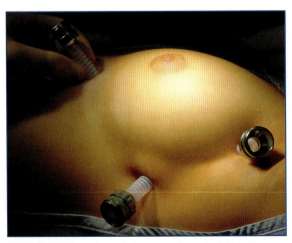

Fig. 21.1 Arrangement of trocars for left sided thoracoscopic thymectomy

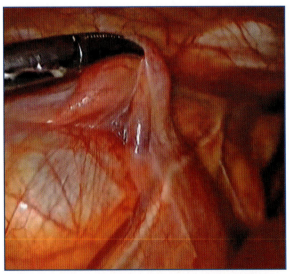

Fig. 21.3 Beginning of preparation at lower-left pole of thymus included the perithymal fat tissue close to phrenic nerve

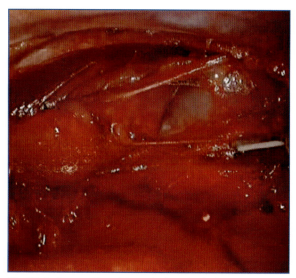

Fig. 21.4 Exposed brachiacephalic vein during preparation of thymus

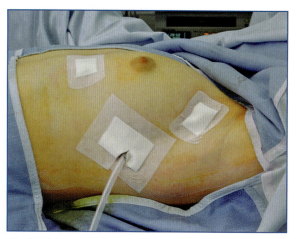

Fig. 21.6 Inserted thoracic drainage

aorta ascendens. Draining thymic veins are divided. The most difficult and critical part of the operation is the dissection of the upper horns of the gland. After dissecting the surrounding fascia the upper horns can be mobilized caudally by applying gentle traction, and dissected free. After that the right pleural cavity is opened for examination of the right-lower thymus (Fig. 21.5). At this point it is possible to visualize the right phrenic nerve beside the cava vein necessary for removing of fat tissue in this region.

The excised specimen is recovered with the aid of a recovery bag, and the procedure is terminated with the placement of a thoracic drain (Fig. 21.6).

Postoperative Treatment

In case of stable postoperative state a prolonged monitoring and stay in the intensive care unit is not necessary. If possible and under condition that there is no myasthenic disorder postoperatively, the patient can be shifted on the first postoperative day to the normal surgical ward. After X-ray chest control and under normal ventilation, the thoracic drainage can be removed on the first postoperative day.

One of the advantages of thoracoscopic thymectomy is the shortness of hospitalization. For the duration of hospitalization no changes in the antimyasthenic medication should be made.

Depending on the clinical situation and postoperative myasthenic signs, an adaptation of medication during the first postoperative half-year could be performed. A definitive estimate of clinical results and success of the thymectomy can be given in the process. That's why a good organized follow-up is necessary for high-quality thymus gland surgery and therapy of myasthenia gravis.

Own Results

Material and Methods

Between August 1997 and December 2007, a total of 263 patients (183 female, 80 male) with stage I-II B myasthenia gravis in the Ossermann/Genkins classification underwent thoracoscopic thymectomy in the Surgical Department of the Oskar-Ziethen Hospital in Berlin-Lichtenberg. Patients with a radiologically demonstrable thymoma having a size of less than 3 cm, and encapsulated and with no evidence of ma-

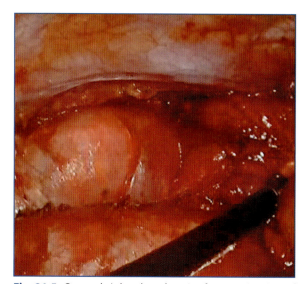

Fig. 21.5 Opened right pleural cavity for examination of right-lower thymus pole

lignancy (Masaoka stage I) were also operated on using the minimally invasive option. The mean age of the patients was 37 years (range: 9 to 84). The indication for thymectomy was established on an interdisciplinary basis with involvement of the patient's neurologist.

In addition to such surgery-related factors as operating time, intraoperative blood loss, morbidity, and mortality, and the histopathology of the surgical specimen, the clinical course over a mean follow-up time of 40.5 months (range: 6 to 84 months) was also analyzed. For this purpose, all the patients were questioned with the aim of eliciting information on possible improvement or worsening of their symptoms, and any modification of their medication, and were then categorized in accordance with the DeFilippi classification [2].

Results

The fully thoracoscopic thymectomy was successfully performed in 241 patients. A conversion to open procedure of thymectomy was performed in 22 (8.3%) cases. In 9 patients, the intraoperative findings raised suspicion of a local metastasized thymus gland carcinoma, which rendered sternotomy with thymectomy and an extended mediastinal resection necessary.

The macroscopic suspicion was confirmed by the findings of the histopathological work-up.

On the occasion of 13 patients a lot of pericardial fatty tissue was found intraoperatively, that supplied to a conversion to sternotomy for complete resection of thymus gland with the surrounding and evenly pericardial fat tissue with ectopic thymus tissue in it.

There was no postoperative mortality. Two patients had to be redrained since removal of the thoracic suction drain was followed by a pneumothorax. After successful extubation in the operating theatre, 4 patients experienced a myasthenic crisis and had to be reintubated and ventilated in the intensive care unit. They were transferred to a neurological unit for further management. From there, following plasmapheresis treatment and optimal drug management, they were discharged to outpatient care with no further complications. In 6 cases a mild postoperative pneumonia was seen and treated with consistent physical therapy and antibiotic medication. This meant that the postoperative morbidity rate was 4.5% overall. Mean duration of operation was 60 min(±8 min).

The histopathological work-up revealed a thymoma in 11.5%, hyperplasia in 66.6%, atrophic gland in 18.1%, and a carcinoma of the thymus gland in 3.7% of the patients. Only 65% of the thymomas were detected by the preoperative diagnostic work-up. With the exception of the patients with carcinoma of the thymus gland, all thymomas were classified Masaoka stage I.

The mean hospital stay was 5.1 days (range: 2 to 17 days). Preoperatively, 77 patients (29.2%) were in stage I, 101 patients (38.4%) were in stage II A and 85 (32.3%) in stage II B (Ossermann/Genkins classification) (Table 21.1).

After a mean follow-up of 40.5 months, 134 patients were seen and investigated by us. 32 patients (23.9%) showed complete remission (stage I), 54 patients (40.3%) were asymptomatic on reduced medication (stage II), in 27 cases (20.1%) symptom severity or medication was reduced (stage III), and 9 patients (6.7%) showed no improvement (stage IV) in the DeFilippi classification. In summary 32 patients (23.8%) experienced complete remission, and 81 (60.4%) experienced an improvement in symptoms or a reduction in medication. In 9 patients (6.7%), medication and/or symptoms remained unchanged post-operatively (Table 21.2).

Most of patients were very satisfied with the short hospitalization and post-operative cosmetic effect (Fig. 21.7).

Discussion

Publications in the literature describe a number of standardized, so far well-worked techniques, such as transsternal, transcervical, or "maximal thymectomy" for treatment strategy of myasthenia gravis [3, 4].

Table 21.1 Preoperative stages of [n = 263] patients with myasthenia gravis before thoracoscopic thymectomy in accordance with Ossermann/Genkins classification (1971)

Stage	Description	Patients [n]	[%]
I	Ocular myasthenia gravis	77	29.2
II A	Mild generalized myasthenia gravis	101	38.4
II B	Mild generalized myasthenia gravis with ocular symptoms	85	32.3

Table 21.2 Clinical results [n = 134 patients] after left-sided thoracoscopic thymectomy and a mean follow up of 40.5 months in accordance with the DeFilippi classification

Stage	Description	Patients [n]	[%]
I	Complete remission	32	23.9
II	Asymptomatic and reduced medication	54	40.3
III	Improved symptoms or reduced medication	27	20.1
IV	Identical symptoms, medication unchanged	9	6.7
V	Worsening of symptoms	12	9.0

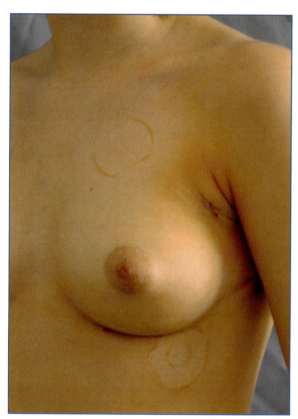

Fig. 21.7 Good cosmetic result after left-sided thoracoscopic thymectomy

Complete thoracoscopic thymectomy is technically feasible, and represents in times of minimal invasive surgery a modern technique for the removal of the thymus gland and mediastinal fatty tissue. Acknowledged benefits for the patient are the low level of surgical trauma and the excellent cosmetic result [3, 5]. These benefits are seen in particular in the case of young patients undergoing thoracoscopic thymectomy – as reports in the literature show [6-8].

As a consequence of the reduced surgical trauma, a lower rate of wound healing disorders, less postoperative thoracic pain and thus a reduction in postoperative pneumonia, have been reported.

Surgical access may be either from the right or left. Yim et al. describe a right-lateral approach, since orientation to the superior vena cava is easier, and the identification of the left brachiocephalic vein is thus facilitated [9, 10]. The pericardial and perithymal fat tissue and that in the aortopulmonary window can be removed completely and any ectopic thymus gland tissue with it [11, 12].

Anatomical studies have shown that ectopic thymus gland may be present both in mediastinal, pericardial, and cervical fatty tissue [13, 14]. With the aim of taking this fact into account, extensive surgical techniques, such a transcervical-transsternal or the extended transsternal approach were developed. This operative approach, however, is associated with a higher level of perioperative morbidity than the minimally invasive procedure. Bulkley et al., for instance, reported a morbidity rate of 33% [15], and Budde et al. 14% [16]. However, since patients with Ossermann and Genkins stage IV myasthenia were also operated on, direct comparability is compromised. In our own patient population, the morbidity rate, at 4.5%, is comparable with that reported by Mack et al. [3].

The surgical literature also reports good long-term results achieved with the purely transcervical approach – another minimally invasive procedure. Brill et al., for instance, reported a long-term remission rate of 45% [17]. Other authors, however, were unable to confirm these excellent results, since on re-operation after the transcervical approach, remnant thymic tissue was found, and symptoms of myasthenia persisted [18].

The reported remission rate for all the established surgical options described above varied between 20% and 40%, and the overall improvement of symptoms or reduction in medication is around 90% (Table 21.3).

It is against these results that those achieved with the thoracoscopic technique have to be measured.

In our own patient population, for example, the remission rate is 23.9%; in the series reported by Mack et al. 19% with more or less identical follow-

Table 21.3 Published results of thymectomy in patients with myasthenia gravis compared with own data

Author (Year)	[n]	Technique	Follow-up [months]	PR [%]	CR [%]
Frist (1994)	46	TS	50	93.6	28.2
Kay (1994)	36	TS	49	72.2	24.5
DeFilippi (1994)	53	TC	51	81.1	17
Masaoka (1996)	375	TS	60	88	45.8
Jaretzki (1988)	95	TS+TC	40	93	38
Stern (2001)	56	TS	82	53	81
Mineo (1996)	31	VATS	39	96	36
Mack (2002)	38	VATS	53	47	14
Own data (2007)	134	VATS	40.5	60.4	23.9

TS, transsternal; TC, transcervical; VATS, Video assisted thoracic surgery; PR, partial remission; CR, complete remission

up times (19.4 and 23 months, respectively) [3]. In the series of operations described by Mineo et al., the remission rate was 36% over the appreciably longer follow-up of 39.6 months [11], in another series published by Loscertales, five of the seven patients operated on profited from the procedure [19]. It may be concluded that the remission rate improves with longer follow-up.

A short disease history, female sex, a milder form of the disease, and hyperplasia of the thymus gland are reported in the literature to be positive prognostic factors for thymectomy [11].

Conclusions

Thoracoscopic thymectomy is a modern, minimally invasive approach to the operative removal of the thymus gland. This technique is just as effective as the above-mentioned conventional surgical techniques. Very low postoperative morbidity, an excellent cosmetic effect, and good early clinical results comparable with those obtained with the conventional methods have resulted in increasing acceptance of the operation by patients and neurologists alike. Thoracoscopic thymectomy therefore represents today in times of minimal invasive treatment first option in the surgical treatment of myasthenia gravis.

References

1. Ossermann KE, Genkins G (1971) Studies in Myasthenia gravis: Review of a twenty-year experience in over 1200 patients. Mt Sinai J Med 38:497-537
2. DeFilippi VJ, Richman DP, Ferguson MK (1994) Transcervical thymectomy for myasthenia gravis. Ann Thorac Surg 57:194-197
3. Mack MJ, Landreneau RY, Yim AP et al (1996) Results of video-assisted thymectomy in patients with Myasthenia gravis. J Thorac Cardiovasc Surg 112(5):1352-1360
4. Mussi A, Lucchi M, Murri L et al (2001) Extended thymectomy in myasthenia gravis: A team-work of neurologist, thoracic surgeon, and anaesthesist may improve the outcome. Eur J Cardiothoracic Surg 19:570-575
5. Yim APC, Lee TW, Izzat MB, Wan S (2001) Place of video-thoracoscopy in thoracic surgical practice. World J Surg 25(2):157-161
6. Kogut KA, Bufo AJ, Rothenburg SS, Lobe TE (2000) Thoracoscopic thymectomy for myasthenia gravis in children. J Pediatr Surg 35(11):1576-1577
7. Kolski H, Vajsar J, Kim PC (2000) Thoracoscopic thymectomy in juvenile myasthenia gravis. J Pediatr Surg 35(5):768-770
8. Tobias JD (2001) Thoracoscopy in pediatric patient. Anaestesiol Clin North Am 19(1):173-176
9. Yim APC, Kay RLC, Ho JKS (1995) Video-assisted thoracoscopic thymectomy for myasthenia gravis. Chest 108:1440-1443
10. Yim APC, Izzat MB, Lee TW, Wan S (1999) Video-assisted thoracoscopic thymectomy. Ann Thoracic Cardiovasc Surg 5(1):18-20
11. Mineo TC, Pompeo E, Lerut TE et al (2000) Thoracoscopic thymectomy in autoimmune myasthenia. Results of left-sided approach. Ann Thorac Surg 69:1537-1541
12. Rückert JC, Czyzewski D, Pest S, Müller JM (2000) Radicality of thoracoscopic thymectomy – An anatomical study. Eur J Cardiothoracic Surg 18:735-736
13. Masaoka A, Nagakoa Y, Kotabe Y (1975) Distribution of thymic tissue at the anterior mediastinum: Current procedure in thymectomy. J Thorac Cardiovasc Surg 70:747-754
14. Jaretzki A, Wolff M (1988) "Maximal" thymectomy for myasthenia gravis. Surgical anatomy and operative techniques. J Thorac Cardiovasc Surg 96:711-716
15. Bulkley GB, Bass KN, Stephenson GR (1997) Extended cervicomediastinal thymectomy in the integrated management of myasthenia gravis. Ann Surg 226:234-235
16. Budde JM, Morris CD, Gal AA et al (2001) Predictors of outcome in thymectomy for myasthenia gravis. Ann Thorc Surg 72:197-202

17. Bril V, Kojic J, Ilse WK, Cooper JD (1998) Long-term clinical outcome after transcervical thymectomy for myasthenia gravis. Ann Thorac Surg 65:1520-1522
18. Mineo TC, Pastore E, Ambrogi V et al (1998) Video-assisted completion thymectomy in refractory myasthenia gravis. J Thorac Cardiovasc Surg 115:252-254
19. Loscertales J, Jimenez Merchan R, Arenas Linares CJ et al (1999) The treatment of myasthenia gravis by video thoracoscopic thymectomy. The technique and the initial results. Arch Bronconeumol 35(1):9-14

CHAPTER 22

Totally Endoscopic Techniques: Right-Sided Thoracoscopic Thymectomy

Gavin M. Wright, Cameron Keating

Introduction

Thymectomy has a history stretching back over a century. Originally removed via a cervical incision, this organ is notable for the variety of methods now described for its removal. From the extensive dissections using combined sternotomy with cervical incision, to basic or extended thymectomy through upper or lower hemi-sternotomy. From small cervical or subxiphoid incisions, unilateral or bilateral thoracoscopic approaches, with or without sternal lift to the use of robotics, the array is as dazzling as the rhetoric of each technique's proponents.

Controlled, but non-randomized studies conclude that the odds of medication-free remission after thymectomy are 2.1 times those who keep their thymus [1]. A randomized controlled trial sponsored by the National Institute of Neurological Disorders and Stroke began recruiting in 2006 to provide conclusive evidence of the benefit of thymectomy. There have only ever been three small (and heterogeneous) randomized trials of thymectomy approaches in myasthenia gravis. Ruckert et al. [2] randomized 20 patients to sternotomy or VATS approach. This study showed that pulmonary function and requirement for narcotics was clearly inferior for the sternotomy group. In the other trial of 50 myasthenic patients, Granetzny et al. [3] demonstrated a lower postoperative ventilation rate and shorter ICU stay for manubriotomy compared with full sternotomy. Chang et al. [4] randomized a total of 33 patients to either bilateral VATS thymectomy or extended transsternal thymectomy in nonthymomatous Osserman class I-III patients. The bilateral VATS approach resulted in longer operating time (4.2 h vs. 1.8 h), less blood loss (74 ml vs. 155 ml), and similar improvement and remission rates. No other evidence-based conclusions can be made about any other approach or its efficacy for any given pathology.

The versatile thoracic surgeon should be able to approach the thymus by a variety of methods. Any single method executed well will be suitable for the majority of cases, and should be the method with which the surgeon is most comfortable, and from which he or she expects to get the best results. In this chapter we will iterate the indications, equipment needed, preoperative work-up, and technical details of the procedure that we perform most commonly.

Indications

By pathology, the indications for thymectomy are identical for right- or left-sided VATS approach with the exception that the right-sided approach allows better access to the highest mediastinal nodes along the right phrenic [5], but less access to the aorto-pulmonary nodes [6]. Each side affords the best view of its respective phrenic nerve. Therefore, a thymoma that is eccentric to the right and adjacent to the nerve needs to be approached from that side to safely obtain the maximum margin without unnecessarily endangering the phrenic nerve. The right side offers more space to maneuver especially if there is any cardiomegaly or chest deformity.

Choice of side is therefore more a product of training, mentoring, and geographic location of the surgeon than any evidence or logic. Safe removal of all intended tissue is the principle goal as in any resectional surgery.

Myasthenia gravis is the most common indication, with the aim of clearing all potential thymic tissue from the neck to the diaphragm [7, 8]. Pathological studies have demonstrated the presence of thymic rests in mediastinal fat away from the macroscopic gland, strongly suggesting that the anterior mediastinum should be completely exenterated [9].

When the indication for surgery is small thymic mass (thymoma, cyst, germ cell tumor) there should be no evidence of fat invasion on CT chest, the lesion should be less than 3 cm in its short axis, and there should be no significant lymphadenopathy or extension to the aorto-pulmonary window.

Oncological principles need to be followed rigorously. Care with tissue, minimal handling of tumor, wide margins, and specimen retrieval in a plastic bag should be the minimum standard. Conversion to an open procedure is more attractive than tumor spillage. There have been two isolated reports of port site recurrence; however, these were for advanced thymic malignancy, which has preponderance for pleural seeding with or without intervention. No technical details were provided for one case [10] and limited details for the other [11].

Equipment

The basic equipment required for right-sided VATS thymectomy is similar to any standard VATS set-up. We also have three bent sponge holders that are useful for grasping tissue in hard-to-reach places and minimizing instrument clash. A set of Kaiser-Pilling graspers is more than adequate for the same purpose. A double-action sponge holder can be useful to grip a thymus through a small port while allowing maximum jaw opening. A long, fine artery forceps or similar instrument to load peanut swabs, and a disposable plastic Yankauer sucker are inexpensive and extremely useful instruments. A 30° telescope is essential for most thoracoscopic operations, and this is not different for thymectomy. The thoracoscopic tower or "stack" should consist of a good quality video monitor and light source, preferably one with a gain function to add light if there is blood in the operative field. We do not believe it is ever necessary (or advisable) to employ CO_2 tension pneumothorax for VATS.

Preoperative Work-up

Myasthenic patients should have optimal therapy to render them as symptom free as possible [12]. As there is no concern about sternal wound healing or infection [13], we use plasma exchange therapy on all but the most minor cases, such as ocular only or minimal bulbar myasthenia [14, 15]. Intravenous gammaglobulin can be used as an alternative when a patient is intolerant of plasma exchange [16].

Other than the usual oncological and surgical work-up, nothing specific is required for other thymectomy indications. If a germ cell tumor is suspected, serum markers including α-fetoprotein, β-HCG and lactate dehydrogenase, and a medical oncology opinion should be sought.

Positioning and Port Placement

Optimal positioning for the thoracoscopic approach must take into consideration many factors, including natural retraction of structures by gravity, optimal exposure of target site, surgeon familiarity with visualized anatomy, and instrument placement. The approach described here has been developed by the authors and successfully used in 100 VATS thymectomies by our group.

Patient Position

Prior to double-lumen endotracheal intubation, the patient is placed on a suction beanbag. After intubation, the patient is rolled 45° toward the left and the beanbag is packed under the right shoulder, hip, and thigh. The left side of the beanbag is used to contain the patient to prevent slippage to the left. A pillow is placed between the legs to protect bony points.

Arm Position

The anesthetist should choose the left arm for monitoring and lines. The right arm is flexed to 90° and the forearm hung above the patient's forehead, suspended on a mastectomy "L"-bar. The latter is fastened to the left side of the table to prevent impingement on the surgeon's arc of activity (Fig. 22.1). The axilla should be shaved at least from the skin crease down. Draping is best accomplished with adhesive tapes to hold the drapes in position, as the field is an awkward shape and orientation.

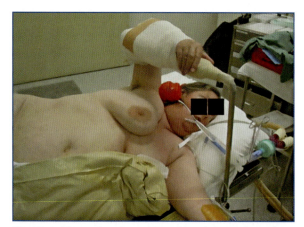

Fig. 22.1 The patient is positioned in a left semilateral position with the right arm on a mastectomy L-bar. A suction beanbag holds the patient securely [17] (reproduced with permission from Springer-Verlag)

Surgeon Position

The surgeon stands on the patient's right side. The assistant surgeon stands to the surgeon's right and the scrub nurse is positioned opposite the assistant. Two video monitors are preferred, so that the scrub nurse can observe proceedings without turning away from the surgeon.

Port Placement

Submammary Port

Depending on the indication, a 25-mm incision is adequate for comfortable removal of even a quite hypertrophic thymus. If the surgery is for thymoma, then the skin incision should be approximately 1.5 times the short axis diameter of the tumor. The incision is made in the submammary fold in the female (Fig. 22.2), and the breast is undermined to allow access to the 4th or 5th intercostal space. In the male, the incision should be just below the nipple, or just lateral and level with the nipple. Diathermy is used to divide a short segment of pectoralis muscle and then intercostal muscle. Hemostasis should be meticulous to avoid breast hematoma, particularly in female patients. The incision is now large enough to accommodate the telescope port and, when necessary, extra graspers or Yankauer sucker at the same time.

Lateral Port

Just behind the anterior axillary line, corresponding to the lateral skin curvature of the breast, and lateral to the pectoralis free edge, a 10-mm port is established in the 4th intercostal space. We make the incision in line with the outer curvature of the breast. This will later serve as the single drain tube site.

Axillary Port

Just below the axillary crease, in the 2nd intercostal space at the mid axillary line, a 5-mm port is inserted. This will only be used for hook diathermy and 5-mm endoscopic grasper, and therefore does not need to be any larger.

Anatomy

Unlike the sternotomy approach, the mediastinum is seen side-on, which actually affords a better view of the anterior mediastinum as a resectable compartment (Fig. 22.3). The anatomical landmarks on the video screen image are as follows:
- Top of screen: Pleural reflection medial to the internal thoracic vessels.
- Left of screen: Arc of internal thoracic vein and origin of superior vena cava.
- Right of screen: Diaphragm and pericardial fat pad.
- Bottom of screen: Right phrenic nerve and pericardiophrenic vessels.

Thymic vein anatomy is not particularly constant. The most common variants are a single vein, which

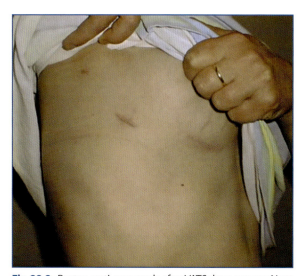

Fig. 22.2 Postoperative wounds after VATS thymectomy. Note that a normal bra would cover the submammary and lower axillary port sites. The remaining 5-mm port is high in the axilla [17] (reproduced with permission from Springer-Verlag)

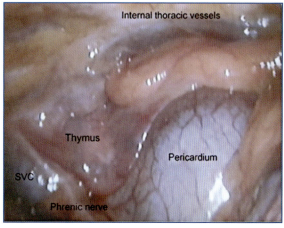

Fig. 22.3 Endoscopic view of thymic anatomy from the right side [17] (reproduced with permission from Springer-Verlag)

drains both lobes in a Y-fashion to the left brachiocephalic vein, or two separate veins draining directly into the brachiocephalic vein [18]. A third vein is not uncommon, and veins may drain into the SVC or right internal thoracic vein from the right lobe and into the left internal thoracic from the left lobe [19]. On one occasion we encountered six discrete veins from the thymus in a patient with other cardiovascular anomalies.

Dissection

With the 30° telescope held by the assistant, alternating between the submammary and lateral port, the surgeon uses a sponge holder or laparoscopic grasper and hook diathermy to commence the pleural incision medial to the internal thoracic vessels. This is continued as close to the diaphragm as possible. At the apex of the pleura, the incision is curved inside the internal thoracic vein course to stop short of the superior vena cava and phrenic nerve. An incision is then made parallel to the phrenic nerve down to the attachment of the mediastinal pleura to the pericardium. This attachment is divided and followed down to the diaphragm, where this incision is joined to the previous pleural incision. This leaves a large disc of pleura to contain the thymus and anterior mediastinal fat as a block.

A peanut swab and diathermy are then alternated to detach the anterior mediastinal fat from the underside of the sternum. This is continued well into the sternal notch. The same maneuvers are then used to separate the thymus from the pericardium. If a thymoma is being resected, extra care should be taken to exclude invasion of pericardium. A disc of pericardium can be excised if in doubt about a small area, but our practice is to perform a sternotomy or thoracotomy if broad-based frank invasion is encountered.

The confluence of the brachiocephalic veins that constitute the origin of the superior vena cava is then dissected with a peanut. Nodal tissue can be swept on to the specimen from under the internal thoracic vein. The left brachiocephalic vein is then identified and is carefully skeletonized anteriorly and inferiorly. Usually the right cervical thymic horn can then be teased down into the mediastinum by dividing the fascial coverings and areolar tissue and pulling carefully "hand over hand" with two graspers. This should expose the thymic vein or veins after further dissection. A multiple firing endoscopic clip applier is then used to double clip the thymic vein(s) proximally. Care must be taken not to injure the brachiocephalic vein or an additional thymic vein by accidentally cutting beyond the clipped vein. The left cervical horn can be pulled down at this time or delayed until the left lobe has been fully mobilized.

The left pleura is identified and deliberately opened in analogous fashion to the right side. This is commenced towards the diaphragm end and proceeds toward the neck by dividing the pleura medial to the left internal thoracic vessels. The reflection at the pericardium is similarly divided. The area around the termination of the left internal thoracic vein is the most difficult area to dissect during this procedure. It is best approached progressively from both the medial side after taking down the left cervical thymic horn, and from the caudal direction, taking care not to injure the vessel itself (Table 22.1).

Table 22.1 Summary of surgical steps

1	Introduce ports Submammary (25mm), AAL/3rd ICS (10mm), MAL/2nd ICS (5mm)
2	Divide mediastinal pleura medial to internal thoracic vein
3	Divide pleura 1cm anterior to phrenic nerve then along attachment to pericardium
4	Brush anterior mediastinum off back of sternum
5	Divide pleural fat near diaphragm and sweep right thymic lobe off pericardium
6	Dissect nodes at brachiocephalic confluence onto mediastinal specimen
7	Skeletonise left brachiocephalic vein and extract right thymic horn from the neck
8	Identify and double clip thymic vein(s)
9	Open left mediastinal pleura medial to left internal mammary vein
10	Sweep left thymic lobe off pericardium
11	Extract left thymic horn
12	Dissect left brachiocephalic nodes onto main specimen
13	Complete the division of left pleura to release the specimen
14	Insert specimen bag beside telescope in submammary port
15	Extract thymus via submammary port
16	Washout blood and place 24 French drain across mediastinum via 10mm port
17	Close submammary incision

Extraction

Once the thymus and mediastinal block is free, it is placed in an EndoCatch (Covidien, USA) or similar specimen retrieval system and removed via the submammary port (Fig. 22.4). After washout, blood should

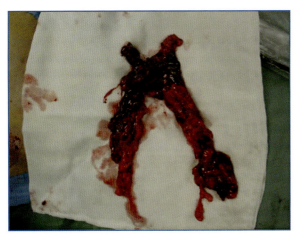

Fig. 22.4 Operative specimen for myasthenia gravis patient [17] (reproduced with permission from Springer-Verlag)

be diligently aspirated from the right posterior pleural cavity. The drain itself is placed across the anterior mediastinum and will not clear this well, especially if clotted. A 24 French-sized intercostal catheter is placed through the lateral 10-mm port and manipulated so that its tip is just in the left pleural cavity, with side holes under the sternum. The submammary incision is closed by approximating the pectoralis muscle (size 1 absorbable suture), then subcutaneous fascia (size 2/0 absorbable suture), and then skin with a subcuticular suture (size 3/0 or 4/0 absorbable suture).

Postoperative Care

Usually the drain tube is removed on the following day, and the patient discharged to home on the day after that. If the patient is symptomatic from myasthenia, hospitalization may have to be tailored to the patient's neuromuscular status. Occasional patients have required inpatient plasma exchange or gammaglobulin therapy. Ventilated intensive care support is not required except for patients with severe generalized or respiratory myasthenia, who have not responded to maximal preoperative therapy including plasma exchange.

Results of VATS Thymectomy

We have previously published our results of VATS thymectomy for 26 cases of myasthenia gravis [7]. We have now performed 100 VATS thymectomies for nonthymomatous myasthenia (57), thymic tumors with/without myasthenia (16/10), diagnostic purposes (13), parathyroid adenomata (2), and teratoma (2).

Our Melbourne group now has long-term follow-up on 71 myasthenic patients who have had right-sided VATS thymectomy. Clinical improvement was achieved in 63 of 71 cases (89%), with 2 unchanged, 1 worse, 3 lost to follow-up, and 2 interim deaths. The crude asymptomatic rate (sum of complete remission, pharmacologic remission and minimal manifestation) was 39 of 71 patients (55%). Long-term complete remission rate for nonthymomatous myasthenia gravis was 41.2% at 8 years using Myasthenia Gravis Foundation of America [9] criteria (Fig. 22.5).

The 26 thymic tumor cases of various subtypes included one squamous cell carcinoma that had an R1 resection. One other patient with invasive thymoma (B2) had an R1 resection despite sterno-thoracotomy and partial resection of SVC. Both of these and all patients with capsular invasion had postoperative radiotherapy.

Five VATS thymectomies in our series had conversion to open surgery (3 right thoracotomies, 1 sternotomy, and 1 sterno-thoracotomy), 3 for bleeding, 1 for technical difficulty early in the series, and 1 for unexpected invasive thymoma. One case started as a right-sided VATS required completion by left-sided VATS approach to avoid injury to the left phrenic nerve, and 1 patient had left-sided VATS (for tumor) from the outset.

The most serious complications have been phrenic nerve palsies in 4 patients. In 2 patients recovery occurred spontaneously within a month. In 1 patient the left phrenic nerve was divided during left-sided VATS to remove a tumor, and the fourth had failed to recover at most recent follow-up. Postoperative pleural and/or pericardial effusions occurred in 3 patients. These were all treated with simple drainage, and then two of the patients were given a pulse of steroid therapy due to raised inflammatory markers. A single case of chylothorax after thymoma resection was treated successfully with VATS pleurodesis and dietary fat restriction.

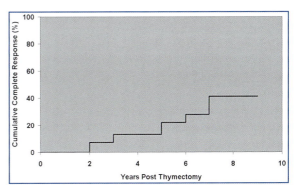

Fig. 22.5 Kaplan-Meier curve of cumulative complete symptomatic remission

Summary

VATS thymectomy is a technically demanding procedure that requires advanced minimally invasive surgery training as well as specific training for the procedure. The right-sided approach is relatively easier due to the larger operating space and the natural curve of the brachiocephalic vein leading straight to the thymic veins. While it can be used to deal with almost all cases, the surgeon must decide when to employ a left-sided VATS approach, cervical approach, or sternotomy, depending on the indication, anatomical/pathological factors, and the patient.

The efficacy of the right-sided approach appears similar to sternotomy approach, with less blood loss, less requirement for narcotic, and less deleterious effects on pulmonary function.

Acknowledgement

The authors wish to thank Mr. Simon Knight from Austin Hospital and Mr. Peter Clarke (retired), formerly of St Vincent's Hospital, in Melbourne for allowing us to include their patients.

References

1. Gronseth GS, Barohn RJ (2000) Practice parameter: thymectomy for autoimmune myasthenia gravis (an evidence-based review): Report of the Quality Standards Subcommittee of the American Academy of Neurology. Neurology 55(1):7-15
2. Ruckert JC, Walter M, Muller JM et al (2000) Pulmonary function after thoracoscopic thymectomy versus median sternotomy for myasthenia gravis. Ann Thorac Surg 70(5):1656-1661
3. Granetzny A, Hatem A, Shalaby A et al (2005) Manubriotomy versus median sternotomy in thymectomy for myasthenia gravis. Evaluation of the pulmonary status. Eur J Cardiothorac Surg 27(3):361-366
4. Chang PC, Chou SH, Kao EL et al (2005) Bilateral video-assisted thoracoscopic thymectomy vs. extended transsternal thymectomy in myasthenia gravis: A prospective study. Eur Surg Res 37(4):199-203
5. Yim AP (1997) Thoracoscopic thymectomy: Which side to approach? Ann Thorac Surg 64(2):584-585
6. Mineo TC, Pompeo E, Lerut TE et al (2000) Thoracoscopic thymectomy in autoimmune myasthesia: Results of left-sided approach. Ann Thorac Surg 69(5):1537-1541
7. Wright GM, Barnett S, Clarke CP (2002) Video-assisted thoracoscopic thymectomy for myasthenia gravis. Intern Med J 32(8):367-371
8. Mack MJ, Landreneau RJ, Yim AP et al (1996) Results of video-assisted thymectomy in patients with myasthenia gravis. J Thorac Cardiovasc Surg 112(5):1352-1359
9. Jaretzki A 3rd, Barohn RJ, Ernstoff RM et al (2000) Myasthenia gravis: Recommendations for clinical research standards. Task Force of the Medical Scientific Advisory Board of the Myasthenia Gravis Foundation of America. Ann Thorac Surg 70(1):327-334
10. Aubert A, Chaffanjon P, Brichon PY (2004) Video-assisted extended thymectomy in patients with thymoma by lifting the sternum: Is it safe? Ann Thorac Surg 77(5):1878
11. Roviaro G, Varoli F, Nucca O et al (2000) Videothoracoscopic approach to primary mediastinal pathology. Chest 117(4):1179-1183
12. Krucylak PE, Naunheim KS (1999) Preoperative preparation and anesthetic management of patients with myasthenia gravis. Semin Thorac Cardiovasc Surg 11(1):47-53
13. Machens A, Emskotter T, Busch C et al (1998) Postoperative infection after transsternal thymectomy for myasthenia gravis: A retrospective analysis of 125 cases. Surg Today 28(8):808-810
14. Juel VC (2004) Myasthenia gravis: Management of myasthenic crisis and postoperative care. Semin Neurol 24(1):75-81
15. Seggia JCB, Abreu P, Takatani M (1995) Plasmapheresis and preparatory method for thymectomy in myasthenia gravis. Arq Neuropsiquiatr 53:411-415
16. Perez Nellar J, Dominguez AM, Llorens-Figueroa JA et al (2001) A comparative study of intravenous immunoglobulin and plasmapheresis preoperatively in myasthenia gravis. Rev Neurol 33(5):413-416
17. Wright G (2006) Timectomia videotoracoscopica con accesso destro. In: Lavini C, Ruggiero L, Morandi U (2006) Chirurgia toracica videoassistita. Principi indicazioni tecniche. Springer-Verlag Italia, Milan, pp 199-204
18. Shiono H, Inoue A, Tomiyama N et al (2006) Safer video-assisted thoracoscopic thymectomy after location of thymic veins with multidetector computed tomography. Surg Endosc 20(9):1419-1422
19. Yune HY, Klatte EC (1970) Thymic venography. Radiology 96(3):521-526

CHAPTER 23
Robotic Techniques

Federico Rea, Giuseppe Marulli

Introduction and History

The left thoracoscopic thymectomy enhanced by the use of robotic system "Da Vinci" allows for a complete removal of thymus and perithymic fat tissue. We adopted this technique to perform the thymectomy in patients affected by nonthymomatous myasthenia gravis, and although it can be safely applied in patients with small thymoma, we prefer a standard sternotomic approach for Masaoka stages II to IV thymoma.

Since 1941, when Blalock [1] first reported results of transsternal thymectomy in patients affected by MG, thymectomy has played a significant role constituting a widely accepted therapeutic option in the integrated management of MG.

Multiple techniques have been described to remove the thymus in MG: transcervical thymectomy (basic or extended) [2], video-assisted thoracoscopic thymectomy (VATS) [3-5] (classic or extended), transsternal thymectomy [6] (standard, extended, or maximal), infrasternal mediastinoscopic thymectomy [7].

Basic techniques for thymectomy enable a radical resection of the thymic gland through a single surgical approach; extended techniques associate more than one access (i.e., transcervical plus transsternal incision for maximal thymectomy proposed by Jaretzki [8]): the rationale of extended techniques is to obtain a complete resection of the visible thymus, the suspected thymus, and cervical-mediastinal fat tissue (in which microscopic foci of thymic tissue may be contained) using a wide exposure.

In the last decade growing interest in minimally invasive surgical techniques has developed. They have also reduced patient morbidity and mortality, infection rate, postoperative hospital stay, and pain medication; moreover, better cosmetic results have led to a greater acceptability of these surgical procedures. Recently, robotic surgery has affirmed itself as an evolution of VATS allowing surgeons to overcome some limitations of classic thoracoscopy (2-D view, limited maneuverability of endoscopic instruments).

The first surgical application of robotic technique was described by Loulmet and Reichenspurner in 1999: they performed a coronary by-pass [9-10].

Subsequently, robotic instruments were applied in other fields too and, in 2001, Yoshino [11] described the first robotic thymectomy in the treatment of small thymoma.

In 2003, Ashton [12] and Rea [13] published a case report on robotic thymectomy in MG using two different approaches: the former surgeon from Columbia University adopted a right-sided approach with completion of the operation through a left-sided approach; the latter, from the University in Padua, used a left-sided approach only. In 2006, Rea et al. [14] reported the first large series of robotic thymectomies.

Description of the "Da Vinci" Robotic System

The "Da Vinci" robotic system consists of an ergonomically designed surgeon's computerized console, a vision system, and a patient-side cart that supports the interactive robotic arms (Fig. 23.1).

The surgeon controls the system sitting at the computerized console far from the patient. The console is connected to the video system and to the robotic-side cart, and it represents the interface between surgeon and robotic system (master/slave system). The surgeon sees the operative field through a binocular localized in the upper part of the console; an infrared system disables the commands when the surgeon is not present. The surgeon's fingers grasp the master controls below the display and realize the movements of robotic instruments. The system translates the 3-D movements of hands and fingers into precise, identical, and real-time movements of surgical instruments inside the patient. A support makes the movements comfortable and is furnished with

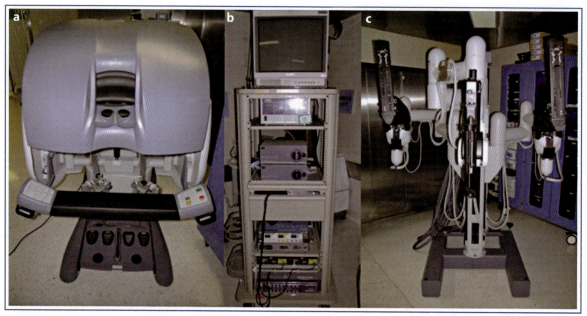

Fig. 23.1a-c The three components of "Da Vinci" robot. **a** The surgeon's console: the surgeon sits at the console far from the patient. He sees the operative field by the binocular and moves the endoscopic instruments by the master controls. **b** The video system with all components, and **c** the patient-side cart that supports the robotic arms (reproduced from [15] with permission of Springer-Verlag Italia)

several buttons for the regulation of various functions like the type of vision (2-D or 3-D view) or the type of optic (0°-30°). Moreover, the system is equipped with a tremor filtering that allows for extremely precise movements. At the bottom of the console a series of 5 pedals permits other controls such as the activation of electrocautery, the variation of focal point of the camera, etc.

The vision system contains the video components: a monitor that allows the personnel in the operating room to view the intervention, and two boxes for control of the video camera and for the balancing of luminosity and contrast of the image. A system for the supply of CO_2 and its intracavitary pressurization can be placed in this tower.

The patient-side cart supports the three or four arms of the robot: the central arm holds the 12-mm-diameter optic. The cylinder contains two distinct optics of 5 mm both equipped with 3 microcameras and their video signal is transferred to the console where the computer synchronizes the information and creates a virtual 3-D image of the operative field.

The left arm is connected with an atraumatic EndoWrist, while the right arm is connected with the electrocautery. The surgical instruments are articulated with the main arm and they are designed with seven degrees of motion and a 360° rotation, which mimics the dexterity of the human hand and wrist.

Operative Technique

The patient is under general anesthesia and has a double-lumen endotracheal tube for selective single lung ventilation during the time of operation.

In the surgical room the patient is positioned left side up, 30° upon a bean bag. The right arm is positioned along the body and the left arm is positioned on a support parallel to the bed; in this manner the axillary region is easily exposed (Fig. 23.2).

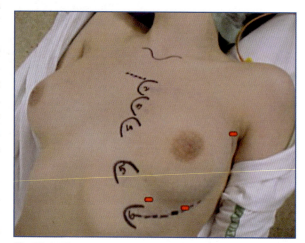

Fig. 23.2 The patient is positioned on the surgical table and the accesses for the ports are evidenced

The robotic console is positioned far from the patient in the operating room; the video column is at the bottom or at the top of the bed depending on the preference of the assistant. The robotic cart is positioned on the right side of the bed with a 45° angle. The arms of the "Da Vinci" surgical system are placed as follows: a camera port for the 3-D 0° stereo endoscope is introduced through a 15-mm incision in the 5th intercostal space in the anterior portion of midaxillary region; two additional thoracic ports are inserted through two additional 5-mm incisions in the 5th intercostal space on the midclavicular line and in the 3rd intercostal space on the anterior portion of midaxillary region (Fig. 23.3a).

Two arms of the Da Vinci system are then attached to the two access points and another arm is attached to the port-inserted endoscope. The left arm has an EndoWrist instrument that grasps the thymus; the right arm is an Endo-Dissector device with electric cautery function used to perform the dissection (Fig. 23.3b).

During surgery the hemithorax is inflated through the camera port with CO_2 ranging in pressure from 6 to 10 mmHg. CO_2 inflation is very useful to obtain a clear view within the chest and to allow an easier dissection as it extends the mediastinal space.

After careful exploration of the mediastinal pleural space, the dissection of the fat tissue starts inferiorly at the left pericardiophrenic angle.

The thymic gland is then divided from the retrosternal area and the left inferior horn of the thymus is subsequently isolated and dissected from the pericardium.

At the top of the mediastinum, the pleura is incised in the area delimited by the mammary vessels in the anterior limit and by the phrenic nerve in the posterior limit. At this point the lower part of the thymus is mobilized upwards and thymic tissue is dissected from the plane of the aorto-pulmonary window. The dissection continues on the right side with the visualization of the right mediastinal pleura and the right inferior horn.

The isolation proceeds up to into the neck until the superior horns are identified and divided from the inferior portion of the thyroid gland by a blunt dissection.

The innominate vein is identified and the dissection continues along the border of the innominate vein up to the point where the thymic veins are identified, clipped, and divided (Fig. 23.4). Through the left access it is also possible to remove the fat tissue in the aorto-pulmonary area (in which ectopic thymic isles can be present) behind the left phrenic nerve, avoiding the risk of nerve injury.

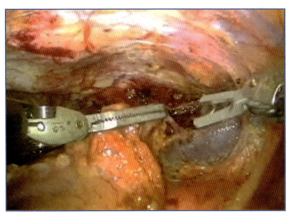

Fig. 23.4 The thymic vein is easily and safely clipped by a clips applicator

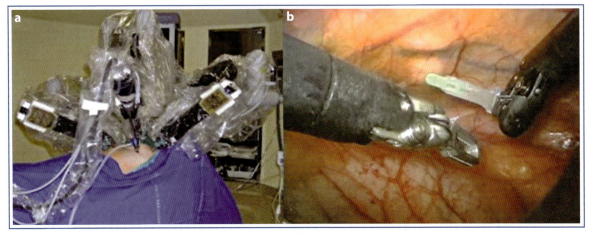

Fig. 23.3a,b **a** The thoracic ports are placed after the identification of the 5th and 3rd intercostal space and the arms of the "Da Vinci" surgical system are attached to the ports and are operative. **b** Endoscopic view of robotic instruments attached to the arms: an EndoWrist on the right arm and an electrocautery on the left arm (reproduced from [15] with permission of Springer-Verlag Italia)

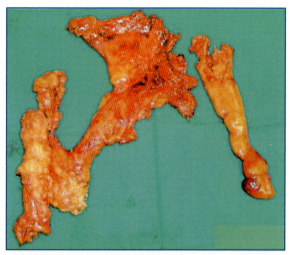

Fig. 23.5 Surgical specimen: the thymic gland and mediastinal fat are removed en-bloc

The thymus gland, the anterior mediastinal, and the neck's fatty tissue are radically resected (Fig. 23.5) and the specimen is placed in an Endo-Bag so it can be removed by trocar incision. After the hemostasis, a 28F drainage tube is inserted through the wound of the 5th intercostal space; the lung is reinflated, and the other wounds are closed.

The patient is extubated in the operating room and, subsequent to an adequate period of observation, returns to the surgical thoracic ward.

The chest drainage tube is removed 24 h after surgery and, if neurological evaluation is satisfactory, the patient is discharged 48-72 h after surgery.

Results

Between April 2002 and December 2007, 65 patients underwent thoracoscopic thymectomy with the "Da Vinci" surgical system at the Division of Thoracic Surgery of Padua. Mean operative time was 120 minutes (ranging from 60 to 240 minutes); no intraoperative mortality or complications were experienced; no conversion to median sternotomy and no more accesses were required. Postoperative complications occurred in three cases (4.6%): one patient had a chilothorax, two patients had a hemothorax caused by bleeding from one access, and both were treated conservatively. Mean time of hospitalization after surgery was 2.5 days (range from 2 to 14 days). In 4 patients histological exam revealed a small (<2 cm) thymoma (Masaoka stage I). All patients judged the cosmetic result as excellent. Clinical results on the first 54 patients with a minimum follow-up of 1 year showed a complete remission in 22.2% of cases and an improvement in 64.8%, for a global benefit rate of 87%.

Conclusions

Thymectomy for MG patients has proven to be an effective therapy leading to good clinical results in terms of improvement or complete remission of symptoms.

The technique of VATS thymectomy has been performed successfully using the left- or right-sided approach. This approach combines the advantages of minimally invasive techniques (fewer complications, minimal thoracic trauma, early improved pulmonary function, a shorter recovery period, and optimal cosmetic results) and an excellent view of the anterior mediastinum, so that an extended thymectomy can be performed, similar to the one in the transsternal approach.

Disadvantages of the VATS technique include a 2-D view of the operative field and the fact that the arms do not articulate, making it difficult to operate in the mediastinum. The development of robotic systems in recent years has permitted surgeons to overcome these limitations. The "Da Vinci" robotic system is equipped with a camera device that allows an intuitive, enhanced 3-D vision of the operative field. The surgical EndoWrist articulates and rotates 360° with a full 7° of freedom; the scale motion with a system for tremor filtering makes the maneuvers more precise. All these characteristics improved, in our experience, the surgical dissection, making it easier than conventional VATS, particularly in remote, fixed, and difficult-to-reach areas of the neck and mediastinum, and enabling a safe and comfortable dissection of vascular and nervous structures. We prefer the left-sided approach as it offers a perfect visualization of the aortic window and reduces the probability of phrenic nerve injury, with a direct vision of the left phrenic nerve, while the right phrenic nerve is partially protected by the superior vena cava. The initial high cost of the robotic system is easily recovered if the robotic instrumentation is used in several different surgical specialties, as in our hospital. Another disadvantage of robotic surgery is its current lack of tactile feedback, but this is compensated by the superior image of the 3-D camera. The learning curve associated with robotic technology could be considered a disadvantage, but learning curves are part of any new technology and, in our experience, determined only an initial increased operative time.

References

1. Blalock A, McGehee HA, Ford FR (1941) The treatment of myasthenia gravis by removal of the thymus gland. JAMA 117:1529
2. Cooper JD, Al-Jilaihawa AN, Pearson FG et al (1988) An improved technique to facilitate transcervical thymectomy for myasthenia gravis. Ann Thorac Surg 45:242-247
3. Mineo TC, Pompeo E, Lerut T et al (2000) Thoracoscopic thymectomy in autoimmune myasthenia: Results of left-sided approach. Ann Thorac Surg 69:1537-1541
4. Mack MJ, Scruggs G (1998) Video-assisted thoracic surgery thymectomy for myasthenia gravis. Chest Surg Clin N Am 8:809-825
5. Novellino L, Longoni M, Spinelli L et al (1994) "Extended" thymectomy without sternotomy, performed by cervicotomy and thoracoscopic techniques in the treatment of myasthenia gravis. Int Surg 79:378-381
6. Masaoka A, Yamakawa Y, Niwa H et al (1996) Extended thymectomy for myasthenia gravis: A 20-year review. Ann Thorac Surg 62:853-859
7. Uchiyama A, Shuji S, Hiroyuki H (2001) Infrasternal mediastinoscopic thymectomy in myasthenia gravis: Surgical results in 23 patients. Ann Thorac Surg 72:1902-1905
8. Jaretzki A, Wolff M (1988) "Maximal" thymectomy for myasthenia gravis. Surgical anatomy and operative technique. J Thorac Cardiovasc Surg 96:711-716
9. Loulmet D, Carpentier A, D'Attelis N et al (1999) Endoscopic coronary artery bypass grafting with the aid of robotic assisted instruments. J Thorac Cardiovasc Surg 118:4-10
10. Reichenspurner H, Damiano RJ, Mack M et al (1999) Use of the voice-controlled and computer-assisted surgical system Zeus for endoscopic coronary artery bypass grafting. J Thorac Cardiovasc Surg 118: 11-16
11. Yoshino I, Hashizume M, Shimada M et al (2001) Thoracoscopic thymomectomy with the Da Vinci computer-enhanced surgical system. J Thorac Cardiovasc Surg 122:783-785
12. Ashton RC, McGinnis KM, Connery CP et al (2003) Totally endoscopic thymectomy for myasthenia gravis. Ann Thorac Surg 75:569-571
13. Rea F, Bortolotti L, Girardi R, Sartori F (2003) Thoracoscopic thymectomy with the Da Vinci surgical system in patient with myasthenia gravis. Interact Cardiovasc Thorac Surg 2:70-72
14. Rea F, Marulli G, Bortolotti L et al (2006) Experience with the "Da Vinci" robotic system for thymectomy in patients with myasthenia gravis: Report of 33 cases. Ann Thorac Surg 81:455-459
15. Lavini C, Ruggiero C, Morandi U (2006) Chirurgia toracica videoassistita. Principi indicazioni tecniche. Springer-Verlag Italia, Milan

CHAPTER 24

Complex Surgical Interventions in Superior Vena Cava Syndrome

Zhen-Dong Gu, Ke-Neng Chen

Introduction

The superior vena cava (SVC) originates from both brachiocephalic veins and returns the blood of upper half body into the right atrium. When the obstruction of SVC happens, blood stasis develops in the head, neck, and upper extremities, then the superior vena cava syndrome (SVCS) shows up. Most of the time, SVCS is associated with malignancies, such as advanced lung cancer, thymic tumors, metastatic solid tumors, and so on [1]. This chapter is dedicated to discussing the treatment, especially the complex surgical interventions, for SVCS.

Anatomy and Collateral Pathways

SVC is a thin-walled low-pressure vascular, unioned by both of the brachiocephalic veins, and descends anterolaterally to the trachea to reach the right atrium. There are some collateral pathways of the SVC system, and when SVCS happens, they will exert an important compensated function to return the blood from the upper body to the heart through the inferior vena cava system. The azygos vein is one of the most important collateral pathways when SVCS shows up, especially when the obstruction is distal to the azygos-SVC junction. The other collateral pathways include the internal mammary veins and superior intercostals veins, both of which, like the azygos vein, can return the venous blood from the upper body into the inferior vena cava (IVC) [2].

Causes of SVCS

SVCS is usually associated with advanced malignant tumors, which account for more than 90% of patients. Of these, lung cancer is the most common (more than 50%). Other tumors include mediastinal tumors, and metastatic disease from carcinoma of breast, colon, kidney, and so on. SVCS associated with thymoma is rare (about 4%). About 5-10% of SVCS are caused by benign disease, such as retrosternal goiters, thrombosis of the SVC and subclavian vein, aortic aneurysms, benign teratomas, and so on [2].

Clinical Presentations

Common clinical presentations of SVCS include dyspnea, swelling of face, neck, and upper extremities, cough, headaches, and dizziness. Uncommon symptoms include chest pain, dysphagia, weight loss, hoarseness, and so on. Physical examination may show edema of the head, neck, and upper torso, dilated superficial veins, sometimes cyanotic or flushed skin over the neck, anterior chest wall, and upper extremities [2]. The severity of such clinical presentations is mainly related to the rate of SVCS progression and the extent of collateral venous pathways. Symptoms will be more significant in acute obstruction and if there are no adequate collateral pathways.

Diagnosis

Chest radiographs and CT scan can show the size and location of the lesion, also the site of obstruction, and relationship with surrounding structures. Contrast-enhanced CT scan can demonstrate the level of obstruction and the development of collateral vessels. Tissue diagnosis should be obtained before initial treatment because the treatment strategies and prognosis can be totally different from each other according to the nature of the tumor [2]. Besides, their complete resection always necessitates simultaneous resection of involved vital organs, and such procedures carry relatively more severe risks [3-5]. Fine needle aspiration is widely used due to its minimal trauma and overall good accuracy [6]. For the patients with enlarged peripheral especially supraclavicular lymph nodes, open lymph node biopsy can be performed. Cervical mediastinoscopy is suitable for patients with malignant anterior mediastinal tumors or enlarged mediastinal lymph nodes. For patients whose thoracotomy is warranted to get the pathological diagnosis, video-assisted thoracic surgery (VATS) is preferred to formal thoracotomy, which may produce disruption of collateral venous pathways and worsening of symptoms [2].

Management

General Management

Initial treatment of SVCS generally includes oxygen supplementation, elevation of the head and upper extremities to promote venous return, and diuretics to reduce peripheral edema. Sometimes the steroids are indicated to decrease laryngeal and cerebral edema [2]. Because the main cause of the SVCS is malignancy, comprehensive treatment that includes chemotherapy, radiotherapy, and surgery are always warranted. Although recent advances in diagnostic techniques have led to more accurate preoperative delineation and histologic diagnoses, determining the appropriate treatment for such complicated tumors accompanied with SVCS remains a challenge for general thoracic surgeons [7, 8].

Surgical Management

For patients with thymic malignancies, the presentation of SVCS always indicates locally advanced disease which may have invaded surrounding tissues, such as major blood vessels, pericardium, lung tissue, and so on, which provide a great therapeutic challenge. However, extensive resection is sometimes indicated, because it may permit long-term survival with good quality of life. Some authors believed that SVCS on its own is very rarely fatal, and the prognosis of the patients mainly related to the histological type and stage of the primary malignancy [9]. Besides, some reports have suggested that en bloc resection and reconstruction of the SVC is technically feasible and in some cases associated with survival benefits [10, 11]. Chen et al. [3] suggested that to prolong the survival of patients with invasive thymic tumors (including malignant thymoma and thymic carcinoma), patients should receive surgery to excise tumor and involved organs. Funakoshi et al. [12] also believed that surgery, based on chemotherapy and radiotherapy, is effective for advanced invasive thymoma. Curran et al. [13] suggested avoiding postoperative radiotherapy if complete resection is achieved with primary surgery. Although there are so many positive points for the role of complex surgical interventions for the treatment of thymic malignancies with SVCS, we should keep it in mind that these published experiences are limited to a small number of case reports and series, containing patients who were highly selected for curative intent surgery. These results suggested that extensive surgical resection is technically feasible, but the appropriate indications for such efforts are often not well delineated [14].

The surgical techniques usually used for the treatment of patient with thymic malignancies accompanied with SVCS included not only tumor resection but also pericardium resection, lung tissue resection, and angio-techniques. Angio-techniques may be the most important, because they allow complete resection in persons who would not otherwise be considered candidates for surgery [3].

The additional angio-techniques which can be used to achieve radical resection include ligation and resection of invaded vein, partial lateral-wall resection of the SVC and simple angioplasty, partial resection of the SVC and angioplasty with a pericardial patch, total resection of the SVC and both innominate veins plus interposition of a single-lumen artificial vessel, and total resection of the SVC and both innominate veins plus reconstruction with a Y-shaped artificial vessel (Fig. 24.1) [3]. Ligation and resection of invaded vein is simple and safe in most circumstances. Due to the slow growth of most thymic tumors, along with the gradual invasion of SVC and presentation of SVCS, the collateral pathways can work more and more efficiently to return the blood from the upper body to the heart through the IVC system. So, to this kind of patients, especially those with severe tumor invasion of the SVC system, clamp of the SVC system during the operation can be tried, and if there is no sign of acute or rapidly progressive SVCS, which indicates that the collateral pathways are efficient for blood return, the invaded vein can be ligated and resected safely. To patients still with patent SVC, especially if the involved vessel's length is less than 2 cm and the circumference is less than half the size of the whole circle, the ligation and resection of SVC is not indicated because it can always induce acute and progressive SVCS. Partial lateral-wall resection of the SVC and simple angioplasty are safe and easily performed in such circumstances. If the SVC is still

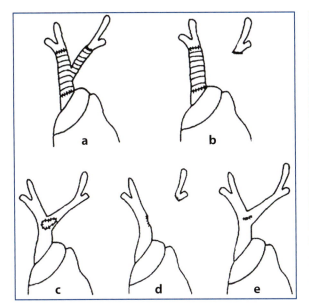

Fig. 24.1a-e Angio-techniques in complex surgical interventions for patients with SVCS. **a** Total resection of the SVC and both innominate veins and reconstruction with a Y-shaped artificial vessel. **b** Total resection of the SVC and interposition with a single-lumen artificial vessel. **c** Partial resection of the SVC and/or innominate veins and angioplasty with a pericardial patch. **d** Left innominate vein was removed and its distal end was ligated. **e** Partial lateral wall of the SVC, innominate vein or both were directly resected and sutured [3] (with kind permission from Springer Science+Business Media)

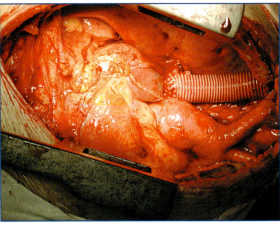

Fig. 24.2 Surgery for patient with SVCS who underwent tumor resection + total resection of SVC + interposition with "single-lumen" artificial vessel [3] (with kind permission from Springer Science+Business Media)

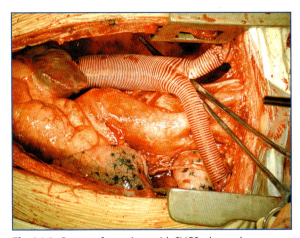

Fig. 24.3 Surgery for patient with SVCS who underwent tumor resection + total resection of SVC and of both innominate veins + reconstruction with Y-shaped artificial vessel [3] (with kind permission from Springer Science+Business Media)

patent with the involved vessel's length more than 2 cm and the circumference more than half the size of the whole circle, resection of the SVC lateral wall and repair with pericardium can be performed. To patients with long-distance invasion of the SVC and presentation of acute or rapidly progressive SVCS after the SVC is clamped during the operation, the resection of the SVC followed by artificial vessel interposition is suggested, which allows the radical resection with the preservation of SVC patency (Figs. 24.2, 24.3) [3].

In angio-techniques, median sternotomy can provide the best exposure of the anterior mediastinal tumor, full length of the SVC and both innominate veins. Surgeons should try to perform an en bloc resection, including the involved vessels, to decrease the possibility of tumor seeding, but if it is hard to perform an en bloc resection, a fractional resection can be considered. When exploring the involved vessel, attention should be paid to tumor emboli, keeping in mind the possible embolism or metastasis. Anticoagulant therapy should be given perioperatively, such as soaking artificial vessels in heparin-salt water, taking eversion sutures to smooth the vascular inner wall, or using heparin followed by aspirin postoperatively [3]. For the graft, many biologic and synthetic materials, such as autologous vein, autologous or bovine pericardial tube, and expanded polytetrafluoroethylene (ePTFE/Gore-Tex) tube have been reported [10, 15, 16]. Some authors prefer autologous spiral saphenous vein graft or superficial femoral vein rather than ePTFE for better graft patency [17]. However, ePTFE has the advantage of being immediately available in length and caliber, and excellent short-term and long-term results have been reported [15, 16].

Other Management

Endovascular Stent

If the life expectancy of the patient with SVCS is short, endovascular stent is preferred to achieve SVC patency, especially in patients who have severe symptoms but are not surgical candidates. It can achieve immediate resolution of symptoms within 24-48 h, and can be frequently repeated according to the need, and does not adversely affect future open surgical reconstruction [17]. Major complications include stent migration, cardiac failure and pulmonary edema from sudden increase in venous return, SVC perforation, and so on [18].

Conclusions

In conclusion, patients, especially tumor patients accompanied with SVCS, should be pathologically identified before initial treatment. Complex surgical interventions for the treatment of thymic malignancies that require vascular resection and reconstruction for curative intent may permit long-term survival with good quality of life. Endovascular stent is preferred for patients with severe symptoms but not surgical candidates. Therefore, a good prognosis for patients with thymic malignancies is possible if a suitable strategy including complex surgical interventions is established.

References

1. Chen JC, Bongard F, Klein SR (1990) A contemporary perspective on superior vena cava syndrome. Am J Surg 160:207-211
2. Deslauriers J, Mehran R (2005) Handbook of perioperative care in general thoracic surgery. Mosby Inc., Philadelphia
3. Chen KN, Xu SF, Gu ZD et al (2006) Surgical treatment of complex malignant anterior mediastinal tumors invading the superior vena cava. World J Surg 30:162-170
4. Wright CD, Mathisen DJ (2001) Mediastinal tumors: Diagnosis and treatment. World J Surg 25:204-209
5. William EW Jr (1995) Thymoma. In: Pearson FG, Deslauriers J, Ginsberg RJ et al (eds) Thoracic surgery. Churchill Livingstone, New York, pp 1419-1427
6. Rosenberger A, Adler O (1978) Fine needle aspiration biopsy in the diagnosis of mediastinal lesions. AJR Am J Roentgenol 131:239-242
7. Bacha EA, Chapelier AR, Macchiarini P et al (1998) Surgery for invasive primary mediastinal tumors. Ann Thorac Surg 66:234-239
8. Yagi K, Hirata T, Fukuse T et al (1996) Surgical treatment of invasive thymoma, especially when superior vena cava is invaded. Ann Thorac Surg 61:521-524
9. Ahmann F (1984) A reassessment of the clinical implications of the superior vena cava syndrome. J Clin Oncol 2:961-969
10. Doty JR, Flores JH, Doty DB (1999) Superior vena cava obstruction: Bypass using spiral vein graft. Ann Thorac Surg 67:1111-1116
11. Dartevelle PG, Chapelier AR, Pastorino U et al (1991) Long-term follow-up after prosthetic replacement of the superior vena cava combined with resection of mediastinal-pulmonary malignant tumors. J Thorac Cardiovasc Surg 102:259-265
12. Funakoshi Y, Ohta M, Maeda H et al (2003) Extended operation for invasive thymoma with intracaval and intracardiac extension. Eur J Cardiothorac Surg 24:331-333
13. Curran WJ Jr, Kornstein MJ, Brooks JJ et al (1998) Invasive thymoma: The role of mediastinal irradiation following complete or incomplete surgical resection. J Clin Oncol 6:1722-1727
14. Park BJ, Bacchetta M, Bains MS et al (2004) Surgical management of thoracic malignancies invading the heart or great vessels. Ann Thorac Surg 78:1024-1030
15. Magnan PE, Thomas P, Giudicelli R et al (1994) Surgical reconstruction of the superior vena cava. Cardiovasc Surg 2:598-604
16. Spaggiari L, Thomas P, Magdeleinat P et al (2002) Superior vena cava resection with prosthetic replacement for non-small cell lung cancer: Long-term results of a multicentric study. Eur J Cardiothorac Surg 21:1080-1086
17. Kalra M, Gloviczki P, Andrews JC et al (2003) Open surgical and endovascular treatment of superior vena cava syndrome caused by nonmalignant disease. J Vasc Surg 38:215-223
18. Pearl ML, Buhl A, DiSilvestro PA et al (2002) Superior vena cava syndrome. Prim Care Update Ob Gyns 9:160-163

CHAPTER 25
Reinterventions for Thymoma Recurrences

Piero Zannini, Giampiero Negri, Monica Casiraghi, Luca Ferla, Paola Ciriaco

Introduction

Surgical resection is considered the gold standard for the treatment of thymomas no matter what the histological type. Even when complete resection is achieved, however, recurrence of thymoma is not uncommon as it occurs in about 10-29% of patients. Recurrences affect subsequent treatment and final outcome but there is still no general consensus on how to manage them. Complete resection of recurrences should be attempted whenever possible to achieve long-term survival. When complete resection is not feasible, an iterative debulking approach may improve survival by reducing the size of these slow-growing tumors. Currently, a multimodality approach combining radiotherapy and/or chemotherapy with surgery may be considered the best treatment for thymoma recurrences.

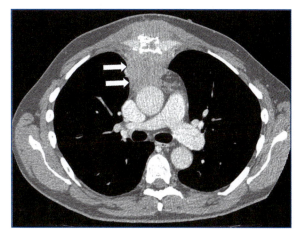

Fig. 25.1 CT scan image showing massive sternal infiltration by a highly invasive thymic carcinoma

State of the Art

Thymic tumors are relatively rare primary tumors originating from the thymic epithelium with an overall incidence of 0.15 cases per 100,000 [1]. These tumors include thymomas, thymic carcinomas, and thymic carcinoids (or neuroendocrine carcinomas). Thymomas represent by far the most common thymic tumor and are the most frequent tumors of the anterior mediastinum, accounting for about 20% of all mediastinal masses in the adult population. They are a heterogeneous group of tumors that include capsulated and benign lesions as well as highly invasive and malignant neoplasms (Fig. 25.1). Their heterogeneity has led to some confusion in distinguishing their clinical behavior and in identifying the most appropriate therapeutic approach. After many years of discussion on the prognostic accuracy of the Masaoka clinical staging system (Table 25.1), new insights have been offered by the recent WHO histological classification system, which divides thymic tumors into six different subtypes (A, AB, B1, B2, B3, and C), based on the morphology of the epithelium cell component (Table 25.2). The WHO classification system establishes a

Table 25.1 Masaoka staging system

Masaoka stage	Criteria
Stage I	Macroscopically completely encapsulated and microscopically no capsular invasion
Stage II	Macroscopic invasion into surrounding fatty tissue or mediastinal pleura, or microscopic invasion into capsule
Stage III	Macroscopic invasion into neighboring organ, i.e., pericardium, great vessels, or lung
Stage IV a	Pleural or pericardial dissemination
Stage IV b	Lymphogenous or hematogenous metastasis

Table 25.2 WHO histological classification system

WHO	Description
Type A	Spindle cell, medullary
Type AB	Mixed
Type B1	Lymphocyte-rich, "organoid," predominantly cortical
Type B2	Cortical
Type B3	Epithelial, atypical, squamoid, well-differentiated thymic carcinoma
Type C	Thymic carcinoma

more reliable correlation between the histological patterns and the clinical course of the disease, thus improving the prognostic value of the clinical Masaoka staging system. Studies applying the WHO classification retrospectively have demonstrated that not only the tumor stage but also the histological subtype could be considered independent prognostic factors [2-4].

Currently the majority of thymomas are considered low-grade malignant tumors with a slow-growing and indolent natural history. However, even if the clinical course is generally benign, these tumors are able to induce local and regional invasion. Up to 33% of thymomas behave aggressively, penetrating the capsule and extending into the mediastinal fat and adjacent organs such as the pleura, pericardium, lung, chest wall, and great vessels. Typical findings are drop metastases into the homolateral pleura and pericardium, whereas lymph node and hematogenous metastases are rare [5-7]. Invasive thymomas may also infiltrate the diaphragm and overrun into the abdomen as well as the retro peritoneum space [8].

Surgical resection is considered the gold standard for the treatment of thymomas no matter what the histological type [9-12]. The mainstay of thymoma treatment is to achieve complete macroscopic resection and microscopic clearance, by removing en bloc all the involved tissue. Several studies have already demonstrated that complete resection of thymomas has a significantly favorable effect on long-term outcome [13-15]. In their retrospective analysis, Strobel et al. [16] found that long-term survival was related to completeness of surgical resection and evidence of recurrence as well as Masaoka tumor stage and WHO histological subtype. However, variables such as patients' age, sex, presence of myasthenia gravis (MG), and tumor size were not statistically correlated with survival.

Recurrence of thymoma is not uncommon even when complete resection is achieved and a long-term follow-up should therefore be envisaged. Thymoma recurrences occur in about 10-29% of patients [17, 18], who therefore require further treatment. Most recurrences occur in the thoracic cavity. In 1997, before the introduction of the WHO classification, Regnard reported a 10% recurrence rate in a series of 285 patients who had undergone complete thymoma resection. Most of the recurrences were intrathoracic and resectable; only two patients had concomitant extrathoracic metastases [15]. Local recurrences may occur in early stage thymoma patients (mainly Masaoka stage I and II) who do not have adjuvant treatment after initial surgery. This reveals that recurrences are likely to occur where microscopic tumor residuals are left in place during surgery [15]. Pleural, pericardial, and pulmonary metastases are more frequent in stage III and IV thymomas even if patients have been treated postoperatively with mediastinal radiation therapy since radiation is able to prevent local mediastinal recurrences but obviously not pleural and pulmonary metastases. Histological subtyping has generated animated discussions during the last decade and it has recently been suggested that the cortical differentiation of the tumor is related to a higher degree of malignancy and consequently with a worse survival. In their retrospective study, Ciccone and Rendina [19] report that all the recurrences in their series occurred in cortical differentiated thymomas (B1, B2, and B3 subtype according to the WHO histological staging system), which may point to an adverse prognostic role of these histological subtypes. Besides, a histological change was noted between primary tumors and the recurrences in about 45% of the patients, mainly towards a higher malignancy, within the cortical differentiation subtypes [19]. Wright et al. [20] showed that recurrence rate, correlated with WHO tumor type, was respectively 27% for B2 thymomas and 50% for B3, demonstrating that WHO and Masaoka stage systems were independent predictors of relapses.

As thymomas are infrequent tumors, there is as yet no well-defined approach to the management of their recurrences, due to the small number of patients in published series [11, 13-15, 21]. Regnard et al. [15] emphasized that the best therapeutic approach for thymoma recurrences was difficult to determine, as no control group was available for comparison. Ruffini et al. [13] demonstrated that the best option for long-term survival was complete surgical resection of recurrences. When resection was necessarily incomplete, it was related to a poor prognosis even if followed by radiation. Haniuda et al. [20] suggest that an iterative debulking approach should be attempted if complete resection is not feasible, to reduce tumor size and improve survival, considering the slow growth of these tumors [21]. Conflicting results are reported by Okumura et al. [22] who found that the overall 10-year survival rate in their reresected patients was significantly higher than in the patients in whom surgical treatment was not performed. Increasingly gaining consensus is the conviction that early stage tumors (stage I) are successfully treated by surgery alone whereas a multimodality treatment is the best approach for unresectable and advanced stage thymomas (stage III or IV), as well as for tumors with a cortical subtype differentiation and for patients with recurrences. Shin et al. [23] showed that locally advanced and unresectable thymoma could be effectively treated by an aggressive multimodal treatment. In a multicenter study Loehrer et al. [24] demonstrated a 50% response rate to chemotherapy treatment in patients with metastatic or recurrent thymomas. Giaccone et al. [25] had similar results. Ciccone and Rendina [19] suggest that adjuvant therapy should also be given to stage I and II thymomas with cortical subtype differentiation, which usually have a poorer prognosis, to decrease recurrence rate and to ensure a longer-term survival. Thymic tumors are sensitive to chemotherapy with a response rate ranging from 30% to 60% in metastatic patients [26]. Chemotherapy may therefore play an important role both as neo-adjuvant treatment for inoperable patients and as adjuvant therapy to improve the long-term, disease-free survival rate for patients who have already undergone surgery. Thymomas are also radioresponsive and radiation may be considered an effective adjuvant therapy that improves local tumor control and survival in patients with invasive thymoma [27]. Postoperative radiotherapy in stage III and IV thymomas has shown a 50-20% reduction in the recurrence rate although its effectiveness in stage II patients is still under discussion [28]. Preoperative and primary radiation alone has not been found to be a valid approach to advanced disease [28].

Recently, new noncytotoxic treatments have been found to be effective in patients with progressive disease [26]. Therapies with corticosteroids for instance have shown a tumor response in patients with advanced disease particularly when combined with chemotherapy [29]. Palmieri et al. [30] reported complete remission of patients affected by thymomas and pure red cell aplasia using octreotide, a synthetic octapeptide somatostatin (SST). On the other hand, interleukin-2 has had a positive response only in phase I studies [31].

In conclusion, multimodal therapies that combine radiotherapy and chemotherapy with surgery, when feasible, are today widely accepted as the best treatment for thymoma recurrences and unresectable advanced thymomas.

Our Experience

We reviewed the records of 81 patients who underwent surgical resection for thymoma in our Unit from January 1994 to December 2007. Fourteen of the 81 patients had a tumor recurrence. Three of these patients were not eligible for reoperation because of their poor performance status. They have therefore been excluded from the present study. The remaining 11 patients underwent surgical resection. All 81 patients were classified on the basis of the Masaoka clinical staging system and the recurrence rate was 7% for stage I, 6% for stage II, 46% for stage III, and 14% for stage IV. The histological specimens (primary and recurrent tumors) of the 11 reoperated patients were retrospectively reviewed and reclassified according to the WHO histological classification system.

At the time of the initial operation, 2 of the 11 patients who developed recurrences were stage I (18%), 2 stage II (18%), 6 stage III (55%), and 1 stage IV (9%). When reclassified according to the WHO histological staging system, no patients had type A thymoma, 2 had type AB (18%), 1 type B1 (9%), 4 type B2 (37%), 3 type B3 (27%), and 1 patient (9%) had a thymic carcinoma (type C). Two patients with a locally advanced thymoma (stage III and IV) received neo-adjuvant chemotherapy at the time of the first operation. All 11 patients had a radical thymoma resection (Tables 25.3, 25.4) and adjuvant treatment

Table 25.3 Group I patients (underwent surgery for thymoma and developed only one recurrence)

	Initial surgery for thymoma					Recurrence of thymoma				
N	Year	Surgical approach	Extention of disease	Radicality	Adjuvant therapy	Year	Surgical approach	Extention of disease	Radicality	Adjuvant therapy
1	1983	Thor	Med fat	+	None	1998	Sternot	Med fat	+	None
2	1993	Thor	Intracapsular	+	None	2006	Sternot	Peri	+	RT
3	1999	Sternot	Pleura	+	RT	2003	Thor	Lung	+	CT + RT
4	1999	Sternot	Pleura	+	CT	2006	Thor	Lung	+	None
5	2003	Sternot	Peri + lung + diaph + med fat	+	RT	2007	Thor	Chest wall + pleura	+	CT
6	2004	Sternot	Med fat	+	RT	2007	Thor	Lung	+	None
7	2006	Sternot	Chest wall	+	CT + RT + tomo	2007	Thor (sequential thor)	Lung	+	CT
8	1972	Thor	Intracapsular	+	None	2007	Sternot	Lung + peri + an vein	+	Delayed for pulmonary embolism

thor, thoracotomy; sternot, sternotomy; med fat, mediastinal fat; peri, pericardium; diaph, diaphragm; an vein, anonymous vein; CT, chemotherapy; RT, radiotherapy; tomo, tomotherapy

Table 25.4 Group II patients (underwent surgery for thymoma and developed more than one recurrence)

		Initial surgery for thymoma				Recurrence of thymoma			
N	Year	Surgical approach	Extention of disease	Radicality	Adjuvant therapy	Year	Surgical approach	Extention of disease	Radicality	Adjuvant therapy
1	1986	Thor	Pl	+	RT	1999 2006	Laparos laparos	Diaph kidney	+ -	None tomo
2	1995	Thor	Peri	+	RT	2004 2004 2004 2007	Lamin thor thor thor-ph- lapar	Spine pl + lung + diaph supra-diaph inf cava	+ - - -	CT CT radiometa- bolic none
3	1997	Sternot	Peri + med fat + lung	+	RT	2002 2003 2004 2005 2006	Lapar thor thor thor thor	Diaph + add a cw + peri + pl + lung pl + lung cw + diaph thor a + lung + diaph	+ + + + -	CT CT CT CT + RT tomo

thor, thoracotomy; sternot, sternotomy; laparos, laparoscopy; lapar, laparotomy; lamin, laminectomy; thor + ph + lapar, thoracophrenolaparotomy; med fat, mediastinal fat; peri, pericardium; diaph, diaphragm; supra-diaph, supra-diaphragmatic; pl, pleura; cw, chest wall; add a, abdominal aorta; thor a, thoracic aorta; inf cava, inferior vena cava; CT, chemotherapy; RT, radiotherapy; tomo, tomotherapy

was administered on the basis of tumor stage. Stage I thymomas had no adjuvant therapy. Of the 2 patients with stage II thymomas, one had no adjuvant treatment and the other had only mediastinal radiotherapy. All stage III and IV patients had adjuvant therapy: 5 had only radiotherapy, 1 chemotherapy, and 1 chemotherapy combined with radiotherapy and subsequently tomotherapy.

Mean time before recurrence was 156 months (range 22 to 420 months). Nine recurrences were asymptomatic and detected at follow-up; 1 recurrence was identified by the onset of chest pain and 1 by neurological symptoms. Two recurrences (18%) had an associated MG. Eight recurrences were confined to the intrathoracic cavity. Only one patient had local mediastinal recurrence; the other 7 developed pleural, pulmonary, pericardial (Fig. 25.2), diaphragmatic, and distant thoracic recurrences (chest wall, thoracic aorta, and dorsal spinal cord) (Fig. 25.3). Three patients had both intrathoracic and extrathoracic metastases. The extrathoracic metastases involved the thoraco-abdominal aorta,

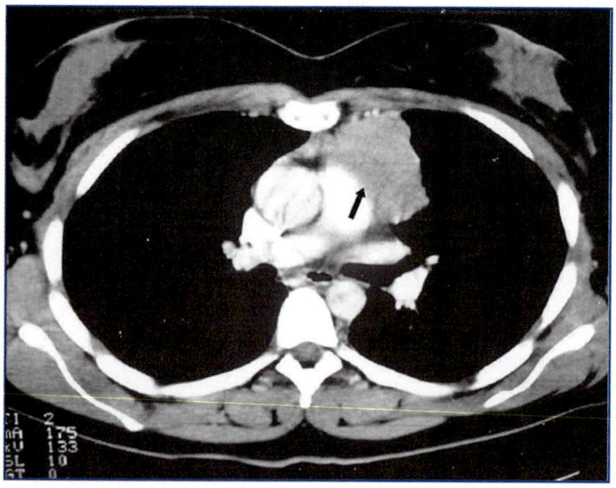

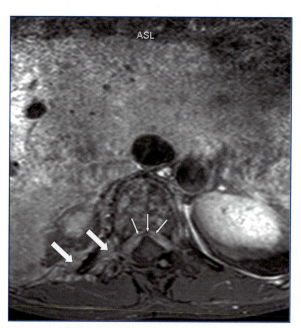

Fig. 25.2 CT scan image showing pericardial infiltration by a thymoma recurrence

Fig. 25.3 RMN image (fat saturated axial T1-weighted after GD injection) showing a thymoma recurrence with spinal cord extension

retroperitoneum (Fig. 25.4), liver, and the inferior vena cava; all were amenable to surgical resection (Tables 25.3, 25.4).

All 11 patients underwent surgical reresection for a total of 20 reoperations. Eight patients were only reoperated once (Group I) whereas 3 patients had multiple reoperation (Group II) (Tables 25.3, 25.4). In Group II patients reresection was performed twice in 1 patient with type AB (stage III) thymoma, 4 times in 1 patient with type B3 (stage III) thymoma, and 5 times in a patient with type B2 thymoma (stage III).

Results

Resection of tumor recurrence was complete in the 8 patients who had a single reoperation. The overall 20 reresections entailed 3 median sternotomies, 12 posterolateral thoracotomies, 1 laparotomy, 1 thoracophreno-laparotomy, 2 laparoscopies, and 1 laminectomy. Tables 25.1 and 25.2 summarize the clinical evolution and treatment of the 11 patients studied.

In Group I, two stage I patients had tumor infiltration of the pericardium; in one of these the tumor extended to the left lung and the anonymous vein. One stage II patient only had a local recurrence whereas the other stage II patient had a pulmonary metastasis. Resections were radical in all stage I and II patients. Three patients with stage III thymomas had a single recurrence with pulmonary metastases, one of whom had bilateral pulmonary recurrences resected by a sequential bilateral thoracotomy. Radical resection was achieved in all patients.

In Group II, 1 patient with stage III thymoma had a diaphragmatic recurrence followed by pararenal metastasis; both recurrences were treated surgically. The remaining two stage III patients developed 5 and 4 recurrences respectively (see Case reports 1 and 2 below). These recurrences often had multiple localizations and were simultaneously present in the thoraco-abdominal region: there were 5 metastases of the diaphragm, 4 lung metastases, 3 recurrences of the pleura, 3 of the great vessels (1 vena cava, 1 thoracic aorta, and 1 abdominal aorta involvement), 2 of the chest wall, 1 of the pericardium, and 1 spinal cord invasion. All three patients had at least one incomplete resection. The only stage IV patient developed pleural and chest wall recurrences which were radically resected.

Patients were restaged after reoperation (Table 25.5). Ten out of the 11 patients with thymoma recurrence had a clinical progression to Masaoka stage III and IV regardless of the initial stage. The eleventh, who was originally stage II, remained stable since the recurrence only involved the mediastinal fatty tissue. None of the patients had a histological progression of the disease. Group I and II received different regimens of therapy, based on the stage of disease, localization of recurrences, extent of infiltration, and preoperative treatment (Tables 25.3, 25.4).

All of the 11 patients were alive at December 2007 with a mean follow-up of 40 months (range 1 month to 115 months) from the time of the first reintervention. This includes the patients in Group II who had an incomplete resection, all of whom are still alive 144 months from the initial surgery.

Table 25.5 Clinical and histological progression of thymoma recurrences

	Initial surgery for thymoma		Recurrence of thymoma	
Case	Stage	WHO	Stage	WHO
1	II	B2	II	B2
2	I	AB	III	AB
3	III	B2	IV	B2
4	III	C	IV	C
5	IV	B3	IV	B3
6	II	B1	IV	B1
7	III	B3	IV	B3
8	I	B2	III	B2
9	III	AB	IV	AB
			IV	AB
				AB
10	III	B3	IV	B3
			IV	B3
			IV	B3
			IV	B3
11	III	B2	IV	B2
			IV	B2
			IV	B2
			IV	B2
			IV	B2

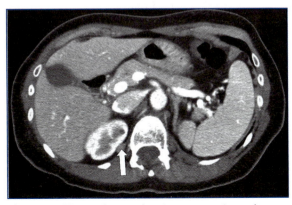

Fig. 25.4 CT scan image showing retroperitoneal recurrence of thymoma closely adherent to the right kidney

Case Reports

We report two extreme cases describing patients who developed multiple recurrences and who subsequently underwent multiple surgical resections and multimodality treatments.

Case Report 1

A 31-year-old woman underwent thymectomy and partial pericardiectomy in 1995 in our Unit of Thoracic Surgery for a cortical thymoma infiltrating the pericardium (stage III Masaoka; WHO B3) followed by radiotherapy on the mediastinum.

Nine years after the primary operation (February 2004), she returned with neurological symptoms and back pain. A total body CT scan showed a voluminous mass localized in the posterior mediastinum with an intraforaminal and intraspinal extension from D7 to D11 associated with two other metastatic lesions, one of which was surrounding the inferior vena cava and descending into the abdomen through the diaphragmatic hiatus (Fig. 25.5). She underwent emergency laminectomy and surgical resection of the intraspinal portion of the lesion to prevent the onset of neurological complications.

After 1 month (March 2004), the patient was readmitted to hospital and underwent right thoracotomy. Surgery disclosed micropulmonary nodules which the previous chest CT scan had not revealed. She therefore underwent debulking procedures on the pulmonary, pleural, and diaphragmatic metastatic lesions. The pericaval lesion was left in place because the patient's condition did not allow extensive thoraco-abdominal surgery. She was therefore treated with adjuvant chemotherapy. However, not only was there no improvement in the caval lesion at CT scan 4 months later but there was obvious evidence of multiple nodules involving the diaphragm and the right costo-phrenic angle.

The nodules were removed through a transthoracic debulking procedure (July 2004). The patient was then referred for radiometabolic therapy with octreotide, which temporarily stopped the progression of the lesion.

Three years after the last reoperation (July 2007), a total body CT scan revealed that the pericaval lesion had increased in size (Fig. 25.6). As the patient had reached a satisfactory overall condition, she was scheduled for the surgical removal of the pericaval lesion via right thoraco-phreno-laparotomy.

At December 2007, 12 years after the primary operation, she is alive with a good performance status although there is radiological evidence of disease in the right hemithorax which has been scheduled for resection.

Case Report 2

A 27-year-old woman was evaluated in our Unit of Thoracic Surgery in November 1997 for a 6-cm mass of the anterior mediastinum displayed at CT scan. She underwent median sternotomy and radical resection of the mass. The tumor infiltrated the pericardium, the left lung, and the left phrenic nerve. The tumor was clinically Masaoka stage III and histologically a cortical differentiated thymoma (WHO

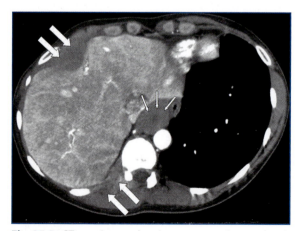

Fig. 25.5 CT scan image showing a metastatic mass localized in the posterior mediastinum with intraforaminal and intraspinal extension from D7 to D11. Two other lesions are evident, one of which surrounding the inferior vena cava and descending into the abdomen through the diaphragmatic hiatus, and the other bordering on the liver

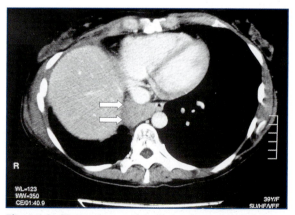

Fig. 25.6 CT scan image showing a thymoma recurrence located in the lower mediastinum interposed between the inferior vena cava and the descending aorta

B2). The patient received adjuvant radiotherapy on the mediastinum after the primary operation.

Five years after initial surgery (May 2002), a total body CT scan showed an abdominal mass involving the left crus of the diaphragm (Fig. 25.7) and extending to the abdominal aorta. A transthoracic needle biopsy of the lesion revealed a recurrence of thymoma. The patient underwent surgical resection, via laparotomy, which appeared to be macroscopically radical. No adjuvant treatment was scheduled.

One year after the first recurrence (May 2003), CT scan revealed a 3-cm lesion localized at the cardio-phrenic angle. At thoracotomy disseminated nodules were found on the pericardium, the left lung, the left parietal pleura, and the left chest wall. All the visible nodules were radically resected and the patient underwent subsequent chemotherapy.

One year after the second reoperation (December 2004), CT scan revealed intrathoracic recurrences. The patient underwent a left rethoracotomy to remove multiple nodules in the left lower lobe and on the chest wall.

One year later (September 2005), she developed a recurrence localized on the left chest wall and infiltrating the diaphragm. She underwent a repeat left thoracotomy to remove all the visible metastases and was given chemo-radiotherapy.

After one year (December 2006) a total body CT scan revealed a recurrence in the left hemithorax with disseminated lesions involving the lung, the diaphragm, and adherence to the thoracic aorta (Fig. 25.8). As a macroscopically radical resection was not accomplished, a tomotherapy was performed on the remnants. Local control was achieved and in December 2007, 10 years after the initial operation, CT scan showed no progression of the disease.

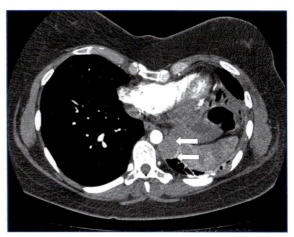

Fig. 25.8 CT scan image showing a thymoma recurrence strictly adherent to the thoraco-abdominal aorta

Conclusions

Surgical resection is the gold standard for the management of thymoma recurrences and should always be attempted even if complete resection cannot always be achieved. Considering the indolent nature of these tumors, an iterative debulking approach is always advisable to reduce the tumor size and improve long-term survival. Early stage tumors (stage I) are successfully treated by surgery alone and multimodality treatments are considered the best approach for advanced stage thymomas (stage III or IV) and for recurrences. Recent data suggest, however, that adjuvant therapy might decrease recurrence rate and ensure longer-term survival in patients with stage I and II cortical subtype thymomas, which usually have a poorer prognosis [19]. Neo-adjuvant chemotherapy is effective for inoperable patients and adjuvant therapy such as chemo- and radiotherapy is reserved for patients who have undergone surgery to improve their long-term, disease-free survival rate. Thus, since thymoma tumors are chemo- and radiosensitive neoplasms, a neo-adjuvant or an adjuvant therapy combined with surgery offers the best management for recurrences and improves patient outcome.

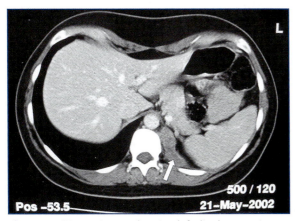

Fig. 25.7 CT scan image showing left diaphragmatic crus thymoma recurrence

References

1. Wright CD, Wain JC, Mathisen DJ et al (2005) Predictors of recurrence in thymic tumors: Importance of invasion, World Health Organization histology, and size. J Thorac Cardiovasc Surg 130:1413-1421
2. Chen G, Marx A, Wen-Hu C et al (2002) New WHO histologic classification predicts prognosis of thymic ep-

ithelial tumors: A clinicopathologic study of 200 thymoma cases from China. Cancer 95:420-429
3. Okumura M, Ohta M, Miyoshi S et al (2002) Oncological significance of WHO histological thymoma classification. A clinical study based on 286 patients. Jpn J Thorac Cardiovasc Surg 50:189-194
4. Rieker RJ, Hoegel J, Morresi-Hauf A et al (2002) Histologic classification of thymic epithelial tumors: Comparison of established classification schemes. Int J Cancer 98:900-906
5. Strollo DC, Rosado-de-Christenson ML, Jett JR (1997) Primary mediastinal tumors. Part 1: Tumors of the anterior mediastinum. Chest 112:511-522
6. Sakai S, Murayama S, Soeda H et al (2002) Differential diagnosis between thymoma and non thymoma by dynamic MR imaging. Acta Radiol 43:262-268
7. Armstrong P (2000) Mediastinal and hilar disorders. In: Armstrong P, Wilson AG, Dee P, Hansell DM (eds) Imaging of diseases of the chest. Mosby, London
8. Verstandig AG, Epstein DM, Miller WT Jr et al (1992) Thymoma–Report of 71 cases and a review. Crit Rev Diagn Imaging 33:201-230
9. Moore KH, McKenzie PR, Kennedy CW, McCaughan BC (2001) Thymoma: Trends over time. Ann Thorac Surg 72:203-207
10. Masaoka A, Monden Y, Nakahara K et al (1981) Follow-up study of thymomas with special reference to their clinical stages. Cancer 48:2485-2492
11. Regnard JF, Magdeleinat P, Dromer C et al (1996) Prognostic factors and long-term results after thymoma resection: A series of 307 patients. J Thorac Cardiovasc Surg 112:376-384
12. Maggi G, Casadio C, Cavallo A et al (1991) Thymoma: Results of 241 operated cases. Ann Thorac Surg 51:152-156
13. Ruffini E, Mancuso M, Oliaro A et al (1997) Recurrence of thymoma: Analysis of clinicopathologic features, treatment, and outcome. J Thorac Cardiovasc Surg 113:55-63
14. Kirschner PA (1990) Reoperation for thymoma: Report of 23 cases. Ann Thorac Surg 49:550-555
15. Regnard JF, Zinzindohoue F, Magdeleinat P et al (1997) Results of re-resection for recurrent thymomas. Ann Thorac Surg 64:1593-1598
16. Strobel P, Bauer A, Puppe B et al (2004) Tumor recurrence and survival in patient treated for thymomas and thymic squamous cell carcinomas: A retrospective analysis. J Clin Oncol 22:1501-1509
17. Blumberg D, Port JL, Weksler B et al (1995) Thymoma: A multivariate analysis of factors predicting survival. Ann Thorac Surg 60:908-913
18. Cohen DJ, Ronnigen LD, Graeber GM et al (1984) Management of patients with malignant thymoma. J Thorac Cardiovasc Surg 87:301-307
19. Ciccone A, Rendina EA (2005) Treatment of recurrent thymic tumors. Semin Thorac Cardiovasc Surg 17:27-31
20. Wright CD, Kessler KA (2005) Surgical treatment of thymic tumors. Semin Thorac Cardiovasc Surg 17:20-26
21. Haniuda M, Kondo R, Numanami H et al (2001) Recurrence of thymoma: Clinicopathological features, reoperation, and outcome. J Surg Oncol 78:183-188
22. Okumura M, Shiono H, Inoue M et al (2007) Outcome of surgical treatment for recurrent thymic epithelial tumors with reference to World Health Organization histologic classification system. J Surg Oncol 95:40-44
23. Shin DM, Walsh GL, Komaki R et al (1998) A multidisciplinary approach to therapy for unresectable malignant thymoma. Ann Intern Med 129:100-104
24. Loehrer PJ, Kim KM, Aisner SC et al (1994) Cisplatin plus doxorubicin plus cyclophosphamide in metastatic or recurrent thymoma. Final results of an intergroup trial. J Clin Oncol 12:1164-1168
25. Giaccone G, Ardizzoni A, Kirkpatrick A et al (1996) Cisplatin and etoposide combination of chemotherapy for locally advanced or metastatic thymoma: A phase II study of the European organization for research and treatment of lung cancer. J Clin Oncol 14:814-820
26. Evans T, Lynch JT (2005) Role of chemotherapy in the management of advanced thymic tumors. Semin Thorac Cardiovasc Surg 17:41-50
27. Ohara K, Tatsuzaki H, Fuji H et al (1998) Radioresponse of thymomas verified with histologic response. Acta Oncologica 37(5):471-474
28. Gripp S, Hilgers K, Wurm R et al (1998) Thymoma: Prognostic factors and treatment outcomes. Cancer 83(8):1495-1503
29. Kirkove C, Berghmans J, Noel H et al (1992) Dramatic response of recurrent invasive thymoma to high doses of corticosteroids. Clin Oncol (R Coll Radiol) 4:64-66
30. Palmieri G, Lastoria S, Colao A et al (1997) Successful treatment of a patient with a thymoma and pure red-cell aplasia with octreotide and prednisone. N Engl J Med 336:263-265
31. Berthaud P, Le Chevalier T, Tursz T (1990) Effectiveness of interleukin-2 in invasive lymphoepithelial thymoma. Lancet 335:1590

CHAPTER 26
Chemotherapy in Thymic Neoplasms

Pier Franco Conte, Fausto Barbieri

Introduction

Thymic neoplasms are chemotherapy-sensitive tumors with a 30-50% 5-year survival in previously untreated patients. Responses in small series have been reported with single-agent doxorubicin, cisplatin, etoposide, ifosfamide, and corticosteroids (Table 26.1).

It should be noted however that corticosteroids and many chemotherapeutic agents are lympholytic; shrinkage of thymic tumors with substantial lymphoid cell infiltration may reflect shrinkage of the nonmalignant components of the tumors rather than the malignant epithelial components. Of uncertainty is whether combination chemotherapy regimens are more effective than single agents; no prospective comparisons have been conducted to date. Moreover, a distinction has to be made in evaluating the results of treatment between thymoma and thymic carcinoma, which presents more often with metastatic spread and/or mediastinal invasion.

Locally Advanced Disease

When a tumor appears unresectable or resectable only at the cost of a great morbidity, then a combined modality approach including induction chemotherapy should be considered.

Neoadjuvant Chemotherapy Followed by Resection

A few studies have reported on the use of chemotherapy followed by surgery with or without radiation therapy for patients with clinically advanced disease.

In a study reported by Macchiarini and colleagues, seven patients with clinically stage III invasive thymoma were given neoadjuvant cisplatin, epirubicin, and etoposide. All seven patients subsequently underwent surgical resection – four complete and three incomplete. Two of the complete resections showed no tumor on subsequent histologic exam [1].

One series of 16 patients with stage III or stage IVa disease were treated with initial ADOC (doxorubicin, cyclophosphamide, vincristine, and cisplatin) chemotherapy. All patients achieved a clinical response to chemotherapy. Eleven patients had residual histologic tumor and received postoperative radiation therapy. The median survival of the entire group was 66 months [2]. At MD Anderson Cancer Center 22 patients received a modified PAC regimen plus prednisone as induction therapy: 77% had a major response and 21 underwent surgical resection followed by radiation in 19. The 7-year overall survival was 79% [3]. In a series of 56 patients with locally advanced thymic tumours treated with cisplatin, epidoxorubicin, and etoposide followed by resection and radiotherapy between 1976 and 2003, Lucchi and coworkers obtained a 10-year survival of 48% and 45.7% for stage III and IVA thymomas, respectively [4]. Recently the results of a single institution experience in multimodality treatment of thymic carcinoma were reported: out of 17 patients treated with preoperative platinum-based chemotherapy 10 (59%) achieved complete surgical resection with a 5-year survival of 80% [5]. It has also been shown that multimodality treatment of patients with neoadjuvant chemotherapy, and surgery, followed by additional adjuvant chemotherapy plus radiotherapy, may improve the survival of patients with locally ad-

Table 26.1 Single agent chemotherapy in thymoma (cumulative data)

Agent	N pts	CR (%)	PR (%)	Durat resp (m)	MS (m)
Cisplatin	48	18	23	1-24	13-24
Doxorubicin	3	–	66	–	–
Ifosfamide	5	40	40	–	–
Steroids	14	14	71	–	–

CR, complete response; PR, partial response; MS, median survival

vanced thymoma [6]. Although multimodality treatment appears effective and may cure locally advanced unresectable malignant thymoma, this is not without risk, and severe postoperative bleeding requiring re-operation has been reported following neoadjuvant chemotherapy for stage III invasive thymoma [7].

Combined Chemotherapy and Radiation Therapy for Unresectable Tumors

An intergroup study of patients with unresectable disease who received the PAC regimen (cisplatin, doxorubicin, and cyclophosphamide) followed by thoracic radiation reported a 5-year survival rate of 52% [8]. Another similar study of 12 patients reported a 92% response rate to the PAC plus prednisone regimen; all patients received postsurgical radiotherapy. At 7 years the overall survival was 100% with a 73% disease-free survival [9]. Finally, in a French study comprising 8 patients treated with chemotherapy followed by surgery and postoperative radiotherapy, 6 were free of disease at 23-77 months from diagnosis [10]. Very rare reports address the use of high-dose chemotherapy in this setting. Iwasaki and coworkers treated 2 patients with 2 cycles of ADOC regimen followed by high-dose etoposide, ICE plus G-CSF and two more cycles of ADOC. Both patients responded to the combination and underwent surgery followed by radiotherapy and remained disease-free for 2 and 5 years [11]. It is to be noticed that although both chemotherapy and radiation have been applied consecutively in patients with malignant thymoma, no extensive investigations focusing on the concurrent application of both treatment modalities have been performed so far.

Metastatic Disease

Chemotherapy is widely used for patients with metastatic disease or progressed after local therapies, such as surgery or radiotherapy. Because of the rarity of these cancers, all series of patients have been relatively small and reflect weak evidence (Table 26.2).

In a study by Highley and colleagues, single-agent ifosfamide was given to patients with stages III and IV disease. Out of 13 patients assessable for response, there were five (38.5%) complete responders and one (7.7%) partial responder. The most frequent toxicities seen were nausea, vomiting, and leukopenia, but all were well tolerated [12]. Combination chemotherapy (mostly platinum-based), however, has been reported to produce complete and partial remissions; some of the complete remissions have been pathologically confirmed at subsequent surgery [13]. In one study, the ADOC regimen (doxorubicin, cisplatin, vincristine, cyclophosphamide) produced a 92% response rate (34 of 37 patients), including complete responses in 43% of patients [14]. One study of combined chemotherapy with cisplatin and etoposide produced responses in 9 of 16 patients treated, with a median response duration of 3.4 years and a median survival of 4.3 years [15]. Nine of 28 patients with invasive thymoma or thymic carcinoma who received four cycles of etoposide, ifosfamide, and cisplatin at 3-week intervals had partial responses. The median duration of response was 11.9 months (range <1 to 26 months), and the median overall survival was 31.6 months. The 1-year and 2-year survival rates were 89% and 70%, respectively [16].

The role of high-dose chemotherapy (CODE regimen) was tested in 2 studies conducted by the Japan Clinical Oncology Group on 53 patients with locally advanced thymoma. Pathologic CR was observed in 3 patients. The median PFS was 9.5 months for stage IV and 4.5 years for stage III diseases. Overall survival at 2 and 5 years were 82% and 57% for stage IV and 96% and 77% for stage III patients [17].

Recurrent Disease

For patients with recurrent disease who are not candidate for re-irradiation, salvage surgery, or progress after steroid therapy, chemotherapy should be taken into account.

Table 26.2 Selected chemotherapy trials in advanced disease

Author	Regimen	Setting	No. pts	RR (%)	CR (%)	Durat. resp (m)
Shin	PAC-Pr	St III-IVA	13	92	23	–
Kim	PAC-Pr	St III-IVB	22	77	14	–
Lohrer & Kim	PAC	Met/Recurrent	30	50	10	11.8
Fornasiero	ADOC	Stage III-IV	37	92	43	12
Lohrer & Jiroutek	VIP	Adv thymic ca.	28	32	0	11.9
Giaccone	EP	Met/Recurrent	16	56	31	40.8

RR, overall response rate; CR, complete response rate; PAC, cisplatin, doxorubicin, cyclophosphamide; Pr, prednisone; ADOC, doxorubicin, cisplatin, vincristin, cyclophosphamide; VIP, etoposide, ifosfamide, cisplatin; EP, etoposide, cisplatin

In a series of 30 patients with stage IV or locally progressive recurrent tumor following radiation therapy, the PAC regimen (cisplatin, doxorubicin, cyclophosphamide) achieved a 50% response rate, including three complete responses, with a median survival of 38 months [18].

In another study, 27 previously treated patients with stage IVA and IVB thymic neoplasms received Pemetrexed 500 mg/sm every 3 weeks (together with vitamin and steroid supplementation): two of these achieved a complete response and two a partial response. The median time to progression was 45 weeks for thymoma and 5 weeks for thymic carcinoma [19]. Moreover, in a study conducted at Indiana University high-dose chemotherapy did not appear to be superior to standard-dose chemotherapy [20].

Octreotide, in combination with prednisone, has been explored as a therapeutic option in thymoma based on the observation that thymomas highly express the somatostatin receptor on their surface and radiolabeled octreotide exhibits high specificity for thymoma compared with thymic hyperplasia and other benign thymic disorders [21]. Thirty-eight patients with advanced thymic cancer (32 thymoma, five thymic carcinoma, one thymic carcinoid) received octreotide (0.5 mg s.c. three times a day) for a maximum of 1 year. If a patient exhibited a complete or partial response at 2 months, octreotide was continued alone, while in case of stable disease at 2 months oral prednisone (0.6 mg/kg per day) was added. Two complete and 10 partial responses were observed, with an overall objective response rate of approximately 32%. Of note, all responses were observed in patients with thymoma. The progression-free survival duration for the combination of octreotide and prednisone was 9.2 months, compared with 2 months for octreotide alone ($p = .039$). The median survival time for patients with thymoma receiving the combination had not been reached and was 46.3 months for those receiving octreotide alone [22].

Occasional responses with docetaxel [23], fluorouracil, ifosfamide, interleukin-2 and, more recently, gefitinib, cetuximab [24], dasatinib [25] and tacrolimus [26] have been reported.

Ongoing Studies (Selection)

Phase I

- BMS-690514 in patients with advanced or metastatic solid tumors
- Sunitinib plus radiation therapy for cancer patients.

Phase II

- Carboplatin combined with paclitaxel in treating patients with advanced thymoma
- Efficacy of octreotide treatment in patients with primary inoperable thymoma
- Erlotinib plus bevacizumab to treat advanced thymoma and thymic cancer.

Conclusions

Thymoma is a rare neoplasm with a largely indolent growth pattern. Because of its potential for invasion and local recurrence, however, a multidisciplinary approach is recommended. Inoperable patients warrant a strategy of induction chemotherapy followed by a surgical reassessment, and adjuvant radiation therapy is often indicated, despite a lack of prospective studies, for any evidence of invasive disease regardless of the degree of resection obtained. Durable responses can be obtained both in the metastatic and recurrent setting, and novel therapies are currently being investigated.

References

1. Macchiarini P, Chella A, Ducci F et al (1991) Neoadjuvant chemotherapy, surgery, and postoperative radiation therapy for invasive thymoma. Cancer 68:706-713
2. Rea F, Sartori F, Loy M et al (1993) Chemotherapy and operation for invasive thymoma. J Thorac Cardiovasc Surg 106(3):543-549
3. Kim ES, Putnam JB Jr, Komaki R et al (2004) A phase II study of a multidisciplinary approach with induction chemotherapy (IC), followed by surgical resection (SR), radiation therapy (RT) and consolidation chemotherapy for unresectable malignant thymoma. Final report. Lung Cancer 44:369-379
4. Lucchi M, Ambrogi MC, Duranti L et al (2005) Advanced stage thymomas and thymic carcinomas: Results of multimodality treatments. Ann Thorac Surg 79(6):1840-1844
5. Huang J, Rizk N, Park B et al (2007) Recent clinical experience with multimodality therapy in thymic carcinoma. Proc ASCO 2007 (absract 18007)
6. Venuta F, Rendina EA, Pescarmona EO et al (1997) Multimodality treatment of thymoma: A prospective study. Ann Thorac Surg 64:1585-1592
7. Venuta F, Rendina EA, De Giacomo T et al (1998) Severe postoperative hemorrhage after neoadjuvant chemotherapy for invasive thymoma. Ann Thorac Surg 66:981-982

8. Loehrer PJ Sr, Chen M, Kim K et al (1997) Cisplatin, doxorubicin, and cyclophosphamide plus thoracic radiation therapy for limited-stage unresectable thymoma: An intergroup trial. J Clin Oncol 15(9):3093-3099
9. Shin DM, Walsh GL, Komaki R et al (1998) A multidisciplinary approach to therapy for unresectable malignant thymoma. Ann Intern Med 129(2):100-104
10. Jacot W, Quantin X, Valette S et al (2005) Multimodality treatment program in invasive thymic epithelial tumor. Am J Clin Oncol 28(1):5-7
11. Iwasaki Y, Ohsugi S, Takemura Y et al (2002) Multidisciplinary therapy including high-dose chemotherapy followed by peripheral blood stem cell transplantation for invasive thymoma. Chest 122:2249-2252
12. Highley MS, Underhill CR, Parnis FX et al (1999) Treatment of invasive thymoma with single-agent ifosfamide. J Clin Oncol 17:2737-2744
13. Hejna M, Haberl I, Raderer M (1999) Nonsurgical management of malignant thymoma. Cancer 85:1871-1884
14. Fornasiero A, Daniele O, Ghiotto C et al (1991) Chemotherapy for invasive thymoma. A 13-year experience. Cancer 68(1):30-33
15. Giaccone G, Ardizzoni A, Kirkpatrick A et al (1996) Cisplatin and etoposide combination chemotherapy for locally advanced or metastatic thymoma. A phase II study of the European Organization for Research and Treatment of Cancer Lung Cancer Cooperative Group. J Clin Oncol 14(3):814-820
16. Loehrer PJ Sr, Jiroutek M, Aisner S et al (2001) Combined etoposide, ifosfamide, and cisplatin in the treatment of patients with advanced thymoma and thymic carcinoma: An intergroup trial. Cancer 91(11):2010-2015
17. Kunitoh H, Tamura T, Fukuda H et al (2006) Dose intensive chemotherapy (Cx) in advanced thymoma: Initial report of Japan Clinical Oncology Group trials (JCOG 9605 and 9606) Proc ASCO 2006 (abstract 7080)
18. Loehrer PJ Sr, Kim K, Aisner SC et al (1994) Cisplatin plus doxorubicin plus cyclophosphamide in metastatic or recurrent thymoma: Final results of an intergroup trial. The Eastern Cooperative Oncology Group, Southwest Oncology Group, and Southeastern Cancer Study Group. J Clin Oncol 12(6):1164-1168
19. Loehrer PJ, Yiannoutsos CT, Dropcho S et al (2006) A phase II trial of pemetrexed in patients with recurrent thymoma or thymic carcinoma. Proc ASCO 2006 (abstract 7079)
20. Hanna N, Gharpure VS, Abonour R et al (2001) High-dose carboplatin with etoposide in patients with recurrent thymoma: The Indiana University experience. Bone Marrow Transpl 28:435-438
21. Palmieri G, Montella L, Martignetti A et al (2002) Somatostatin analogs and prednisone in advanced refractory thymic tumors. Cancer 94:1414-1420
22. Loehrer PJ Sr, Wang W, Johnson DH et al (2004) Octreotide alone or with prednisone in patients with advanced thymoma and thymic carcinoma: An Eastern Cooperative Oncology Group phase II trial. J Clin Oncol 22:293-299
23. Tetsuya O, Horoyuki A, Kato D et al (2004) Efficacy of docetaxel as a second-line chemotherapy for thymic carcinoma. Chemotherapy 50:279-282
24. Farina G, Garassino MC, Gambacorta M et al (2007) Response of thymoma to Cetuximab. Lancet Oncol 8:449-450
25. Chuah C, Lim TH, Lim AS et al (2006) Dasatinib induces a response in malignant thymoma. J Clin Oncol 34:56-58
26. Taguchi T, Suehiro T, Toru K et al (2006) Pleural dissemination of thymoma showing tumor regression after combined corticosteroid and tacrolimus therapy. Eur J Int Med 8:575-577

CHAPTER 27
Radiotherapy in Thymic Neoplasms

Tony Y. Eng, Aidnag Z. Diaz, Join Y. Luh

Introduction

The role of adjuvant radiotherapy in thymic tumors has not been explicitly defined. Since epithelial thymic tumors are relatively radiosensitive, many clinicians advocate the use of adjuvant radiation therapy in all cases, in addition to those cases where there is extension beyond the capsule [1-4]. Justification for adjuvant radiation is based on studies showing decreased recurrence rates for stage II disease with adjuvant therapy from 30% to 5% [5, 6]. Other groups suggest that, due to the low incidence of local recurrence after complete resection of stage II thymomas, radiation therapy should be reserved for selected patients [7-10]. Schmidt-Wolf [11] proposed that adjuvant external-beam radiotherapy should be considered only for stages II and III disease where there were extensive adhesions between tumor and pleura, microscopic pleural infiltration, or macroscopic invasion of the pericardium, large vessels, or lung. In addition, Chen [12] noted that completely resected stage II thymomas of WHO subtype A, AB, and B-I may not require adjuvant therapy. There is general agreement, however, that incompletely resected or primary unresectable thymomas of all stages should be treated with radiation with or without chemotherapy [13, 14].

Although surgery remains the first choice of treatment for stage I to III thymomas [15-17], there still is controversy concerning the optimum adjuvant treatment of thymoma after complete resection. For stage I thymoma, most studies report no or very few relapses after surgery without any adjuvant therapies [5, 6, 18]. Nevertheless, it has been reported that local recurrence occurs as frequently as pleural dissemination, even after complete resection of thymoma [5, 19, 20]. Postoperative mediastinal irradiation seems to be the most effective adjuvant therapy for reducing the risk of local recurrence and prolonging survival in patients with locally advanced thymoma [21, 22].

Stage I

Stage I thymomas have an excellent prognosis after complete resection. Most groups accept that there is no need for irradiation after surgery for stage I thymomas. In the Memorial Sloan Kettering experience, 25 stage I patients underwent complete resection with one recurrence and 95% 5-year survival and 86% 10-year survival rates [23]. Fujimura and colleagues [17] reported no recurrences in 31 stage I thymomas after total resection alone. Ten-year survival rate was 74.3%. The Massachusetts General Hospital experience between 1939 and 1990 included 52 stage I patients who were all treated with thymectomy alone. No patient relapsed or died of thymoma [24]. In 1988, Curran and colleagues [5] reported no recurrences in 43 stage I thymomas after total resection, with only 1 patient receiving neoadjuvant radiotherapy. Despite a relapse-free survival of 100%, the 5-year survival was only 67% due to a high frequency of severe myasthenia gravis in this patient population.

In the MD Anderson experience, between 1962 and 1987, Pollack and colleagues [25] presented 11 stage I patients who underwent total resection (5 patients who received postoperative radiotherapy, 50 Gy at standard fractionation, and 6 who did not). There were two recurrences (one in each group). A series from Osaka University Medical School presented 38 stage I patients, 26 who underwent irradiation, and 12 who were not radiated [22]. There were no recurrences in the radiated group, but one recurrence (8%) in the nonradiated group.

In a study by Masayuki [26], no recurrence was observed in patients with stage I thymoma after surgery with or without mediastinal irradiation. These results suggest that routine postoperative mediastinal irradiation is not indicated for patients with stage I thymoma after complete resection. However, 21.6% and 25% of stage II and stage III patients respectively suffered from recurrences. In those groups mediastinal irradiation did not have a significant effect on recurrence rate when stratified by the clinical stage. These results suggest that it is very hard to select the patients who need the additional therapy based solely on clinical staging. Local invasion has been recognized as the most important clinical parameter for thymoma, particularly in stage II patients [19, 27]. To avoid the disadvantages of clinical staging, Masayuki proposed classification based on pleural and pericardial invasion [6]. Data from Singhal et al. [10] reinforces the trend to refrain from radiating patients with completely resected stage I thymoma. It documents a single recurrence out of 27 stage I patients treated by resection alone and no significant difference between patients treated by resection alone versus resection plus irradiation. For stage I thymoma complete resection by an experienced surgical team is sufficient to maintain local control.

Stage II

It is well accepted that factors influencing prognosis in thymoma are completeness of the surgical resection, Masaoka stage, and WHO histological classification. The prognostic significance of these factors has been largely demonstrated in some recent series in the international literature [1, 18, 28-31]. Although completely resected, about 10% of stage II thymoma manifest local or pleural recurrence even after many years [28-30]. This observation and the demonstrated relative high sensitivity of thymoma to radiation therapy leads to recommendations advocating radiation therapy for all patients with stage II thymoma irrespective of resection status. The consistency of such recommendations is not clear [32]. Whereas the true indication of radiation therapy for stage II thymomas is still controversial, late local morbidity associated to mediastinal and lung irradiation are well-known (cardiac morbidity such as valve fibrosis, pericarditis with pericardial effusions, increased frequency of coronary artery disease; radiation pneumonitis and chronic pulmonary fibrosis; esophageal strictures, dismotility and malignancies; mediastinal fibrous and hematopoietic malignancies) [33-36].

During the past decades, some authors have advocated postoperative radiation therapy [5, 21, 37] whereas few studies have argued against it [23, 38]. Nakahara et al. [22] in 1988 reported a 29% (2 of 7) recurrence rate for patients with stage II thymoma submitted to surgery only, whereas 8% (2 of 25) patients have disease relapse after surgery and postoperative radiotherapy. The patients in this cohort received between 30 Gy in 3 weeks and 50 Gy in 6 weeks. Ogawa and colleagues [37] presented 61 Masaoka stage II patients who underwent postoperative mediastinal radiotherapy. Despite all patients receiving radiotherapy, 6 patients (10%) still experienced recurrence (2 mediastinal and 4 pleural). Their conclusion was that radiotherapy prevents mediastinal recurrence for patients with completely resected thymoma but is insufficient to avoid pleural-based recurrence. Blumberg et al. [23] reported about 30 patients submitted to surgery and irradiation ($n = 17$) or to surgery alone ($n = 13$): the recurrence and survival rates were similar for the two groups.

In some cases, the association of radiation therapy to surgery for the treatment of stage II thymomas seems to negatively affect long-term survival. Quintanilla-Martinez et al. [24] in 1994 presented 32 stage II patients submitted to surgery. Seven of them received postoperative irradiation. Recurrence rates were 28% and 8% for patients undergoing surgery and radiotherapy and surgery alone, respectively (difference was not significant). In a previous study, Ruffini et al. [38] showed a significantly lower recurrence rate in a cohort of patients treated with surgery alone compared with patients who underwent surgery and irradiation (the difference was significant $p = 0.02$): the effect of postoperative radiotherapy seemed potentially harmful. A significant portion of the literature does not perform disease-free or disease-specific survival analysis for stage II thymoma; most concentrate on overall survival.

The evaluation of the real impact of radiotherapy on long-term survival of completely resected stage II thymoma patients is difficult due to the relative indolent natural history of these tumors. The use of overall survival data as an endpoint in the literature has falsely lowered the expected long-term survival of thymoma patients. Progression-free survival and disease-related death seem to be better endpoints in the evaluation of this disease due to the long natural history and confounding factors such as the high incidence of myasthenia gravis.

More recently, two papers focused on the value of postoperative radiotherapy in stage II completely resected thymomas. Mangi et al. [39] updated their 27-year experience and presented 49 completely resected stage II patients. Thirty-five patients were submitted to surgery alone, whereas 14 patients underwent surgery and irradiation. The addition of adjuvant irradiation did not affect long-term disease control. Disease-specific survival for stage II thymoma patients was 100% with and without RT ($p = 0.87$).

Between February 1992 and 2002, Singhal et al. [10] performed 167 resections for thymoma. Of these, 70 patients were believed to have tumors in stage IIb or less intraoperatively, and all of these patients underwent complete resection. They reviewed the histopathology of 62 of 70 patients. Thirty thymomas demonstrated less than complete transcapsular microscopic invasion (stage I) and 40 thymomas demonstrated microscopic transcapsular invasion or macroscopic invasion into surrounding fatty tissue (stage II). Forty-seven patients underwent surgery without postoperative mediastinal radiotherapy. Dosages in the 23 radiated patients (3 stage I and 20 stage II) consisted of 45-55 Gy at standard fractionation. Median follow-up was 70.3 months. Stage II patients who were radiated ($n = 20$) and those who were not radiated ($n = 20$) consisted of identical proportions in stages IIa and IIb. Two patients recurred (1 unradiated stage I patient and 1 radiated stage IIb patient). Overall 5-year survival rate was 91%. All who died were free of recurrence at time of death. Log-rank test showed no difference in Kaplan Meier survival curves ($p = 0.32$) between the radiated and unradiated groups.

Between 1988 and 2000, Rena et al. [40] performed 197 resections for thymoma. Thirty-two patients underwent complete surgical resection (14 stage IIA and 18 stage IIB); 26 patients underwent complete resection and subsequent mediastinal irradiation (11 stage IIA and 15 stage IIB). Dosages of radiation were 45-54 Gy, in 25-30 fractions. With a median follow-up of 91 months (range 9 to 170), five intrathoracic recurrences occurred. Disease-free survival rate at 5- and 10-years were 94% and 87%, respectively. Log-rank test showed no difference in Kaplan-Meier survival curves ($p = 0.432$) between radiated and nonradiated patients. These data support the concept that radical surgical resection alone, resulting in complete resection of the tumor, should be considered sufficient treatment for Masaoka stage II thymoma. Of course, the patients were referred for radiation therapy on the basis of a subjective assessment of risk of recurrence.

For stage II thymomas, the results in the literature do not give clear guidelines about indications for postoperative radiotherapy. Adjuvant radiation therapy has been used postoperatively by most surgeons when an incomplete resection is performed. For completely resected stage II tumors, some studies have argued against radiotherapy [23, 38, 40, 41] while other studies have advocated postoperative therapy [5, 21, 37].

Several authors have felt that radiotherapy should follow surgery. In the experience of Curran and colleagues [5], 19 patients underwent complete resection for stage II thymoma. No further pathologic elaboration was available. One patient received postoperative irradiation. One third of patients (6 of 18) who did not receive radiotherapy experienced local recurrence. No relapse was noted in the patient who was radiated. The authors concluded that resection without radiotherapy was inadequate but statistical analysis was not possible because only 1 patient underwent surgery and adjuvant radiotherapy. A series from Osaka University Medical School reported an increased recurrence rate for patients with resected stage II thymomas who did not undergo adjuvant radiotherapy, as compared with those who did receive postoperative radiotherapy. They concluded radiotherapy was indicated for any patient who had any capsular microinvasion or where the margin status was not assessed [21]. Other authors have felt adjuvant radiotherapy should be performed only with certain caveats or not at all. A report from Memorial Sloan Kettering described 26 stage II thymoma patients between 1949 and 1993 who underwent complete resection, 17 of whom received adjuvant irradiation and 9 of whom were without radiotherapy. Recurrence rates ($p = 0.21$) and survival rates ($p = 0.14$) of the two groups were similar [23]. Ruffini and colleagues [38] from University of Torino presented an interesting report of 58 stage II patients, 13 of whom underwent adjuvant irradiation. Four patients (31%) recurred despite adjuvant radiotherapy, and 2 patients (4%) recurred without postoperative treatment. They demonstrated with statistical significance ($p = 0.02$) that the effect of postoperative irradiation was potentially harmful. However, they admitted to a possible selection bias toward patients who were selected for radiotherapy based on what appeared to be clinically advanced disease.

The Massachusetts General Hospital experience presented 32 stage II patients who underwent thymectomy [24]. Seven of them received postoperative irradiation. In stage II patients, one of the 16 minimally invasive (stage IIa) tumors recurred, compared with 3 of 16 grossly invasive (stage IIb) tumors. Two of seven patients (28.3%) who received adjuvant radiotherapy relapsed at 6 and 16 years, and 2 of 24 patients (8%) who received no adjuvant treatment relapsed at 5 and 13 years.

In this series the Massachusetts General Hospital group attempted to correlate the pathologic extent of disease and histologic classification with outcome [24]. There was no clear effect of irradiation on outcome. However, none of the 12 patients with medullary or mixed thymoma relapsed, whereas 4 of 19 patients with predominantly cortical (2 of 13) or well-differentiated thymic carcinoma (2 of 6) relapsed. On the basis of these results, they recommended that stage II medullary and mixed thymomas be spared adjuvant therapy but that stage II cortical thymomas receive a postoperative treatment regimen. If one is inclined to radiate, the experience of the Massachusetts General Hospital indicates that the addition of histologic subtyping is a reasonable approach to fine-tuning this decision [24].

More recently, the Massachusetts General Hospital updated its 27-year experience and presented 49 completely resected stage II patients [39]. Fourteen stage II patients underwent postoperative irradiation and 35 did not. The addition of adjuvant radiotherapy did not alter local or distant recurrence rates. Disease-specific survival at 10 years in stage II patients was 100% with and without RT ($p = 0.87$).

Kundel et al. [42] retrospectively reviewed the files of 47 patients with thymic tumors treated by adjuvant radiation at Tel Aviv University from 1984 to 2003. All patients underwent thoracotomy followed by either total macroscopic resection (n = 42) or biopsy (n = 5). The radiation dose ranged from 26 to 60 Gy. Median duration of follow-up was 10.6 years. Overall 5-year survival was 73% (60-88%): 77% for thymoma (n = 35/45) versus 33% for thymic carcinoma (n = 2/6) ($p = 0.14$). Better survival was associated with lower disease stage (II vs. III/IVA, $p = 0.01$), resection ($p = 0.0004$), myasthenia gravis at presentation ($p = 0.04$), and higher radiation dose (≤45 vs. >45 Gy, $p = 0.02$); sex, smoking, tumor size, pathology, and margin status had no effect. Locoregional relapse occurred in 11 patients and distant metastasis in 4. The 5-year disease-free survival was 67% (52-86%), with a median time to recurrence of 8.3 years. The better overall survival and disease-free survival associated with higher doses of radiation were also true for stage II patients. On multivariate analyses after adjusting for age, higher disease stage and lower radiation dose were found to adversely affect overall survival and disease-free survival. Thymic carcinoma had an impact only on disease-free survival. They concluded that postoperative radiation therapy to doses above 45 Gy may improve the disease-free and overall survival of patients with invasive thymoma, especially stage II, and that thymic carcinoma has a worse prognosis.

Stage III

Forty-five stage III patients underwent resection and in 36 it was complete. Thirty-eight stage III patients received radiation therapy. Baseline prognostic factors between radiated and nonradiated groups were similar. The addition of adjuvant radiotherapy did not alter local or distant recurrence rates in patients with stage III thymoma. Disease-specific survival at 10 years in stage III patients who did not receive radiation was 75% (95% confidence interval, 32-100%) and in patients who did receive radiation therapy it was 79% (95% confidence interval, 64-94%) ($p = 0.21$). The most common site of relapse was the pleura [43].

Thymoma is a difficult condition to study because of its rarity, indolent natural history, and high mortality due to unrelated causes [44-46]. The 5-year survival rate for thymoma approximates 60% and has not changed over the past three decades [5, 23, 47-50] despite advances in operative management, radiotherapy, and chemotherapy. Surgery remains the mainstay of clinical management. Generally accepted 5-year and 10-year overall survival rates for stage III thymoma are 60-80% and 50-75%, respectively [1, 51].

There is neither consensus statement nor randomized trial data to support the use of adjuvant radiation therapy in the care of patients with stage III thymoma. The current standard of care appears to involve adjuvant radiation for the majority of stage III patients, but the criteria for administering adjuvant radiation therapy to patients with stage III thymoma vary from institution to institution and are controversial. Currently, postoperative radiation is offered either to all thymoma patients [18, 21, 22, 48], to those with invasive features on pathologic examination of the specimen, or to patients with tumors greater than 5 cm in size [23]. It may be that patients who do not require radiation will receive it, unnecessarily subjecting them to the risks of that modality.

Despite the evenly balanced prognostic factors in the two treatment groups, Mangi et al. [43] could not demonstrate an advantage to adjuvant RT in stage III thymoma. Most centers consider the addition of postoperative radiation therapy as the standard of care for stage III thymoma patients, and would recommend the routine referral of these patients for adjuvant radiation therapy [32, 51] even though there is no clear data supporting this clinical course.

Radiation therapy to the chest is not benign. Several reports of late consequences such as hematopoietic malignancies, esophageal malignancies, dysmotility and strictures, or radiation pneumonitis and chronic pulmonary fibrosis [33-36, 52-56] have emerged. In addition, a recent study has detailed a variety of late postradiation injuries to the heart that include entities such as restrictive cardiomyopathy, cardiac valve fibrosis, conduction defects (manifested by monotonous heart rate, persistent tachycardia, and blunted hemodynamic responses to exercise), pericardial effusions, reduced peak oxygen uptake during exercise (an independent predictor of premature death), and accelerated coronary artery disease [57]. Given the potential for serious consequences from radiation therapy, a policy of selective radiation therapy for patients with stage III thymoma should be considered. A consensus on this subject is made difficult by the indolent natural history of this disease, and by the large numbers of patient deaths from unrelated causes. These reasons also make a prospective randomized study investigating the possible benefits of radiation therapy as unlikely to ever be undertaken.

To evaluate the role of radiation therapy in the management of stage III thymoma, Mangi et al. [43] reviewed seven articles in which at least 10 stage III patients were studied and in which patients both received and did not receive adjuvant radiation therapy after complete resection. They then compared the two groups. Six of the seven authors [1, 8, 23, 26, 37, 38] were unable to demonstrate any advantage to adjuvant radiation therapy in terms of either local control or survival. Local recurrence rates ranged from 19% to 31% after radiation (median, 22%) and from 4% to 45% without radiation (median, 23%). These differences did not reach statistical significance, except in the study by Ruffini and colleagues [38] who demonstrated a significant advantage to not receiving adjuvant radiation ($p = 0.02$).

Mangi et al. [43] reported the disease-specific survival at 10 years was 79% in the group receiving radiation and 75% in the group not receiving radiation ($p = 0.21$). Patients receiving radiation had a recurrence rate of 32%, and those not receiving radiation had a recurrence rate of 29%, similar to those reported in the literature. This difference did not reach statistical significance. Because the recurrence rate is not influenced by the addition of radiation therapy, and because the majority of patients with stage III disease can safely undergo complete resection, it is difficult to recommend the routine use of postoperative radiation for patients with stage III disease who undergo complete resection. Radiation therapy has a role for patients who could not possibly have a complete resection, and it may have a role for patients whose surgeon suspected a close margin. Such a paradigm has been established and followed for most intrathoracic neoplasms [58]. Stage III patients may also benefit from a cisplatin-based course of adjuvant chemotherapy because most recurrences are pleural rather than mediastinal [43].

Neoadjuvant Radiation Therapy

One group of patients that may benefit from neoadjuvant therapy is the group who displays clear evidence of invasion of adjacent structures by bulky tumors on preoperative imaging. Neoadjuvant radiation therapy as outlined by Myojin et al. [51] may be of benefit in downsizing the tumor and enhancing resectability. The decision to proceed with a neoadjuvant regimen needs to be undertaken by the treating physician on a case-by-case basis. If review of the preoperative imaging does not remove doubts about resectability, computed tomographic-guided core needle biopsy, an anterior mediastinotomy, and open biopsy or video-assisted thoracoscopic examination of the chest should be undertaken for diagnosis. Care must be taken at that time not to disturb tumor planes in order to prevent widespread pleural dissemination. If pleural disease is present, or if tumor planes are disrupted at the time of operation, there may be a benefit to intrapleural administration of platinum-based chemotherapeutic agents that have been reported to be useful in thymic tumors with pleural spread [59]. Mangi et al. [43] do not favor routine video-assisted thoracoscopic biopsy of advanced thymomas for fear of causing pleural dissemination. They find the video-assisted approach most useful to document stage IVA pleural disease.

A neoadjuvant chemotherapy strategy for patients with stage III thymoma that appears to hold promise has recently been described by Venuta and colleagues [60]. This group has prospectively described a regimen of induction chemotherapy including cisplatin (51 mg/m^2), adriblastin (50 mg/m^2), and cyclophosphamide (500 mg/m^2) administered three times every 3 weeks in which treatment was made by protocol. Ninety-three percent of patients successfully completed therapy. One patient demonstrated complete remission (7%), 2 had a complete response (13%), 8 had partial responses (53%), and 5 had stable disease (33%). Twenty percent of patients were downstaged to stage II, and 67% of patients initially believed to be unresectable were rendered resectable by the administration of neoadjuvant chemotherapy. Unresectable patients and resected patients were referred for chemoradiation therapy. The administration of neoadjuvant chemotherapy improved 10-year survival from 71% (no induction therapy) to 90%, but this did not reach statistical significance. Therefore a combined neoadjuvant approach with both chemotherapy and radiation therapy deserves further analysis in a prospective fashion. Given the rarity of this disease a prospective clinical trial will need the participation of multiple institutions and may be best undertaken under the auspices of a national trials oncology group.

Yagi et al. [61] treated 41 patients with invasive thymoma, including 34 stage III, 5 stage IVa, and 2 stage IVb thymomas. Thirty-eight patients received radiotherapy, 11 preoperatively to shrink the tumor volume and render the lesion more amenable to surgical resection. Both IVb patients were dead within 30 months of surgery. Twelve patients with invasion of the superior vena cava or innominate vein had angioplasty or reconstruction performed as part of the surgical procedure. The overall 5-year survival rate for the cohort was 77% and the 10-year survival rate was 59%. In the stage III group patients, there was a significant difference in survival between those with complete and those with incomplete resection. Ten of the 12 patients who had angioplasty with or without reconstruction of the superior vena cava or innominate vein survived without recurrence of the tumors. The authors concluded that aggressive surgery with angioplasty and vascular reconstruction are recommended because successful treatment for invasive thymomas depends on complete resection of the tumors. Neoadjuvant radiotherapy may render some inoperable tumors operable and thus improve the chances of tumor control by allowing for a more complete resection [61].

Pleural Invasion

Uematsu et al. [62] retrospectively reviewed forty-three patients with invasive thymoma treated with surgery and radiation therapy between 1978 and 1993. All 43 patients underwent a complete surgical resection and were judged to have Masaoka's stage II-III invasive thymoma. Of these, 23 patients received entire hemithorax and mediastinal radiotherapy (EH-MRT) and the remaining 20 received mediastinal radiotherapy (MRT). Of the 23 patients with EH-MRT, 11 were stage II and 12 stage III. Of the 20 with MRT, 11 were stage II and 9 stage III. In most cases, the entire hemithorax received 15 Gy in 15 fractions over 3 weeks (without lung compensation calculation). In both the EH-MRT and MRT group, the total radiation doses to the mediastinum were similar with a median of 40 Gy. The median follow-up time after surgery was 63 months and no patients were lost to follow-up. Only one of the 23 patients with EH-MRT relapsed. On the other hand, 8 of the 20 with MRT relapsed, 6 of whom died of disease. The pleura was the most common site of failure. At 5 years, the relapse-free rate was 100% for those receiving EH-MRT and 66% for those with MRT ($p = 0.03$); the overall survival rate was 96% for those with EH-MRT, and 74% for those with MRT (p: not significant). The most significant treatment-related complication was radiation pneumonitis requiring treatment, in 1 patient who received MRT and 3 who received EH-MRT, including one death of a 72-year-old man and a 68-year-old woman with severe lung fibrosis [62, 63].

Radiotherapy Techniques

The radiotherapy techniques used in the treatment of thymic tumors is best described by Eng et al. [64] and it resembles that of other thoracic tumors (see Fig. 27.1). It uses high energy (>10 MV) X-rays generated by a linear accelerator. CT scans are used to

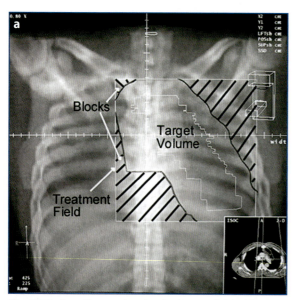
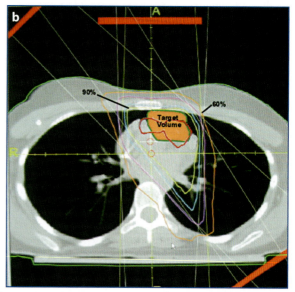

Fig. 27.1a,b **a** Conventional radiotherapy field with custom block (*black lines*) covering the tumor bed and mediastinum (with permission from [64]). **b** Treatment plan showing isodose lines around the target volume

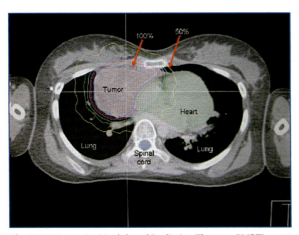

Fig. 27.2 Intensity Modulated Radiation Therapy (IMRT) treatment plan with isodose lines conforming to the shape of target volume in the mediastinum (with permission from [68])

delineate the target volume. Surgical clips placed during resection are very useful to mark positive margins and/or areas of residual disease as well as the extent of initial disease in completely resected tumors where the surgeon suspects residual microscopic or subclinical disease. Although still a matter of controversy, the adequate planning target volume should include the surgical bed, any gross residual tumor, and areas of suspicious subclinical disease such as the mediastinal lymph nodes with a 1.5- to 2-cm margin as seen in Fig. 27.1. The San Antonio group [64] recommends moderate levels of radiation doses between 45 and 55 Gy at standard fractionation, and 1.8 to 2 Gy per fraction for microscopic residual disease using three-dimensional treatment planning to minimize the dose to adjacent critical organs, such as the lung. The M.D. Anderson group [25] noted a 50% in-field local failure rate in stage III and IVa patients treated with less than 60 Gy using standard fractionation after varying degrees of surgical resection. Others have recommended doses of 60 Gy or higher in patients who have unresectable disease or are left with gross residual disease after surgical resection [9, 50, 64]. The use of modern radiotherapeutic techniques, such as intensity modulated or image guided radiotherapy, are currently emerging for the treatment of most thoracic tumors including thymoma [65-67] (Fig. 27.2). It allows more sparing of adjacent critical structures.

Other Thymic Tumors

Like thymoma, thymic carcinoma also arises in the thymic epithelium, but with a higher propensity for capsular invasion and metastases. Low-grade thymic carcinomas, though, are characterized by relatively favorable clinical courses with a lower incidence of local recurrence and metastasis [64]. Owing to the paucity of cases, optimization of therapeutic regimens has yet to be elucidated. A prescriptive dose range has yet to be defined, with most studies using 40-70 Gy with standard fractionation scheme (1.8-2.0 Gy/fraction). Thymic carcinoid tumors, also known as neuroendocrine tumors of the thymus, are extremely rare, accounting for less than 5% of all neoplasms of the anterior mediastinum. They often invade locally, commonly metastasizing to regional lymph nodes [69]. Distant metastases to bone, liver, or skin can occur in 30-40% of cases [70] and may be seen in 70% of patients within 8 years from initial diagnosis [71]. Complete surgical resection is the preferred method of treatment, although recurrence is common. Despite a lack of evidence, incomplete resections followed by radiation (and/or chemotherapy) have been used, and may improve local control without significant increased morbidity and mortality [71]. Despite aggressive treatments, most patients do poorly. Overall 5-year survival according to one report was 31%, with all 14 patients dead after about 9 years [72]. Other rare thymic tumors include fibrolipomas and liposarcomas. The main distinction between thymofibrolipoma and thymoliposarcoma is the presence of atypical lipoblasts in the latter [73]. The absence of atypical stromal cells is of paramount value to distinguish thymofibrolipomas from thymoliposarcomas. Thymofibrolipomas are composed of broad fibrous bands that traverse both adipose and thymic components. Thymofibrolipomas are considered to be a histologic variant of thymolipoma. Hence, they are benign with no sexual predilection, and may occur at any age [74]. These tumors are usually well circumscribed, being soft and white in color. They are usually surrounded by normal thymus tissue. Treatment primarily consists of surgical resection.

Radiation Treatment Results

The local control rates after a complete resection and adjuvant radiation therapy have ranged approximately from 65% to 85% and lower for incomplete resection and radiation therapy [25, 41, 49]. Table 27.1 summarizes some of the selected radiation treatment results. As all studies are retrospective in nature, bias in patient selection is unavoidable. In general, patients who were subjectively referred for adjuvant radiation therapy often had worse prognostic factors. Even after complete resection, invasive thymomas still carry a poorer prognosis than noninvasive tumors [41-44].

Table 27.1 Summary of selected radiation treatment results for thymoma

Authors/year	No. patients(stage)	XRT regimen	Radiation dose (Gy)	Local control (%)	5-year survival rate (%)	Comments
Rena et al. 2007 [40]	25 (IIa) 33 (IIB)	32 surg only 26 postop	45–54	94% surg only 88% postop	94 (DFS) (87% at 10 yrs) No difference in survival	XRT not needed after complete radical resection for stage II thymoma
Kundel et al. 2007 [42]	33 (II) 12 (III) 2 (IVa)	Postop (42 after gross resection and 5 biopsy)	26–60	77%	77 (thymoma) 33 (Thymic Ca) 74 (DFS, thymoma) 0 (DFS, thymic Ca) 86 (II) 50–45 (III/IVa)	Higher XRT dose (>45 Gy) was better. Other prognostic factors were stage, resection, myasthenia gravis
Bretti et al. 2004 [75]	43 (III) 20 (IVa)	Preop/postop +/− chemo	24–30 preop 45–55 postop	–	Median PFS 59 m (III) 21 m (IVa)	Preop XRT improved resection rate
Kondo et al. 2003 [8]	522 (I) 247 (II) 201 (III) 101 (IV)	+/− postop +/− chemo	– 43.7+/−7.7 (II) 45.4+/−8.4 (III) –	99.1 (I) 95.9 (II) 71.6 (III) 65.7 (IV)	100 (I) 98 (II) 89 (III) 71 (IV)	Largest study. No difference in recurrence w/ or w/o XRT in stage II and III patients. High complete resection rates
Latz et al. 1997 [76]	10 (II) 14 (III) 19 (IV)	Postop +/− chemo	10–72 (median 50)	81	90 (II) 67 (III) 30 (IV)	Uncertain XRT benefit for completely resected stage II
Mornex et al. 1995 [9]	21 (IIIa) 37 (IIIb) 32 (IVa)	Preop and postop +/− chemotherapy	30–70 (median 50)	86 (IIIa) 59 (IIIb/IVa)	64 (IIIa) 39 (IIIb)	Great impact of XRT on local control. Recommends >50 Gy for incomplete resection
Cowen et al. 1995 [77]	13 (I) 46 (II) 58 (III) 32 (IVa)	Preop/postop +/− chemo	22–50 preop 30–70 postop (median 40–55)	78.5 (overall) 100 (I) 98 (II) 69 (III) 59 (IVa)	59.5 (DFS) (49.5% at 10 yrs)	Stage and extent of resection influenced local control and survival
Haniuda et al. 1992 [6]	70 (II/III)	Postop	40–50	100 (IIp1)* 70 (III)	74 (II) 69 (III)	XRT benefited patients w/ pleural adhesion w/o microinvasion
Pollack et al. 1992 [25]	11 (I) 8 (II) 10 (III) 7 (IV)	Postop; primary XRT (22 pts)	50 Gy (median)	59 (overall)	74 (I) 71 (II) 50 (III) 29 (IV)	Incompletely resected patients did worse. Recommends multimodality treatment for these patients
Urgesi et al. 1990 [41]	59 (III) 18 (IVa)	Pre- and postop	39.6–60	85–90	78 (III) (58% at 10 yr)	Most relapses were out of XRT fields
Hug et al. 1990 [78]	44 (II–IV)	Preop/postop	40 (median)	89 (II/III)	92 (II) 62 (III)	High failure rates in surgery only patients
Jackson et al. 1991 [79]	28 (II/III)	Postop (after Bx or subtotal)	32–60 (mean 42)	61	53 (OS) (44% at 10 yrs)	High XRT complications of 11% w/2 deaths
Curran et al. 1988 [5]	43 (I) 21 (II) 36 (III) 3 (IV)	Postop for II–IV	32–60	100 (II/III-total resection) 79 (II/III-subtotal resection/biopsy)	100 (I)(DFS) 58 (II) 53 (III)	No recurrence for stage I after surgery only; XRT improved local control for stage II/III
Nakahara et al. 1988 [22]	45 (I) 33 (II) 48 (III) 12 (IVa) 3 (IVb)	Postop (73% received XRT)	30–50	–	100 (I) 91.5 (II) 87.8 (III) 46.6 (IV) 97.6 (complete resection) 68.2 (subtotal) 25 (biopsy)	Complete resection + XRT resulted in best survival

* Fibrous adhesion to the mediastinal pleura without microscopic invasion; *XRT* radiation therapy; *Chemo* chemotherapy; *PFS* progression free survival; *DFS* disease free survival; *OS* overall survival; *Ca* carcinoma; *w/* with; *w/o* without (adapted with permission from [64])

Five-year survival rates for invasive thymomas range from 53% to 70% [5, 22, 31]. Survival rates continue to fall with long-term follow-up and 10-year survival rates may be considerably lower [80].

Summary

Thymoma is a radiosensitive tumor for which complete resection appears to provide adequate local control and long-term survival. For Masaoka stage I thymoma complete resection by an experienced surgical team is sufficient to maintain local control. Radiation therapy can improve local control in those patients whose tumors are not completely resected. Treatment doses between 40 and 55 Gy at standard fractionation seem to be sufficient to enhance the chances of local control in most cases. In patients with gross residual or unresectable disease doses of 60 Gy or higher may be needed. Despite the availability of adjuvant therapy, every attempt should be made to achieve complete tumor resection as this confers the best chance for local control and long-term survival irrespective of stage, without the added toxicity of chest irradiation. Neoadjuvant radiotherapy with or without chemotherapy may be beneficial in downstaging selected patients with Masaoka stage III tumors and improve the chances for a complete resection. Patients with pleural invasion may not benefit from local radiotherapy since their disease is most likely disseminated throughout the pleura. In fact, 38% of those with pleural invasion in Ogawa's series developed pleural dissemination, suggesting that this population will recur throughout the pleura regardless of choice of local therapy. For this group of patients, the use of hemithoracic irradiation, 10 to 17 Gy in 2 to 3 weeks, in conjunction with a mediastinal boost of an additional 40 Gy should be considered to improve loco-regional control, taking into account that there is a significantly increased risk of pneumonitis. Patients with advanced local disease, stage IVa disease, will have a poor prognosis irrespective of the local treatment modality used. For now, primary surgery and the educated, judicious use of radiation therapy, with or without chemotherapy, will offer our patients with thymomas the best hope of disease control and possibly cure.

References

1. Regnard JF, Madgeleinat P, Dromer C et al (1996) Prognostic factors and long term results after thymoma resection: AP series of 307 patients. J Thorac Cardiovasc Surg 112:376-384
2. Gripp S, Hilgers K, Wurm R et al (1998) Thymoma: Prognostic factors and treatment outcomes. Cancer 83:1495-1503
3. Thomas CR, Wright CD, Loehrer PJ (1999) Thymoma: State of the art. J Clin Oncol 17:2280-2289
4. Wang LS, Huang MH, Lin TS et al (1992) Malignant thymoma. Cancer 70:443-450
5. Curran WJ Jr, Kornstein MJ, Brooks JJ, Turrisi AT III (1988) Invasive thymoma: The role of mediastinal irradiation following complete or incomplete surgical resection. J Clin Oncol 6:1722-1727
6. Haniuda RA, Morimoto M, Nishimura H et al (1992) Adjuvant radiotherapy after complete resection of thymoma. Ann Thorac Surg 54:311-315
7. Abeel A, Mangi A, Wright CD et al (2002) Adjuvant radiation therapy for stage II thymoma. Ann Thorac Surg 74:1033-1037
8. Kondo K, Yasumasa M (2003) Therapy for thymic epithelial tumors: A clinical study of 1,320 patients from Japan. Ann Thorac Surg 76:878-884
9. Mornex F, Resbeut M, Richaud P et al (1995) Radiotherapy and chemotherapy for invasive thymomas: A multicentric retrospective review of 90 cases. The FNCLCC trialists. Fédération Nationale des Centres de Lutte Contre le Cancer. Int J Radiat Oncol Biol Phys 32:651-659
10. Singhal S, Shrager JB, Rosenthal DI et al (2003) Comparison of stages I-II thymoma treated by complete resection with or without adjuvant radiation. Ann Thorac Surg 76:1635-1642
11. Schmidt-Wolf IG, Rockstroh JK, Schuller H (2003) Malignant thymoma: Current status of classification and multimodality treatment. Ann Hematol 82:69-76
12. Chen G, Marx A, Wen-Hu C et al (2002) New WHO histologic classification predicts prognosis of thymic epithelial tumors: A clinicopathologic study of 200 thymoma cases from China. Cancer 95:420-429
13. Agrawal S, Datta NR, Mishra SK et al (1999) Adjuvant therapy in invasive thymoma: An audit of cases treated over an 8-year period. Indian J Cancer 36:46-56
14. Loehrer PJ (1999) Current approaches to the treatment of thymoma. Ann Med 31:73-79
15. Wilkins EW Jr, Castleman B (1979) Thymoma: A continuing survey at the Massachusetts General Hospital. Ann Thorac Surg 28:252-256
16. Maggi G, Giaccone G, Donadio M et al (1986) Thymomas: A review of 169 cases, with particular reference to results of surgical treatment. Cancer 56:765-776
17. Fujumura S, Kondo T, Handa M et al (1987) Results of surgical treatment for thymoma based on 66 patients. J Thorac Cardiovasc Surg 93:708-714
18. Maggi G, Casadio C, Cavallo A et al (1991) Thymoma: Results of 241 operated cases. Ann Thorac Surg 51:152-156
19. Uematsu M, Kondo M (1986) A proposal for treatment of invasive thymoma. Cancer 58:1979-1984
20. Lewis J, Wick MR, Scheithauer BW et al (1987) Thymoma: A clinicopathologic review. Cancer 60:2727-2743

21. Monden Y, Nakahara K, Iioka S et al (1985) Recurrence of thymoma: Clinicopathological features, therapy, and prognosis. Ann Thorac Surg 39:165-169
22. Nakahara K, Ohno K, Hashimoto J et al (1988) Thymoma: Results with complete resection and adjuvant postoperative irradiation in 141 consecutive patients. J Thorac Cardiovasc Surg 95:1041-1047
23. Blumberg D, Port JL, Weksler B et al (1995) Thymoma: A multivariate analysis of factors predicting survival. Ann Thorac Surg 60:908-914
24. Quintanilla-Martinez L, Wilkins EW, Choi N et al (1994) Thymoma: Histologic subclassification is an independent prognostic factor. Cancer 74:606-617
25. Pollack A, Komaki R, Cox JD et al (1992) Thymoma: Treatment and prognosis. Int J Radiat Oncol Biol Phys 23:1037-1043
26. Haniuda M, Miyazawa M, Yoshida K et al (1996) Is postoperative radiotherapy for thymoma effective? Ann Surg 224(2):219-224
27. Verley JM, Hollmann KH (1985) Thymoma: A comparative study of clinical stages, histologic features, and survival in 200 cases. Cancer 55:1074-1086
28. Okumura M, Ohta M, Tateyama H et al (2002) The World Health Organization histologic classification system reflects the oncologic behavior of thymoma. A clinical study of 273 patients. Cancer 94:624-632
29. Kondo K, Yoshizawa K, Tsuyuguchi M et al (2004) WHO histologic classification is a prognostic indicator in thymoma. Ann Thorac Surg 77:1183-1188
30. Rena O, Papalia E, Maggi G et al (2005) World Health Organization histologic classification: An independent prognostic factor in resected thymomas. Lung Cancer 50:59-66
31. Masaoka A, Monden Y, Nakahara K et al (1981) Follow-up study of thymoma with special reference to their clinical stages. Cancer 48:2485-2492
32. Kohman LJ (1997) Controversies in the management of thymoma. Chest 112:296-300S
33. Kleikamp G, Schnepper U, Korfer R (1997) Coronary artery disease and aortic valve disease as a long-term sequel of mediastinal and thoracic irradiation. Thorac Cardiovasc Surg 45:27-31
34. Shulimzor T, Apter S, Weitzen R et al (1996) Radiation pneumonitis complicating mediastinal radiotherapy postpneumonectomy. Eur Respir J 9:2697-2699
35. Yeoh E, Holloway RH, Russo A et al (1996) Effects of mediastinal irradiation on esophageal function. Gut 38:166-170
36. Cionini L, Pacini P, De Paola E et al (1984) Respiratory function tests after mantle irradiation in patients with Hodgkin disease. Acta Radiol Oncol 23:401-409
37. Ogawa K, Uno T, Toita T et al (2002) Postoperative radiotherapy for patients with completely resected thymoma: A multi-institutional, retrospective review of 103 patients. Cancer 94:1405-1413
38. Ruffini E, Mancuso M, Oliaro A et al (1997) Recurrence of thymoma: Analysis of clinicopathologic features, treatment and outcome. J Thorac Cardiovasc Surg 113:55-63
39. Mangi AA, Wright CD, Allan JS et al (2002) Adjuvant radiation therapy for stage II thymoma. Ann Thorac Surg 74:1033-1037
40. Rena O, Papalia E, Oliaro A et al (2007) Does adjuvant radiation therapy improve disease-free survival in completely resected Masaoka stage II thymoma? Eur J Cardio Thorac Surg 31:109-113
41. Urgesi A, Monetti U, Rossi G et al (1990) Role of radiation therapy in locally advanced thymoma. Radiother Oncol 19:273-280
42. Kundel Y, Yellin A, Popovtzer A et al (2007) Adjuvant radiotherapy for thymic epithelial tumor: Treatment results and prognostic factors. Am J Clin Oncol 30(4):389-394
43. Mangi AA, Wain JC, Donahue DM et al (2005) Adjuvant radiation of stage III thymoma: Is it necessary? Ann Thorac Surg 79:1834-1839
44. Boonen A, Rennenberg R, van der Linden S (2000) Thymoma-associated systemic lupus erythematosus, exacerbating after thymectomy: A case report and review of the literature. Rheumatology 39:1044-1046
45. Wilkins KB, Sheikh E, Green R et al (1999) Clinical and pathologic predictors of survival in patients with thymoma. Ann Surg 230:562-572
46. Welsh JS, Wilkins KB, Green R et al (2000) Association between thymoma and second neoplasms. JAMA 283:1142
47. Moore KH, McKenzie PR, Kennedy CW et al (2001) Thymoma trends over time. Ann Thorac Surg 72:203-207
48. Wilkins EW, Grillo HC, Scannell G et al (1991) Role of staging in prognosis and management of thymoma. Ann Thorac Surg 51:888-892
49. Krueger JB, Sagerman RA, King GA (1988) Stage III thymoma results of postoperative radiation therapy. Radiol 168:855-858
50. Ciernik IF, Meier U, Lutolf UM (1994) Prognostic factors and outcome of incompletely resected invasive thymoma following radiation therapy. J Clin Oncol 12:1484-1490
51. Myojin M, Choi NC, Wright CD et al (2000) Stage III thymoma pattern of failure after surgery and postoperative radiotherapy and its implication for future study. Int J Rad Onc Biol Phys 46:927-933
52. Veeragandam RS, Golden MD (1998) Surgical management of radiation-induced heart disease. Ann Thorac Surg 65:1014
53. Carlson RG, Mayfield WR, Normann S et al (1991) Radiation-associated valvular disease. Chest 99:538-545
54. Sherrill DJ, Grishkin BA, Galal FS et al (1984) Radiation-associated malignancies of the esophagus. Cancer 54:726-728
55. Velissaris TJ, Tang AT, Millward-Sadler GH et al (2001) Pericardial mesothelioma following mantle field radiotherapy. J Cardiovasc Surg (Torino) 42:425-427
56. Johansson S, Svensson H, Denekamp J (2000) Timescale of evolution of late radiation injury after postoperative radiotherapy of breast cancer patients. Int J Radiat Oncol Biol Phys 48:745-750

57. Adam MJ, Lipsitz SR, Colan SD et al (2004) Cardiovascular status in long-term survivors of Hodgkin's disease treated with chest radiotherapy. J Clin Onc 22:3139-3148
58. PORT Meta-analysis Trialists Group (1998) Postoperative radiotherapy in non-small-cell lung cancer systematic review and meta-analysis of individual patient data from nine randomized controlled trials. Lancet 352:257-263
59. Refaely Y, Simansky DA, Paley M et al (2001) Resection and perfusion thermochemotherapy: A new approach for the treatment of thymic malignancies with pleural spread. Ann Thorac Surg 72:366-370
60. Venuta F, Rendina EA, Longo F et al (2003) Long-term outcome after multimodality treatment for stage III thymic tumors. Ann Thorac Surg 76:1866-1872
61. Yagi K, Hirata T, Fukuse T et al (1996) Surgical treatment for invasive thymoma, especially when the superior vena cava is invaded. Ann Thorac Surg 61:521-524
62. Uematsu M, Yoshida H, Kondo M et al (1996) Entire hemithorax irradiation following complete resection in patients with stage II-III invasive thymoma. Int J Radiat Oncol Biol Phys 35(2):357-360
63. Yoshida H, Uematsu M, Itami J et al (1997) The role of low-dose hemithoracic radiotherapy for thoracic dissemination of thymoma. Radiation Medicine 15(6):399-403
64. Eng TY, Thomas CR Jr (2005) Radiation therapy in the management of thymic tumors. Sem Thorac Cardiovasc Surg 17(1):32-40
65. Fox T, Simon EL, Elder E et al (2007) Free breathing gated delivery (FBGD) of lung radiation therapy: Analysis of factors affecting clinical patient throughput. Lung Cancer 56(1):69-75
66. Willoughby TR, Forbes AR, Buchholz D et al (2006) Evaluation of an infrared camera and X-ray system using implanted fiducials in patients with lung tumors for gated radiation therapy. Int J Radiat Oncol Biol Phys 66(2):568-575
67. Berson AM, Emery R, Rodriguez L et al (2004) Clinical experience using respiratory gated radiation therapy: Comparison of free-breathing and breath-hold techniques. Int J Radiat Oncol Biol Phys 60(2):419-426
68. Eng TY et al 2007 The thymus. In: Everyone's guide for cancer therapy, 5th edn. Andrew McMeel Pub, Kansas City, MO
69. Fukai I, Masaoka A, Fujii Y et al (1999) Thymic neuroendocrine tumor (thymic carcinoid): A clinicopathologic study in 15 patients. Ann Thorac Surg 67(1):7-9 (Comment); Ann Thorac Surg 67(1):208-211
70. Wick MR, Rosai J (1991) Neuroendocrine neoplasms of the mediastinum. Sem Diagn Pathol 8:35-51
71. Asbun HJ, Calabria RP, Calmes S et al (2003) Thymic carcinoid. Ann Surg 57:442, 1991 Case report. Am J Clin Oncol 26(3):270-272
72. De Montprevill V, Macchiarini P, Dulmet E (1996) Thymic neuroendocrine carcinoma (carcinoid): A clinicopathologic study of fourteen cases. J Thorac Cardiovasc Surg 111:134-141
73. Sung MT, Ko SF, Hsieh MJ et al (2003) Thymoliposarcoma. Ann Thorac Surg 76(6):2082-2085
74. Moran C, Handan Z, Koss M (1994) Thymofibrolipoma: A histologic variant of thymolipoma. Arch Pathol Lab Med 118:281-282
75. Bretti S, Berruti A, Loddo C et al (2004) Piemonte Oncology Network. Multimodal management of stages III-IVa malignant thymoma. Lung Cancer 44(1):69-77
76. Latz D, Schraube P, Oppitz U et al (1997) Invasive thymoma: Treatment with postoperative radiation therapy. Radiol 204:859-864
77. Cowen D, Richaud P, Mornex F et al (1995) Thymoma: Results of a multicentric retrospective series of 149 non-metastatic irradiated patients and review of the literature. FNCLCC trialists. Fédération Nationale des Centres de Lutte Contre le Cancer. Radiother Oncol 34(1):9-16
78. Hug E, Sobczak M, Choi N et al (1990) The role of radiotherapy in the management of invasive thymoma. Int J Radiat Oncol Biol Phys 19(Suppl 1):161-162
79. Jackson MA, Ball DL (1991) Postoperative radiotherapy in invasive thymoma. Radiother Oncol 21:77
80. Park HS, Shin DM, Lee JS et al (1994) Thymoma. Cancer 73:2491

Complementary Treatments in Thymic Neoplasms: Steroids and Octreotide

Liliana Montella, Giovannella Palmieri

Background

Permanent control of disease in heavily pretreated patients with metastatic thymic tumors can be difficult to obtain [1]. Alternative treatment strategies have been tested. Following, we will focus on the basic knowledge supporting clinical treatment with steroids and/or somatostatin analogs in thymic epithelial tumors (TET).

Role of Steroids in the Treatment of Thymic Neoplasms

Traditionally, TET have been classified into four categories, i.e., predominantly spindle cell, predominantly lymphocytic, predominantly mixed lymphocytic and epithelial, and predominantly epithelial thymoma on the basis of the lymphocyte epithelial cell ratio and the shape of epithelial cells [2]. Recently, the World Health Organization (WHO) Committee adopted a new classification system based on the cytological features of the thymic epithelial cells and proportion of lymphocytes with prognostic implications [3]. This classification distinguishes medullary (type A), cortical (type B1, B2 and B3), mixed (type AB) thymomas and thymic carcinomas (type C). Thymoma were distinguished in A and B depending on whether the neoplastic cells have a spindle or oval shape or whether they have a dendritic or epithelioid appearance. Type B thymomas were differentiated into B1, B2, and B3 according to the increasing epithelial/lymphocytic ratio and the emergence of atypia of the neoplastic epithelial cell. Paraneoplastic myasthenia gravis occurs only in A and B type thymomas. Given the frequent association of thymomas with paraneoplastic syndromes requiring steroids, tumor response to this therapy was often incidentally recognized [4-7].

Glucocorticoids exert antiproliferative effects in various cell types, have a lymphocytolytic effect, and induce apoptosis in thymocytes. Although they act mainly on the lymphocytic component of the tumor, their effectiveness is apparently unrelated to thymoma cell type [8, 9].

Glucocorticoid receptors were identified in both human and murine cultured thymic epithelial cells [10] and glucocorticoid hormones modulate thymic epithelial cell proliferation and production of thymic hormones [11].

Investigation on glucocorticoid receptor (GR) expression on neoplastic TECs and the effects of glucocorticoids in vitro on the cell cycle progression of tumor cells was performed [12]. Thymoma specimens were obtained during surgery from 21 patients. Three of the specimens with glucocorticoid therapy were examined using the TdT-mediated dUTP-biotin nick-end labeling method. Primary tumor specimens from ten untreated thymomas were examined for GR expression by immunohistochemistry. Isolated neoplastic TECs from the remaining eight untreated thymomas were examined using immunohistochemistry, flow cytometric, and cell cycle analysis. GR resulted to be expressed on neoplastic TECs as well as on nonneoplastic thymocytes in thymomas, regardless of WHO histological classification. Glucocorticoids caused an accumulation of TEC in G0/G1 phase in all cases examined (n = 6), and also induced apoptosis in the three with the lowest levels of Bcl-2 expression.

Several reports of effective treatment of thymic tumors with steroids were reported [4-7, 13-17]. Glucocorticoids were able to produce response in thymic tumors refractory to chemotherapy [7, 13]. High doses of corticosteroids were used in some cases [14-16]. In one case high dose methylprednisolone (1,000 mg on days 1-5 and 500 mg on days 6 and 7) with chemotherapy cisplatin (80 mg/m^2 on day 1) and adriamycin (40 mg/m^2 on day 1) was used in an invasive thymoma. The treatment with three courses of this combined chemotherapy resulted in the improvement and regression of all clinical signs and symptoms [15]. This regimen confirmed to be effective in a series of 14 patients with advanced invasive thymoma [16]. Seventeen untreated patients with invasive thymoma underwent glucocorticoid therapy prior to surgical resection [17]. The steroid pulse consisted of 1 g of methylprednisone each day for 3 days. Overall response rate was 47.1% (8 of 17). B1 thymoma was the most responsive histotype. Moreover, a marked reduction in the CD4+8+ double-positive immature thymocytes that expressed higher levels of glucocorticoids receptor was shown. Tumor shrinkage is conditioned by the presence of CD4+CD8+ double-positive immature lymphocytes, which are more present in B1 thymomas than in the other histotypes. Apoptotic changes were observed not only in lymphocytes, but also in neoplastic epithelial cells. Oral prednisone (50 mg/d) for 6 months was able to produce a complete response in a metastatic B3 thymoma, being progressed after 6 months of octreotide alone at the dose of 10 mg in every 28 days [18]. In some cases the need for prolonged use of steroids was highlighted [8, 19, 20].

Role of Somatostatin-based Therapy in Thymic Neoplasms

Somatostatin (SS) is originally identified as a small peptide inhibiting the release of growth hormone and was accidentally found during studies concerning the distribution of growth hormone-releasing factor in the hypothalamus of rats [21]. Somatostatin is synthesized as part of a large precursor molecule that is rapidly cleaved. Two important bioactive peptides are known: somatostatin-14 and somatostatin-28.

The various actions of somatostatin are mediated through interaction with specific membrane receptors. These receptors are different for pharmacological properties, i.e., binding to different somatostatin analogs, tissue distribution, regulation, and signaling [22]. Five subtypes named sst_{1-5} have been identified all with a high affinity for somatostatin 14 and 28. The sst_2 gene product is alternatively spliced to encode two receptor proteins, sst_{2A} and sst_{2B}, differing in their carboxy-terminal sequence. All five subtypes are functionally linked to adenylate cyclase through a coupling mechanism involving guanine nucleotide-binding (G) protein. Binding of somatostatin to the receptor results in a reduction of the intracellular levels of cyclic AMP and ionized calcium and an increase in the tyrosine phosphatase activity. Each somatostatin receptor subtype seems to be linked to a specific biological function, this latter being triggered by a signaling mechanism related to a specific subtype. Moreover, the expression of somatostatin receptors can be regulated by its own ligand. One of the mechanisms of this regulation is receptor-mediated internalization. Treatment with somatostatin analogs may induce either down- or up-regulation of receptors.

Somatostatin is widely distributed throughout the body and acts on several target cells mainly in the central nervous system, endocrine and exocrine glands, and gastrointestinal tract. Many human tumors express more than one somatostatin receptor subtype, with sst_2 being predominant. Generally, somatostatin displays inhibitory effects on secretive and proliferative processes. Multiple somatostatin receptor subtypes can be expressed by the same tissue and this makes it difficult to define their individual functional role.

Somatostatin receptors (ssts) are expressed by several normal tissues and a wide range of malignancies, strictly neuroendocrine [23] or not [24-26]. Lymphoid cells, especially when activated, also express ssts [27], thus enabling in vivo visualization of inflammatory diseases by somatostatin receptor scintigraphy (SRS). Somatostatin has a plasma half-life shorter than 3 min. For this reason, metabolically stable analogs with a longer half-life have been synthesized for clinical application. The most-used analogs in clinical practice are octreotide and lanreotide, which bind to sst_2, sst_3, and sst_5, but not to sst_1 and sst_4. A long-acting octreotide formulation (octreotide acetate LAR) which consists of octreotide incorporated into microspheres of the biodegradable polymer poly(DL-lactide-co-glycolide glucose) has been developed with the goal to preserve octreotide activity with improved patient convenience and quality of life because of reduced administrations.

Somatostatin and SS analogs inhibit tumor cell proliferation both directly and indirectly. Direct antitumor activities include blockade of synthesis/production of autocrine/paracrine growth-promoting hormones and growth factors, inhibition of growth factor-mediated mitogenic signals and induction of apoptosis [28]. Several mechanisms have been reported to be involved in cell growth arrest induced by somatostatin and analogs including stimulation of tyrosine phosphatases, regulation of MAP kinases, inhibition of Na^+-H^+ exchanger and modulation of nitric oxide production [28]. Induction of apoptosis may be mediated through sst_3. Indirect control of tumor by somatostatin is related to inhibition of angiogenesis. Endothelial cells express sst_2 and sst_3 [29]. Several experimental results indicate that somatostatin and analogs inhibit angiogenesis in vitro and in vivo.

The identification of ssts is generally considered the rationale for therapeutic application of SS analogs. The expression of somatostatin receptors has been studied firstly at the mRNA level by in situ hybridization and reverse transcriptase polymerase chain reaction (RT-PCR). Recently, immunohistochemistry performed with polyclonal antibodies specific for each subtype have been used to study protein expression in rat and human tissues.

Focusing on thymus, several hormones and neuropeptides have been detected in thymic cells and the expression of specific receptors has been reported on both thymic epithelial cells and thymocytes [30, 31]. Somatostatin and their receptors are expressed by the immune and the hematopoietic cells [30, 32].

In 1989, Fuller and Verity demonstrated somatostatin gene expression in the rat thymus and suggested that it exerted a possible paracrine role in modulating T-lymphocyte development [33]. Intrathymic production of somatostatin has been shown [34].

Reubi et al. identified somatostatin receptors in normal thymus and in thymic carcinoids, but not in thymomas [35, 36]. Furthermore, none of the patients submitted to somatostatin receptors scintigraphy had uptake in normal thymus [35]. SS-binding sites visualized by autoradiography were located in the thymic medulla where thymic epithelial cells are the predominant cell type. However, the diffuse and homogeneous labeling pattern suggested that also other types of cells express somatostatin receptors [35]. Ferone et al. studied somatostatin receptors expression both in normal and neoplastic thymus [30, 37]. Normal human thymus expresses somatostatin mRNA and somatostatin receptors subtypes (ssts) sst_1, sst_{2A}, and sst_3, and cultured thymic epithelial cells expressing sst_1 and sst_{2A} mRNA do not proliferate under SS treatment.

Specific [^{125}I-Tyr^3]-octreotide binding on cryostat sections from thymic tissues confirmed that the binding was mainly localized in the medulla [37].

Low doses of dexamethasone enhance the expression of the somatostatin gene in the thymic gland [38]. However, studies concerning the combined effect of glucocorticoids and octreotide on thymic epithelial cells are still lacking.

A combined evaluation by in vitro techniques demonstrated expression of sst_1, sst_2, and sst_3 in a B1 (cortical) thymoma [39] and of sst_2 and sst_3 in a A (medullary) thymoma [40] which were both previously detected by SSR scintigraphy. Further evaluation of somatostatin receptor expression was performed by immunohistochemistry. Sst_{2A} and sst_3 expression was evaluated on tissue specimens of 14 thymic tumors (1 B1 thymoma, 6 B2 thymomas, 1 B3 thymoma, 1 combined B2+B3 thymoma, 3 C thymoma, 2 small cell neuroendocrine carcinoma) [41].

Four tumors stained positive for both sst_{2A} and sst_3; two tumors for sst_{2A} and five tumors for sst_3 only; three tumors were completely negative. Overall, 11 out of 14 (approximately 78% of the cases studied) expressed at least one of these somatostatin receptor subtypes. The staining was highly heterogeneous and the sst_{2A} and sst_3 expression was associated to different cell-types. Sst_3 expression was predominantly associated with thymocytes and sst_{2A} expression confined to malignant epithelial cells or within stromal structures.

SSR expression in thymic epithelial tumor could also represent a sort of neuroendocrine differentiation of a neoplasm originating from an organ containing neuroendocrine cells. The expression of somatostatin receptors in thymic tumors fits well with the increasing recognition of neuroendocrine features in these tumors [42, 43].

The evidence of somatostatin receptors expression by thymic tumors was demonstrated in vivo prior to most in vitro studies previously mentioned. A high in vivo indium-labeled octreotide (^{111}In-DTPA-D-Phe^1-octreotide) uptake in thymic tumors, but not in adult patients with histologically diagnosed benign thymic hyperplasia [44, 45]. ^{111}In-DTPA-D-Phe^1-octreotide specifically binds to sst_2 with high affinity. In detail, Lastoria et al. studied 18 patients including 13 cases of thymic tumors, one thoracic, lymphangioma and four benign thymic hyperplasia. Tumors were clearly identified in all 13 patients with primary or metastatic lesions. Following this evidence, a patient affected by malignant thymoma and pure red cell anemia was treated with octreotide (1.5 mg per day) plus prednisone (0.6 mg/kg/day) and showed a significant tumor shrinkage and resolution of the anemia, while the single drugs used alone were ineffective [20]. These results prompted a phase II study involving sixteen patients from the same institution with advanced thymic tumors, unresponsive to conventional chemotherapeutic regimens [46]. The schedule included administration of somatostatin analog octreotide (1.5 mg/day subcutaneously) associated with prednisone (0.6 mg/kg/day orally for 3 months, 0.2 mg/kg/day orally during follow-up). In 8 cases, octreotide was replaced by the long-acting analog lanreotide (30 mg/every 14 days intramuscularly). Treatment was prolonged until progression of disease was documented. The overall response rate among 16 evaluable patients was 37%. One patient (6%) had a complete response, 5 (31%) had a partial response, 6 obtained a stabilization of disease, and 4 progressed during the treatment. After a median follow-up of 43 months, the median survival was 15 months, and median time to progression was 14 months. Treatment was generally well tolerated with acceptable toxicity: cholelithiasis (1 patient), Grade 2 cushingoid appearance (3 patients), Grade 1 diarrhea (5 patients), Grade 2 hyperglycemia (3 patients). Figure 28.1 shows a prolonged stabilization of disease in a chemorefractory patient.

The most important study following this report was reported by Loehrer et al. who tried to better establish the role of octreotide and prednisone in advanced thymic tumors [47]. This was a multicenter study concerning 38 assessable patients that were treated with octreotide alone and after 2 months continued the same treatment or changed to the association of octreotide and prednisone according to response. Octreotide was administered at a dose of 0.5 mg subcutaneously t.i.d. for a maximum of 1 year and prednisone at a dose of 0.6 mg per day. They reported four partial responses with octreotide alone (4/38, 10.5%) and two complete responses and six partial responses (8/38, 21%) with octreotide associated with prednisone. As the Authors recognize, the study design does not allow definitive conclusions on the activity of octreotide alone. In fact, some later responses were reported in patients exhibiting minor response at the 2-month evaluation. The short duration of therapy could have conditioned the results reported. Somatostatin analogs act differently from conventional chemotherapeutic drugs, thus producing more frequently slow shrinkage of tumor and stable disease rather than significant responses after 2 months of therapy.

The eligibility criteria of ECOG study harbor a potential confounding factor: all patients receiving corticosteroids for myasthenia gravis received the same dosage after entering into the study. This means that myasthenic patients were administered steroids also during the supposed 2 months of octreotide alone.

Management of thymic tumors is often difficult because of concomitant association of various paraneoplastic syndromes. This peculiar feature outlines a profound involvement of the immune system in the development and outcome of this tumor.

Immune system alterations in patients with thymic tumors are increasingly recognized both at a biological and clinical level [48, 49]. Somatostatin and steroid interference with immune system functions are known and they are probably important in the control not only of tumor cells, but also of the thymoma-related immune disorders. In human lymphoid cells (lymphocytes, monocytes) somatostatin has been shown to modulate both secretion processes (i.e., immunoglobulin and cytokine production) and cell growth. Somatostatin has a "biphasic" effect on the function of immune cells, either on secretion or on cell proliferation with maximal inhibitory effects at nanomolar concentrations, and lower or absent effects at higher (micromolar) concentrations [32]. The biphasic response of immune cells to so-

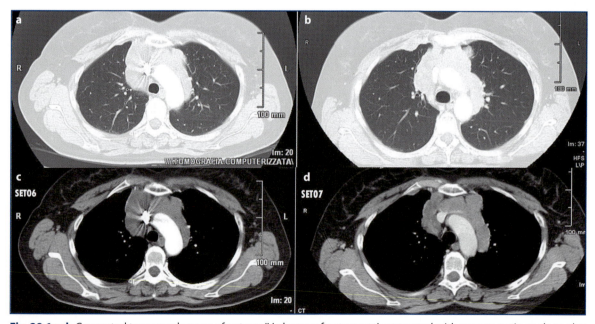

Fig. 28.1a-d Computed tomography scan of a stage-IV-chemorefractory patient treated with somatostatin analogs plus prednisone. The mediastinal mass and intrascissural pleural nodules remained unchanged after 1 year of treatment

matostatin is important when we consider the possible implications of a somatostatin-based treatment on immune system functions. Actually, there are no data on the relationship between the therapeutic concentrations of somatostatin analogs and the effects on immune response of the patients.

With such complexity of interactions to be seen in the development and progression of this rare neoplasm, together with the complex immune alterations, the final effect of somatostatin analogs on the outcome is difficult to define.

Conclusions

Significant evidence support a role for steroids and somatostatin in the management of thymic tumors. Given the rarity of this neoplasm along with the complex interferences between different histotypes and distinct clinical features, it is very difficult to define the exact role of these unconventional treatments. Further insights into biological mechanisms underlying tumor development and growth and well-designed large trials combining biological and clinical data will probably give a real significance to the intriguing results reported.

References

1. Thomas CR, Wright CD, Loehrer PJ (1999) Thymoma: State of the art. J Clin Oncol 17:2280-2289
2. Müller-Hermelink HK, Marx A (1999) Pathological aspects of malignant and benign thymic disorders. Ann Med 31(Suppl 2):5-14
3. Rosai J, Sobin LH (1999) Histological typing of tumors of the thymus. In: Word Health Organization, International Histological Classification of Tumors, Germany, Heidelberg, pp 1-65
4. Almog C, Pik A, Weisberg D, Herczeg E (1978) Regression of malignant thymoma with metastases after treatment with adrenocortical steroids. Isr J Med Sci 14:476-480
5. Mizuno T, Hashimoto T, Yamakawa Y et al (1992) A case of small thymoma associated with myasthenia gravis in which the tumor was reduced by corticosteroid therapy. Nippon Kyobu Geha Gakkai Zasshi 40:975-977
6. Fujiwara T, Mizobuchi T, Shibuya K et al (2007) Rapid regression of stage IVb invasive thymoma under palliative corticosteroid administration. Gen Thorac Cardiovasc Surg 55:180-183
7. Barratt S, Puthucheary ZA, Plummeridge M (2007) Complete regression of a thymoma to glucocorticoids, commenced for palliation of symptoms. Eur J Cardiothorac Surg 31:1142-1143
8. Hu E, Levine J (1986) Chemotherapy of malignant thymoma. Case report and review of the literature. Cancer 57:1101-1104
9. Suda T, Sugimura S, Hattori Y et al (1998) High-dose methylprednisolone-containing chemotherapy in advanced invasive thymoma-report of three cases. Nippon Kyobu Geha Gakkai Zasshi 46:115-120
10. Dardenne M, Itoh T, Homo-Delarche F (1986) Presence of glucocorticoid receptors in cultured thymic epithelial cells. Cell Immunol 100:112
11. Dardenne M, Savino W (1990) Neuroendocrine control of the thymic epithelium: Modulation of thymic endocrine function, cytokeratin expression and cell proliferation by hormones and neuropeptides. Progr Neuro Endocrin Immunol 3:18-25
12. Funakoshi Y, Shiono H, Inoue M et al (2005) Glucocorticoids induce G1 cell cycle arrest in human neoplastic thymic epithelial cells. J Cancer Res Clin Oncol 131:314-322
13. Tandan R, Taylor R, Di Costanzo DP et al (1990) Metastasizing thymoma and myasthenia gravis. Favorable response to glucocorticoids after failed chemotherapy and radiation therapy. Cancer 65:1286-1290
14. Kirkove C, Berghmans J, Noel H, van de Merckt J (1992) Dramatic response of recurrent invasive thymoma to high doses of corticosteroids. Clin Oncol (R Coll Radiol) 4:64-66
15. Hayashi M, Taira M, Yamawaki I, Ohkawa S (2006) High-dose methylprednisolone with chemotherapy for invasive thymoma: A case report. Anticancer Res 26(5B):3645-3648
16. Yokoi K, Matsuguma H, Nakahara R et al (2007) Multidisciplinary treatment for advanced invasive thymoma with cisplatin, doxorubicin, and methylprednisolone. J Thorac Oncol 2:73-78
17. Kobayashi Y, Fujii Y, Yano M et al (2006) Preoperative steroid pulse therapy for invasive thymoma: Clinical experience and mechanism of action. Cancer 106:1901-1907
18. Tiseo M, Monetti F, Ferrarini M et al (2005) CASE 1. Complete remission to corticosteroids in an octreotide-refractory thymoma. J Clin Oncol 23:1578-1579
19. Green JD, Forman WH (1974) Response of thymoma to steroids. Chest 65:114-116
20. Palmieri G, Lastoria S, Colao A et al (1997) Successful treatment of a patient with a thymoma and pure-red cell aplasia with octreotide and prednisone. N Engl J Med 336:263-265
21. Krulich L, Dhariwal APS, McCann SM (1968) Stimulatory and inhibitory effect of purified extracts on growth hormone release from rat pituitary in vitro. Endocrinology 83:783-790
22. Schonbrunn A (1999) Somatostatin receptors present knowledge and future directions. Ann Oncol 10(Suppl 2):17-21
23. Eriksson B, Oberg K (1999) Summing up 15 years of somatostatin analog therapy in neuroendocrine tumors: Future outlook. Ann Oncol 10(Suppl 2):S31-S38

24. Schultz S, Schultz S, Schmitt J et al (1998) Immunocytochemical detection of somatostatin receptors sst1, sst2A, sst2B and sst3 in paraffin-embedded breast cancer tissue using subtype-specific antibodies. Clin Cancer Res 4:2047-2052
25. Nilsson S, Reubi JC, Kalkner KM et al (1995) Metastatic hormone-refractory prostatic adenocarcinoma expresses somatostatin receptors and is visualized in vivo by [111In]-labeled DTPA-D-[Phe1]-octreotide scintigraphy. Cancer Res 55:5805s-5810s
26. Reubi JC, Waser B, van Hagen PM et al (1992) In vivo and in vitro detection of somatostatin receptors in human malignant lymphomas. Int J Cancer 50:895-900
27. van Hagen PM, Hofland LJ, ten Bokum AMC et al (1999) Neuropeptides and their receptors in the immune system. Ann Med 31(Suppl 2):15-22
28. Guillermet-Guilbert J, Lahlou H, Cordelier P et al (2005) Physiology of somatostatin receptors. J Endocrinol Invest 28(Suppl 11):5-9
29. Adams RL, Adams IP, Lindow SW et al (2005) Somatostatin receptors 2 and 5 are preferentially expressed in proliferating endothelium. Br J Cancer 92:1493-1498
30. Ferone D, van Hagen PM, Colao A et al (1999) Somatostatin receptors in the thymus. Ann Med 31(Suppl 2):28-33
31. Dardenne M (1999) Role of thymic peptides as transmitters between the neuroendocrine and immune system. Ann Med 31(Suppl 2):34-39
32. Hofland LJ, van Hagen PM, Lamberts SWJ (1999) Functional role of somatostatin receptors in neuroendocrine and immune cells. Ann Med 31(Suppl 2):23-27
33. Fuller PJ, Verity K (1989) Somatostatin gene expression in the thymus gland. J Immunol 143:1015-1017
34. Savino W, Arzt E, Dardenne M (1999) Immunoneuroendocrine connectivity: The paradigm of the thymus-hypothalamus/pituitary axis. Neuroimmunomodulation 6:126-136
35. Reubi JC, Waser B, Horisberger U et al (1993) In vitro autoradiographic and in vivo scintigraphic localization of somatostatin receptors in human lymphatic tissue. Blood 82:2143-2151
36. Reubi JC, Horisberger U, Kappeler A et al (1998) Localization of receptors for vasoactive intestinal peptide, somatostatin, and substance P in distinct compartments of human lymphoid organs. Blood 92:191-197
37. Ferone D, van Hagen PM, van Koetsveld PM et al (1999) In vitro characterization of somatostatin receptors in the human thymus and effects of somatostatin and octreotide on cultured thymic epithelial cells. Endocrinology 140:373-380
38. Timsit J, Savino W, Safieh B et al (1992) Growth hormone and insulin-like growth factor-I stimulate hormonal function and proliferation of thymic epithelial cells. J Clin Endocrinol Metab 75:183-188
39. Ferone D, van Hagen PM, Kweekkeboom DJ et al (2000) Somatostatin receptor subtypes in human thymoma and inhibition of cell proliferation by octreotide in vitro. J Clin Endocrinol Metab 85:1719-1726
40. Ferone D, Kwekkeboom DJ, Pivonello R et al (2001) In vivo and in vitro expression of somatostatin receptors in two human thymomas with similar clinical presentation and different histological features. J Endocrinol Invest 24:522-528
41. Lastoria S, Palmieri G, Ferone D et al (2001) In vitro and in vivo detection of somatostatin receptors in thymic tumors. 9th European Congress of Endocrinology, Torino
42. Lauriola L, Erlandson RA, Rosai J (1998) Neuroendocrine differentiation is a common feature of thymic carcinoma. Am J Surg Pathol 22:1059-1066
43. Hishima T, Fukayama M, Hayashi Y et al (1998) Neuroendocrine differentiation in thymic epithelial tumors with special reference to thymic carcinoma and atypical thymoma. Hum Pathol 29:330-338
44. Lastoria S, Vergara E, Palmieri G et al (1998) In vivo detection of malignant thymic masses by Indium-111-DTPA-d-Phe^1-octreotide scintigraphy. J Nucl Med 39:634-639
45. Lastoria S, Palmieri G, Muto P, Lombardi G (1999) Functional imaging of thymic disorders. Ann Med 31(Suppl 2):63-69
46. Palmieri G, Montella L, Martignetti A et al (2002) Somatostatin analogs and prednisone in advanced refractory thymic tumors. Cancer 94:1414-1420
47. Loehrer PJ, Wang W, Johnson DH, Ettinger DS (2004) Octreotide alone or with prednisone in patients with advanced thymoma and thymic carcinoma: An Eastern Cooperative Oncology Group phase II trial. J Clin Oncol 22:293-299
48. Masci AM, Palmieri G, Vitiello L et al (2003) Clonal expansion of CD8+ BV8 T lymphocytes in bone marrow characterizes thymoma-associated B-lymphopenia. Blood 101:3106-3108
49. Montella L, Masci A, Merkabaoui G et al (2003) B-cell lymphopenia and hypogammaglobulinemia in thymoma patients. Ann Hematol 82:343-347

CHAPTER 29
Thymus-related Myasthenia Gravis. Multimodal Therapy and Follow-up

Riccarda Gentile, Loredana Capone, Rudolf Schoenhuber

Introduction

Over the last 30 years Myasthenia Gravis (MG) has become amenable to successful treatment, primarily from the remarkable advances in our understanding of the biology of neuromuscular transmission and of pathogenic processes underlying the disorder [1-5]. With treatment, today, most patients can expect to lead normal or nearly normal lives. Some cases of MG may go into remission temporarily, and muscle weakness may disappear so that medications can be discontinued.

How the autoimmune response mediated by specific antibodies to the acetylcholine receptor (AChR) is initiated and maintained in MG is not completely understood. However, the thymus appears to play a role in the process: it is abnormal in approximately 75% of patients with MG; in about 65% thymus is hyperplasic, with active germinal centers, while 10% of patients have thymus tumors (thymoma) [3-5].

In 85% of generalized cases and in more than 50% of ocular cases the antibodies are against the AChR. Of the 15% of generalized MG patients without AChR antibodies, 20-50% have antibodies against another synaptic antigen, muscle-specific tyrosine kinase (MuSK). The remaining patients probably have antibodies against unknown antigens at the neuromuscular junction. The relatively few patients with thymoma often have antibodies against additional striated muscle antigens such as titin, and ryanodine receptors.

The anti-AChR antibodies reduce the number of available AChRs at neuromuscular junctions, several distinct mechanisms decreasing the efficiency of neuromuscular transmission. Failure of transmission at many neuromuscular junctions results in fatigue and weakness [2-5].

History of MG Treatments

MG has been one of the prototypes of the development of rational therapeutic interventions, based on scientific hypotheses, supported by the tremendous development of immunology, and confirmed by clinical studies, including randomized controlled trials, In 1960, Simpson first proposed that MG was an autoimmune disease and hypothesized that it resulted from an antibody-dependent block in neuromuscular transmission. Investigations in the 1970s demonstrated the deficiency of AChR at the neuromuscular junction in MG, the production of animal models by immunization with AChR, the passive transfer of the disease between species with immunoglobulin G, and the presence of antibodies to AChR in most patients with MG. Subsequently, the immunopathogenic and electrophysiological mechanisms involved in the disease were elucidated [6-7].

Coincident with these discoveries, effective treatments were developed, including acetyl cholinesterase (AChE) inhibitors in the 1950s, and by the 1970s, prednisone and other immunosuppressive medications were available. In the 1970s, thymectomy (TE) – first described as a treatment modality in 1936 – became an increasingly accepted form of therapy. In the 1980s, both plasma exchange (PE) and intravenous immunoglobulin (IVIG) were used to treat MG, particularly in patients with life-threatening illness [8].

However, problems and questions remain. On one side the mortality rate for MG has decreased over the last 50 years; reports suggesting that the documented increased prevalence of MG is due to better survival more likely reflect improved case ascertainment in the elderly. On the other side, most of these treatments have considerable side effects so that the treatment of MG may involve trading one disease for another.

Disease Management for MG

In this chapter we will address some problems the clinician is confronted with today in dealing with patients suffering from MG.

MG is typically managed according to the clinical presentation symptoms. Ocular MG is usually first seen and treated by ophthalmologists, who within the usual work-up of patients with ptosis and diplopia consider neuroimaging with MRI of the brain and orbit and a neurological consultation. A patient with vague symptoms of fatigability of the oropharyngeal muscles is most often seen by an ENT physician, who in the absence of focal lesions sends the patient to a neurologist. Most patients with symptoms of generalized fatigue are first seen by their primary physician and finally sent to a neurologist with an expertise of neuromuscular diseases. Only the few patients with the symptoms of a mediastinal syndrome or those with the occasional detection of mediastinal mass are sent directly to the pneumologist or the thoracic surgeon, the main readership of this volume. The thoracic surgeon will be asked for consultation for almost all patients, since, particularly in North America, a thymectomy will be considered for all MG cases.

MG is a disease for which a multidisciplinary approach is essential. The competences needed are found in several medical and surgical subspecialties: ophthalmology, neurology, immunology, pathology, radiology, thoracic surgery, oncology, radiotherapy, anesthesiology, ENT, rehabilitation, and clinical psychology. Only very few centers are able to comprehensibly treat MG patients, but most patients are successfully managed by a neurologist with competence in neuromuscular diseases and a skilled thoracic surgeon experienced with the particularities of MG, particularly with the problems arising in the perioperative phase. The surgeon himself usually manages patients with a thymoma and no signs and symptoms of MG, but also in these cases a neurological consultation before surgery and at follow-up is reasonable.

In this chapter the clinical management of patients with MG will be mainly addressed from the point of view of the thoracic surgeon who comes in contact for one reason or another with MG patients and asks himself what kind of work-up is reasonable to exclude or confirm MG in a patient with an apparently asymptomatic mediastinal mass and what treatment options are available for patients with MG.

Diagnostic Work-up and Clinical Follow-up of a Patient with a Mediastinal Mass But No Clinical Signs of MG

Even if there are anecdotic reports of patients who have developed signs and symptoms of MG at various time intervals following a thymectomy (TE), most patients with thymoma do not have MG at diagnosis nor develop it later. However, due to the variable course of MG, subtle symptoms go often unrecognized.

MG should be screened for by a careful anamnesis, a neurological examination with a scoring system quantifying the patient's disability [9], and the determination of AChR-antibodies. Neurophysiologic tests are not necessary, since their predictive value is low. Single fiber electromyography (SFEMG) is more sensitive, but it is very time consuming, and therefore expensive and not widely available [10].

In case of minimal signs of fatigue, a test with edrophonium chloride should be performed and the patient should be stabilized clinically before surgery. The anesthesiologist must be informed of the diagnosis of MG. The following treatment depends on the clinical progression of the disease [11-14].

Every patient with a thymoma must be informed about the possibility of developing MG, in order to timely recognize symptoms as diplopia, ptosis, dysarthria, dysphagia, and respiratory symptoms, and be made aware of drug-induced MG. Information material can be downloaded from the National Institutes of Health and from several national patient organizations [15].

Treatment of Patients with Clinical Signs and Symptoms of MG

Considerable progress has been made in reducing morbidity and mortality in MG by different treatment approaches, both symptomatic aimed at reducing the effects of the antibody attack and immune-directed treatments aimed at suppressing the pathogenic antibody production or controlling the damage induced by them.

Mortality has also been reduced by improved methods in critical care.

Symptomatic Treatment of MG

The bedrock of symptomatic treatment of autoimmune MG are the ACh-esterase (AChE) inhibitors, especially pyridostigmine. These agents inhibit the breakdown of ACh at the neuromuscular junction, with consequent increase of available ACh sufficient to stimulate AChR and facilitate muscle activation and contraction. These drugs are purely symptomatic and are used as first-line therapy in newly diagnosed MG patients, and as sole long-term treatment of milder forms of generalized MG and especially in ocular MG [12-13].

Adverse effects are caused by the increased concentration of ACh at both nicotinic and muscarinic synapses. The common muscarinic effects are gut hypermotility (stomach cramps, diarrhea), increased sweating, excessive respiratory and gastrointestinal secretions, and bradycardia. The main nicotinic adverse effects are muscle fasciculations and sometimes cramps.

Based on case reports, case series, and daily clinical experience it is commonly agreed that an anti-AChE drug should be the first-line treatment for all forms of MG (good practice point), even if the systematic review of the few placebo controlled randomized trials failed to formally confirm its effectiveness [16].

Pyridostigmine is usually well tolerated at standard doses of up to 60 mg given at 4-h intervals 4 or 5 five times per day. In most cases at night no medication is necessary. The optimal dose is found by slowly increasing from initial 30 mg 4 times a day and depends on the balance between clinical improvement and adverse effects. It can vary over time and with concomitant treatment and must, therefore, be adjusted accordingly.

Immune Directed Treatments for MG

If symptomatic treatment with AChE inhibitors is not effective enough, more aggressive treatment strategies must be considered [11-14]. This is particularly true in MG patients with a thymoma or those with anti-titin and anti-ryanodine antibodies, since they usually have a more severe disease. The aim is to induce and then maintain remission of symptoms by suppressing the autoimmune response either by reducing the production of pathogenic antibodies or the damage induced by them. Over the years this has been done surgically by removing the thymus or pharmacologically with steroids or other immunosuppressive drugs, or by removing antibodies with plasma exchange or interfering with their effects with intravenous immunoglobulin.

Immunosuppression and thymectomy are routinely used for all patients with MG except for those with less severe forms of ocular MG, even if the studies supporting this approach are so far scanty and methodologically inadequate to clearly answer the relevant questions. Most evidence is still anecdotal or comes from case series, from which the greater efficacy of combined immunosuppressive treatments has been shown. As with other rare diseases, randomized controlled trials with comparable patient groups of sufficient size to give reliable answers are very difficult to organize. Complementary to these big trials, which are still needed and some of which are under way, are the systematic reviews of smaller, yet qualitatively sound studies, whose cases are combined in a meta-analysis to increase the power by reducing the variance of the response.

Corticosteroids

A Cochrane review by Schneider-Gold et al. (2005) reports the data available on the treatment of MG with steroids [17]. The autoimmune nature of MG and the beneficial effects of this group of drugs in other autoimmune diseases are the rationale for using steroids and other immunosuppressive drugs in MG. Corticosteroids activate T helper cells and increase the proliferation of B-cells, activated T-cells and antigen-presenting cells.

Simon (1935) reported the beneficial effect of adrenocorticotrophic hormone (ACTH), while Soffler observed the shrinking effect of ACTH on thymus (1948). Von Reis (1966) first documented exacerbation of myasthenic symptoms, sometimes with lethal outcome when respiratory and swallowing difficulties increase at the beginning of high-dose corticosteroid treatment. Warmholts (1971) reported the beneficial effect of high dose alternate-day administration. Seybold and Drachman overcame this problem in 1974 by gradually increasing doses [6].

Because of the heterogeneity of clinical trials, with their different primary and secondary outcomes, despite the 70-year long experience of steroid therapy for MG, there is still no clear formal evidence that corticosteroids are efficacious in treating MG. However, numerous observational studies strongly support the efficacy of corticosteroids for the treatment of MG, suggesting corticosteroids as the mainstay of the treatment for MG, in particular in mild and moderately severe forms [13].

In the last 20 years several retrospective studies have reported very good efficacy of prednisone used with different dosages. A very high rate of remission or marked improvement was reported in generalized MG by many authors. In these observational studies, remission or marked improvement is seen in 70-80% of MG patients treated with oral corticosteroids, usually prednisone (class IV evidence), but the efficacy has never been studied in double blind, placebo-controlled trials [17].

Corticosteroids have several advantages; they have a short onset of action (1-3 months) and can be used in pregnancy, while there can be transient initial severe exacerbation, usually after 1-3 weeks (2-5%), and there are many well-known long-term side effects.

Side effects of varying severity, including osteoporosis, diabetes mellitus, infections, glaucoma, gastric ulcers, psychic disturbances, weight gain, and aseptic bone necrosis, were found in 52.2% of patients. The risk of osteoporosis is reduced by giving bisphonate (class IV evidence), and antacids may prevent gastrointestinal complications.

It is a good practice point to use oral prednisolone as first choice drug when immunosuppressive drugs are necessary in MG. Still unclear is the most appropriate dosage (starting with high doses or gradually increasing doses; daily or alternate-day regimen; the best way of tapering treatment; when to start; the use in association with other immunosuppressive drugs).

Since a high starting dose can precipitate a myasthenic crisis after 4-10 days, alternatively treatment can be started with 10-25 mg on alternate days increasing the dose gradually to 60-80 mg on alternate days. To achieve a rapid response in critically ill MG patients high daily steroid dosages are used in combination with PE or IVIG as short-time treatments to overcome the temporary worsening. At remission, usually after 4-16 weeks, the dose is slowly tapered to the minimum effective dose, possibly given on alternate days (good practice point).

Plasma Exchange

In PE antibodies are removed from patient sera by membrane filtration or centrifugation. Improvement starts within the first week and the effect lasts for 1-3 months. Gajdos et al. (2006) in their Cochrane review on short-term benefits of PE conclude: "There are no adequate randomized controlled trials, but many case series report short-term benefit from plasma exchange in MG, especially in myasthenic crisis" [18]. The NIH consensus of 1986 states: "the panel is persuaded that PE can be useful in strengthening patients with MG before TE and during the postoperative period. It can also be valuable in lessening symptoms during initiation of immunosuppressive drug therapy and during an acute crisis". In these cases this procedure is probably more effective than IVIG.

PE is, therefore, recommended as a short-term treatment in MG, especially in severe cases to induce remission and in preparation for surgery [12-13]. The most common regimen is that of 5 exchanges over 9-10 days.

Intravenous Immunoglobulin

Intravenous immunoglobulin (IVIG) has been used for the same indications as PE; rapidly progressive disease, preparation of weak patients for surgery including TE, and as an adjuvant to minimize long-term side effects of oral immunosuppressive therapy. The results did not show a significant difference between the two treatments for MG exacerbations. Nonrandomized evidence consistently suggests that they are equally effective [19-20].

The use of IVIG is technically easier than plasma exchange and the administration of IVIG is associated with a less than 5% rate of mild and self-limited adverse events.

Gajdos, Chevret, and Toyka in their Cochrane review in 2006 report that in severe exacerbations of MG there is not a significant difference between IVIG and PE. Furthermore, they showed no significant difference in efficacy between administrating 1 g/kg and 2 g/kg of intravenous immunoglobulin over 2-5 days. In chronic MG, there is insufficient evidence for the efficacy of IVIG [19].

The use of IVIG, at the usual dosage 1 g/kg (over 2-5 days), should probably be reserved to severe exacerbations, for strengthening patients with MG before TE and during the postoperative period. It can also reduce symptoms during initiation of immunosuppressive drug therapy and during an acute crisis, like PE, having probably less side effects [12-13].

Thymectomy

In 1939 Alfred Blalock et al. reported the remission of generalized myasthenia in a 21-year-old woman following the removal of a cystic thymus tumor. Blalock and colleagues proceeded to perform TE in nonthymoma patients, reporting improvement in at least half the cases, so that in the 1970s TE had been accepted as a form of therapy for MG [2, 5, 6]. However, there has never been clear evidence to support this treatment modality, so the role of TE in the management of MG remains uncertain. A systematic review made in 2000 by the American Academy of Neurology shows that patients undergoing TE were twice as likely to attain medication-free remission, 1.6 times as likely to become asymptomatic and 1.7 times as like to improve [21]. The interpretation of these data is difficult, since MG patients undergoing TE were younger, more often women, and were more likely to have generalized and severe MG. Severe MG patients undergoing TE had larger relative rates of better outcome when compared with severe MG patients not undergoing TE. Since it cannot be excluded that MG patients undergoing TE received also more aggressive medical therapy than MG patients not receiving TE, the positive TE-favorable outcome reflects probably the effects of a more aggressive therapeutic approach, both medical and surgical.

So far the benefit of TE in nonthymomatous autoimmune MG has not definitely been established [21]. It is not surprising that the indication for TE for nonthymomatous MG varies within and between different countries [22]. TE may increase the probability of remission or improvement in patients with severe MG, but only a randomized controlled trial of sufficient potency will allow to confirm the conviction of all surgeons and most neurologists that TE is really useful for MG patients. So far, TE should be considered as one of the multiple therapeutic options for all patients with generalized MG, as a "rescue" therapy in nonthymomatous patients with severe MG [12-13].

In MG patients with a thymoma the main aim of TE is to treat the tumor more than for having any effect on the MG. Once thymoma is diagnosed, TE is indicated irrespective of the severity of MG (good practice point) [12-13]. Thymoma is a slow-growing tumor and TE should be performed only after stabilization of the MG. The prognosis depends on early and complete tumor resection.

The incidence with which MG occurs in patients with thymoma increases with the age of the patient. In men older than 50 and women older than 60, the incidence appears to be greater then 80%. The majority of patients with MG do not have thymoma. The incidence is 10-42% depending on the reporting medical center. Men with MG are 1.8-2 times more likely to have a thymoma than women. Because of the significant association between thymoma and MG, an evaluation of the mediastinum with CT or MRI is recommended in all patients with MG.

Other Immunosuppressive Drugs

If symptomatic therapy with cholinesterase inhibitors and immunosuppression with glucocorticosteroids are insufficient to control the symptoms of MG, after having considered TE, PE, and IVIG further treatment options include azathioprine, cyclosporine, methotrexate, mycophenolate mofetil, tacrolimus, or cyclophosphamide [12-13]. They have all been tried anecdotally as an add-on therapy. Several randomized controlled trials are under way. So far, their effectiveness cannot be proven [23].

Azathioprine, a commonly used immunosuppressant, is metabolized to 6-mercaptopurine, which inhibits DNA and RNA synthesis and interferes with T-cell function. The onset of therapeutic response may be delayed for 4-12 months, and maximal effect is obtained after 6-24 months. Azathioprine is usually well tolerated but idiosyncratic flu-like symptoms or gastrointestinal disturbances including pancreatitis occur in 10%, usually within the first few days of treatment. Some patients develop hepatitis with elevations of liver enzymes. Leucopenia, anemia, thrombocytopenia, or pancytopenia usually respond to drug withdrawal. Blood cell effects and hepatitis often do not recur after cautious reintroduction of the drug. Careful monitoring of full blood cell count and liver enzymes is mandatory and the dosage should be adjusted according to the results. About 11% of the population are heterozygous and 0.3% homozygous for mutations of the thiopurine methyltransferase gene and have an increased risk of azathioprine-induced myelosuppression. One large double-blind randomized study has demonstrated the efficacy of azathioprine as a steroid-sparing agent with a better outcome in patients on a combination of azathioprine and steroids than in patients treated with steroids alone (class I evidence). In patients where long-term immunosuppression is necessary, azathioprine should be started together with steroids to allow tapering the steroids to the lowest dose possible, while maintaining azathioprine (level A recommendation). Azathioprine is prescribed at the initial dose of 2.5-3 mg/kg daily; the maintenance dose is 1.5-2.5 mg/kg qd.

Cyclosporine has an immunosuppressive effect in both organ transplantation and autoimmune disorders. It is an inhibitor of T-cell function through inhibition of calcineurin signaling. Cyclosporine is effective in MG, has significant side-effects of nephrotoxicity and hypertension and should be considered only in patients intolerant or unresponsive to azathioprine, when long-term immunosuppression and relatively rapid response (1-3 months) is needed and especially when prednisone cannot be used or is ineffective. The risk of using this drug is the high nephrotoxicity (dose-related), increased risk of malignancy, teratogenicity, and drug interactions with NSAIDs, Amphotericin B, and nephrotoxic drugs. The usual initial dose is 2.5 mg/kg bid and is then gradually reduced to the clinically lowest effective dose, since it may be effective below "therapeutic range" in serum.

Mycophenolate mofetil's active metabolite, mycophenolic acid, is an inhibitor of purine nucleotide synthesis and impairs lymphocyte proliferation selectively. A few studies including a small double-blind placebo controlled study of 14 patients have shown that mycophenolate mofetil is effective in patients with poorly controlled MG and as a steroid sparing medication (class III, class IV evidence). Mycophenolate mofetil should be tried in patients intolerant or unresponsive to azathioprine or in patients in whom steroids are ineffective or cannot be used. The advantages are the moderate onset of action (12 months) and the few side effects (diarrhea, insomnia, urinary tract infections, low risk of late malignancies, no major organ toxicity). It is an immunosuppressive agent developed and originally used to prevent acute rejection of solid-organ transplantation: there is still little experience in the treatment of MG [24-25].

Methotrexate can be tried in very selected MG patients who do not respond to the immunosuppressive drugs, because, although it is well studied in other autoimmune disorders, there is no evidence of efficacy in MG.

Cyclophosphamide is an alkylating agent with immunosuppressive properties. It is a strong suppressor of B-lymphocyte activity and antibody synthesis and at high doses it also affects T-cells. In a randomized, double blind, placebo-controlled study including 23 MG patients, those on treatment had significantly improved muscle strength and a lower steroid dose compared with the placebo group. Intravenous pulses of cyclophosphamide allowed reduction of systemic steroids without deterioration of muscle strength or serious side-effects (class II evidence). However, the relative high risk of toxicity including bone marrow suppression, opportunistic infections, bladder toxicity, sterility, and neoplasm limits the use of this medication to MG patients intolerant or unresponsive to steroids plus all other currently used immunosuppressive drugs.

Tacrolimus (FK506) is a macrolide molecule of the same immunosuppressant class as cyclosporine. It inhibits the proliferation of activated T-cells via the calcium-calcineurin pathway. FK506 also acts on ryanodine receptor mediated calcium release from sarcoplasmic reticulum to potentiate excitation-contraction coupling in skeletal muscle. Case reports and a small open trial all showed a useful improvement of MG with minor side effects. Interestingly, patients with anti-RyR antibodies (and potential excitation-contraction coupling dysfunction) had a rapid response to treatment indicating a symptomatic effect on muscle strength in addition to the immunosuppression. FK506 should be tried in MG patients with poorly controlled disease, especially in RyR antibody-positive patients (level C recommendation).

Monoclonal antibodies against different lymphocyte subsets such as anti-CD20 (rituximab) (B-cell inhibitor), and anti-CD4 (T-cell inhibitor) have been reported to improve cases of refractory MG [26]. These treatment strategies are promising, but more evidence is needed before any recommendations can be given.

Training, Weight Control, Lifestyle Modifications, Pregnancy, and Breast-Feeding

The importance of reducing weight and modification of activities of daily living has been suggested, but there is no hard scientific evidence to support this. There are reports that show some benefit of respiratory muscle training in MG and strength training in mild MG. Physical training can be carried out safely in mild MG and produces some improvement of muscle force.

The course of MG during pregnancy is unpredictable: 20% worsen, 20% improve, 60% don't change; exacerbations are most common in the first trimester and first postpartum month. There is no correlation between severity of MG before pregnancy and the course during pregnancy.

The treatment during pregnancy is not very different: drugs like AChE, corticosteroids, PE, and IVIG are safe. There is a minor risk in using azathioprine. Drugs like cyclosporine A are associated with more spontaneous abortions and preterm deliveries, while drugs like methotrexate, and mycophenolate should probably not be used during pregnancy.

During breast feeding immunosuppressants should be avoided because they can induce immunosuppression in the neonate [27].

A Practical Approach to the Management of MG Patients

Evidence-based medicine (EBM) is the conscientious, explicit, and judicious use of current best evidence in making decisions about the care of individual patients. The practice of EBM means integrating individual clinical expertise with the best available external clinical evidence from systematic research. Today's healthcare professionals cannot avoid demonstrating the effectiveness and the efficiency of their clinical decisions, also in cases for which there is insufficient data or for diseases with a highly variable unpredictable course, such as MG.

This means that we must take into account all available evidence, coming from systematic reviews [16-18, 20, 21, 23], from guidelines [13], from reviews and textbooks [11-12], and original papers, but also from informal professional contacts with more experienced colleagues and from personal experience. We must also consider the patient's values and expectations, particularly risk aversion in case of still-unproven treatments or treatments with possible late adverse effects, in case of participation in randomized controlled trials. Integrated into EBM is also our scientific knowledge of the pathogenesis of MG and the nature of the autoimmune process, even if for most aspects there is not enough formal evidence, as for the effectiveness of PE and IVIG [18, 20].

Keeping these general principles of EBM in mind, for any patient with MG, once the diagnosis of MG is established, symptomatic therapy with an AChE inhibitor should be tried. Every thymoma patient should be treated with TE. Depending on the clinical course and the localization (ocular or generalized) of the MG related disability decisions have to be made together with the patient and in his best interest.

Ocular MG

Treatment of patients with MG localized to the ocular district has two goals: to return the person to a clear vision by reducing ptosis and double vision and to prevent the generalization of the disease.

AChE inhibitors improve visual disability in 20-40% of people with ocular MG, but do not reduce the risk of generalization of the disease that usually starts within the first 2 years of the disease, while steroids limit the symptoms in ocular MG and seem to reduce the risk of generalization. Azathioprine has been used with success to spare steroids, while other immunosuppressants, commonly used in generalized MG, and TE are not routinely used in ocular MG [12-13, 28-31].

Patients with a pure ocular form are first treated with anti-AChE; in case of excessive side effects or lack of effectiveness steroids are added [28-29]. Patients are then closely (at 3-month intervals) followed in the first 2 years in order to timely recognize generalization of the disease.

Generalized MG

Patients with generalized MG and insufficient response to pyridostigmine therapy should be considered for TE, ideally within 1 year of disease onset [12-13].

If this is not sufficient, the patient is started on high-dose daily prednisone (commonly 1 mg/kg daily), with the goal of inducing a remission.

If there is no remission several facts must be considered before starting a more aggressive treatment [14]: inappropriate patient and physician expectations, a wrong diagnosis, misinterpretation of persisting symptomatology on treatment (concomitant autoimmune diseases as Grave's, Lambert-Eaton's), inappropriate use of pyridostigmine (wrong dosage, wrong timing), and incorrect use of prednisolone (insufficient dose and duration, steroid myopathy).

A steroid-sparing agent, such as azathioprine or mycophenolate mofetil, is added if steroid treatment is expected to be needed for more than a year. To prevent steroid-induced osteoporosis bisphosphonate is indicated. Any other side effects of prednisone or of the other immunosuppressants are treated as they appear.

Once remission is established, the tapering of the prednisone is begun, aimed at an alternate-day dosing schedule, with the goal to reach the minimum dose of prednisone that will keep the patient in remission. A common schedule is to first reduce prednisone every other day by 5 mg every 2 weeks. The AChE inhibitors are tapered as tolerated. The slow tapering of the prednisone is continued.

If MG symptoms return during the tapering phase, the dose of prednisone at that time is held steady for a few weeks to allow spontaneous recovery. If there is no stabilization within a few weeks or if the patient worsens, a full course of IVIG or PE is indicated, otherwise a drastic increase in the steroid dose are required to re-establish the remission, since minor dose increases to last previously effective dose is usually not effective.

Possible causes of failure, or apparent failure, of MG to respond to conventional treatment have again to be considered [14]. Beyond the inappropriate expectations, wrong diagnosis, misinterpretation of persisting symptomatology on treatment, inappropriate use of pyridostigmine, incorrect use of prednisone, also inappropriate dose and expectations of azathioprine (or other immunosuppressants) and the patient's compliance must be addressed.

Once the patient is again in remission, the prednisone is even more slowly tapered, to zero or to the lowest effective dose. Then also other immunosuppressants are very slowly reduced. In case of symptom recurrence, immunosuppression is started again, usually with prednisone combined with the previously effective immunosuppressant.

The patient must always be informed not only on the rationale and expected effect of treatment, but also on the risks. Decisions must be taken according to the patient's expectations and values. The patient's understanding of the disease process is essential. It increases his compliance to therapy, but also allows him to immediately recognize and report life-threatening symptoms, such as dysphagia and dyspnoea, which – if not treated immediately – lead to respiratory insufficiency, responsible for the mortality of MG.

References

1. Grob D, Brunner N, Namba T, Pagala M (2008) Lifetime course of myasthenia gravis. Muscle Nerve 37:141-149
2. Conti-Fine BM, Milani M, Kaminsk HJ (2006) Myasthenia gravis: Past, present, and future. J Clin Invest 116:2843-2854
3. Hirsch NP (2007) Neuromuscular junction in health and disease. Br J Anaesth 99:132-138
4. Mahadeva B, Phillips LH, Juel VC (2008) Autoimmune disorders of neuromuscular transmission. Semin Neurol 28:212-227
5. Juel VC, Massey JM (2007) Myasthenia gravis. Orphannet J Rare Dis 2:44
6. Keesey JC (2004) A history of treatments for myasthenia gravis. Semin Neurol 24:5-16
7. Pascuzzi RM (1994) The history of myasthenia gravis. Neurol Clin 12:231-242
8. Hughes T (2005) The early history of myasthenia gravis. Neuromuscul Disord 15:878-886
9. Jaretzki A, Barohn RJ, Ernstoff RM et al (2000) Myasthenia gravis: Recommendations for clinical research standards. Ann Thorac Surg 70:327-334
10. Benatar M (2006) A systematic review of diagnostic studies in myasthenia gravis. Neuromusc Dis 16:459-467
11. Richman DP, Agius MA (2003) Treatment principles in the management of autoimmune Myasthenia Gravis. Ann NY Acad Sci 998:457-472
12. Hilton-Jones D, Palace J (2005) The management of myasthenia gravis. Pract Neurol 5:18-27
13. Skeie GO, Aposolski S, Evoli A et al (2006) Guidelines for the treatment of autoimmune neuromuscular transmission disorders. Eur J Neur 13:691-699
14. Hilton-Jones D (2007) When the patient fails to respond to treatment: myasthenia gravis. Pract Neurol 7:405-411
15. National Institute of Neurological Disorders and Stroke. http://www.ninds.nih.gov/disorders/myasthenia_gravis/myasthenia_gravis.htm, http://www.myasthenia.org/
16. Mendiratta MM, Kuntzer T, Pandey S (2008) Anticholinesterase treatment for myasthenia gravis (Protocol). Cochrane Databases of Systematic Reviews, Issue 1
17. Schneider-Gold C, Gajdos P, Tojka KV, Hohlfeld RR (2005) Corticosteroids for myasthenia gravis. Cochrane Databases of Systematic Reviews, Issue 2
18. Gajdos P, Chevret S, Toyka K (2002) Plasma exchange for myasthenia gravis (review). Cochrane Databases of Systematic Reviews, Issue 1
19. Gajdos P, Tranchant C, Clair B et al (2005) Treatment of myasthenia gravis exacerbation with intravenous immunoglobulin. A randomized double-blind clinical trial. Arch Neurol 62:1689-1693
20. Gajdos P, Chevret S, Toyka K (2006) Intravenous immunoglobulin for myasthenia gravis (review). Cochrane Databases of Systematic Reviews, Issue 1
21. Gronseth GS, Barohn RJ (2000) Practice parameter: Thymectomy for autoimmune myasthenia gravis (an evidence based review). Neurology 55:7-15
22. Shahrizaila N, Pacheco OA, Vidal DG et al (2005) Thymectomy in myasthenia gravis: Comparison of outcome in Santiago, Cuba and Nottingham, UK. J Neurol 252:1262-1266
23. Hart IK, Sathasivam S, Sharshar T (2007) Immunosuppresive agents for myasthenia gravis. Cochrane Databases of Systematic Reviews, Issue 4
24. Ciafaloni E, Massey JM, Tucker-Lipscomb B, Sanders DB (2001) Mycophenolate mofetil for myasthenia gravis: An open-label pilot study. Neurology 56:97-99
25. Meriggioli MN, Ciafaloni E, Al-Hayk KA et al (2003) Mycophenolate mofetil for myasthenia gravis. An analysis of efficacy, safety and tolerability. Neurology 61:1438-1440
26. Kakoulidou M, Bjelak S, Pirskanen R, Lefvert AK (2007) A clinical and immunological study of myasthenia gravis treated with infliximab. Acta Neurol Scand 115:279-283
27. Hoff JM, Daltveit AK, Gilhus NE (2007) Myasthenia gravis in pregnancy and birth: Identifying risk factors, optimising care. Eur J Neurol 14:38-43
28. Agius MA (2000) Treatment of ocular myasthenia with corticosteroids. Arch Neurol 57:750-751
29. Kaminski HJ, Daroff R (2000) Treatment of ocular myasthenia. Steroid only when compelled. Arch Neurol 57:752-753
30. Benatar M, Kaminski H (2006) Medical and surgical treatment for ocular myasthenia. Cochrane Databases of Systematic Reviews, Issue 1
31. Benatar M, Kaminski HJ (2007) Evidence report: The medical treatment of ocular myasthenia (an evidence-based review). Neurology 68:2144-2149

CHAPTER 30
Thymus Transplantation

M. Louise Markert, Blythe H. Devlin, Elizabeth A. McCarthy, Ivan K. Chinn, Laura P. Hale

History

Thymus transplantation was first attempted in the 1960s and 1970s using fetal thymus tissue [1, 2]. The results overall were disappointing [3-6]. In part the poor outcomes related to the lack of reagents needed to characterize and identify the patients into those who were truly athymic (complete DiGeorge anomaly) and those who had bone marrow stem cell problems (severe combined immunodeficiency). It is also possible that the fetal thymus tissue was too small to reconstitute a human infant [7]. The use of fetal thymus carried the risk of fatal graft versus host disease since mature T-cells can be found in the human thymus by the end of the first trimester [3]. By 1986, in a review of 26 infants treated with fetal thymus transplantation, 22 had died; the other 4 patients had achieved a 3-year survival [6].

Important research was conducted in animals in the 1970s and 1980s which would provide the background for improved outcomes. Hong and colleagues showed that thymus transplantation from completely mismatched mouse strains could reconstitute T-cells in nude mice [8]. In the 1980s and 1990s Haynes and colleagues performed animal experiments in which postnatal human tissue was transplanted into mice [9]. Dr. Haynes had reported in the early 1990s [9] that fragments of postnatal human thymus (readily available as discarded tissue from exposure of the heart in congenital cardiac surgery) could be transplanted in the SCID/human mouse model. If the mice were pretreated with an antibody against murine NK cells and macrophages, the human thymus tissue remained viable and murine T-cells colonized the thymus within 1-3 months. Human thymopoiesis did not develop as there was not a source of human stem cells.

In addition to the animal experiments that were essential for the development of the current thymus transplantation trials, other advances in the 1980s and 1990s allowed for critical advancement of the field. Dr. Haynes and other investigators developed monoclonal antibody reagents that identified components of the human thymus [10-12] and the earliest stages of human thymocyte development [13, 14]. In the 1990s, the ability to stain the cultured tissue for cytokeratin and other thymic elements allowed Markert and Haynes to develop culture conditions that maximized the viability of the cultured thymus slices [15]. Other monoclonal antibodies were developed to identify naïve T-cells [16]. This progress allowed accurate determination of the presence of thymically derived T-cells. At the same time the underlying immunodeficiencies were better defined. In particular, the difference between partial and complete DiGeorge anomaly was clarified, with the partial DiGeorge anomaly patients having a small thymus versus the complete DiGeorge anomaly patients having no thymus at all [17-19]. The former had some thymic-derived T-cells that could reject transplants. The latter did not have thymically derived T-cells; thus engraftment was facilitated.

Patient Population

The target population for thymus transplantation is the group of athymic infants with complete DiGeorge anomaly. DiGeorge anomaly is characterized by defects in organs derived from the 3rd and 4th pharyngeal pouches and the intervening 4th pharyngeal arch [20]. The parathyroid, thymus and heart are variably affected [19, 21-25]. Most infants have some parathyroid deficiency and require calcium replacement [26]. Typical heart defects include interrupted aortic arch type B and truncus arteriosus, although some patients have no cardiac defect at all [23, 26]. In complete DiGeorge anomaly, the thymus is absent. Other common problems in infants with complete DiGeorge anomaly include speech delay, aspiration, gastroesophageal reflux, rib or vertebral anomalies, renal abnormalities, atypical facies, developmental delay, hearing or visual deficits, 7th nerve palsies, and cleft palate. Approximately half of children with complete DiGeorge anomaly have 22q11 hemizygosity [26-28]; approximately 20% have CHARGE association (*c*oloboma, *h*eart defect, choanal *a*tresia, growth or developmental *r*etardation, *g*enital hypoplasia, and *e*ar anomaly or deafness) [26, 29, 30] often with CHD7 mutations [31]; approximately 15% are infants of diabetic mothers [26, 32, 33]; and the remaining infants have no genetic or syndromic associations [26]. All athymic infants have a fatal condition and succumb to infection within the first 2 years of life because of their profound immunodeficiency [17].

Complete DiGeorge anomaly may present with two different phenotypes. The majority of infants have "typical" complete DiGeorge anomaly. These infants usually have very few T-cells (<50/mm^3) and always have fewer than 50 naïve T-cells/mm^3. Naïve T-cells are recent thymic emigrants that co-express CD45RA and CD62L [16]. Almost all of these infants will lack a proliferative response to the mitogen phytohemagglutinin (PHA) [17]. These infants do not have a rash. At some point after birth many infants with complete DiGeorge anomaly will develop circulating oligoclonal T-cells associated with rash and lymphadenopathy [34-36]. This phenotype is called "atypical" complete DiGeorge anomaly [34]. Patients with atypical complete DiGeorge anomaly resemble those with Omenn's syndrome [37-39]. The skin on biopsy shows spongiotic dermatitis with T-cell infiltration [34]. The T-cells appear to have developed without having been "educated". The oligoclonal T-cells seem to attack the infant and do not protect against opportunistic infections. These T-cells have infiltrated the liver, associated with hepatomegaly and elevated liver transaminases (unpublished). Strikingly, the oligoclonal T-cells can expand to very high numbers such as 40,000/mm^3 (unpublished). Despite the high T-cell numbers, less than 5% are naïve in phenotype. The peripheral T-cells may or may not proliferate in response to PHA. The two phenotypes of complete DiGeorge anomaly must be distinguished because the atypical patients can reject thymus transplants. Atypical patients require peritransplantation immunosuppression.

Screening of Recipients for Transplantation

Currently in the USA, an Investigator New Drug (IND) application with the Food and Drug Administration (FDA) is required for thymus transplantation. Because thymus transplantation is an experimental procedure, all transplantation is conducted under Institutional Review Board (Ethics Committee)-approved and FDA-reviewed protocols. Informed consent is obtained from parents of the donors and recipients prior to thymus transplantation.

The recipients are screened prior to transplantation to confirm the diagnosis of athymia and to better characterize the subject. For the diagnosis of athymia, the subject must have fewer than 50/mm^3 naïve T-cells in the peripheral blood on flow cytometry. In atypical complete DiGeorge patients with oligoclonal T-cells, less than 5% of circulating T-cells can be naïve in phenotype. Stimulation of peripheral blood mononuclear cells with the mitogen phytohemagglutinin is done to characterize the patient's T-cell response and determine if immunosuppression will be required. Every subject is tested for 22q11 hemizygosity.

In infants with rash and circulating T-cells, additional studies are performed. The clonality of the T-cells is assessed by flow cytometry and spectratyping [40]. T-cell receptor rearrangement excision circles (TREC) are quantified [41]. TRECs are episomes of DNA that form when the V, D, and J segments of DNA come together to encode the variable portion of the T-cell receptor chains. Absence of TRECs confirms the diagnosis of athymia made by the flow cytometry showing a lack of naïve T-cells.

In the atypical patients, maternal engraftment [42] and graft versus host disease (GVHD) from unirradiated blood transfusions must be ruled out. DNA is obtained from the infant's buccal swab and from the mother. The DNA samples are compared using molecular methods to DNA extracted from T-cells isolated from the infant's peripheral blood. GVHD from a blood transfusion is a life-threatening complication. The only infant who presented with GVHD in our series died despite intensive therapy to try to suppress the third party T-cells. Maternal cells are rarely seen in atypical complete DiGeorge anomaly. Their affect on transplant outcomes is not known at this time.

To prepare for transplantation, standard testing is conducted to assess the medical condition of the infant. Testing includes electrolytes, liver transaminases, renal function (creatinine, blood urea nitrogen, urinalysis, renal ultrasound), and HLA typing. A cardiac evaluation is performed to assess suitability for surgery. As for other transplant recipients, the subjects are screened for HIV-1 and hepatitis B and C. Subjects are also screened for human herpes virus 6 (HHV6), Epstein Barr virus (EBV), and cytomegalovirus (CMV). HHV6 may have a detrimental affect on thymus development [43]. EBV and CMV are worrisome infections for infants with profound immunodeficiency as they can cause severe disease and may also be associated with lymphoproliferative disease [44-47]. Parents are counseled during the informed consent process that these infections may affect outcomes. If EBV or CMV is present, anti-viral therapy is instituted.

Infants are screened for autoimmune disease with complete blood counts, thyroid studies, Coombs antibody test, a urinalysis, and anti-HLA antibodies. If the subject has anti-HLA antibodies, the thymus used for transplantation cannot have the specific HLA antigens detected by the anti-HLA antibodies.

Donor Screening for Thymus Transplantation

The thymus tissue is obtained as tissue discarded during cardiac surgery. The surgeon removes thymus tissue to access the surgical field to improve the cardiac surgical outcome. The transplant team is called for all discarded thymuses. If an infant is awaiting thymus transplantation, the transplant team requests permission to approach the parents to obtain consent to use the discarded tissue for transplantation, to obtain blood and urine from the donor infant, and to obtain blood from the donor's mother.

The thymus donors are extensively screened for infectious diseases. The guidelines published by the FDA in the Code of Federal regulations are followed [48]. Thymus tissue is screened for hepatitis B, hepatitis C, EBV, and CMV by PCR. The thymus donor is screened for CMV infection by urine culture and by PCR of the blood. The donor is also screened for EBV by PCR of the blood. For donors over 1 month of age, additional screening is performed for HHV6 and West Nile Virus by PCR. All standard donor screening [48] is conducted on blood, including testing for hepatitis B and C, HIV-1, HIV-2, HTLV-1, HTLV-2, and syphilis.

The immune status of the donor infant is tested by flow cytometry to confirm normal percentages of total T, CD4, CD8, naïve CD4, naïve CD8, and B and NK-cells. Testing for 22q11 and HLA typing is performed on thymocytes that are harvested at the time of tissue slicing. Hemizygosity for 22q11 excludes a thymus donor.

The donor's parents are asked about autoimmune disease in themselves and the donor's siblings. Exclusion criteria include type I diabetes, thyroid disease, common variable immunodeficiency, lupus erythematosis, Crohn's disease, ulcerative colitis, and rheumatoid arthritis.

The donor's mother is tested for the same infections as the donor plus toxoplasmosis and Chagas disease. If the mother is IgG positive for toxoplasmosis, the infant is tested as well. The mother is tested for antibodies to CMV and EBV. Results consistent with acute infection lead to exclusion of the donor. In addition, extensive questionnaires are reviewed with the donor's parents to review risk factors for Creutzfeldt-Jacob disease, small pox exposure, severe acute respiratory syndrome (SARS) exposure, and West Nile disease exposure. Lastly, the mother is asked a series of lifestyle questions, including a sexual history to assess risk for HIV-1 and hepatitis.

Tissue Processing and Tissue Screening for Thymus Transplantation

The thymus tissue is brought to the laboratory and sliced aseptically using a Stadie-Riggs microtome [49] (Fig. 30.1). The slices are approximately 0.5-1 mm thick. Slices are placed on Millipore filters on surgical sponges which serve as rafts. Four filters are placed in each cell culture dish (Fig. 30.1) in thymus organ medium. The medium contains fetal calf serum, Hams F12, and HEPES [26]. The medium is aspirated daily and new medium is dripped onto the filters. This practice helps remove the T-cells from the tissue slices. All procedures are performed under Good Tissue Practices [50] under Standard Operating Procedures.

Donor tissue, thymocytes, and nucleic acid samples are stored on the day of harvest. These samples include DNA that can be used later to evaluate the recipient for graft versus host disease. Samples of tissue are stored frozen. Formalin fixed tissue is embedded in paraffin.

The identity of the tissue as thymus is confirmed by visual inspection and by immunohistochemistry from frozen or formalin fixed sections on the day of harvest, a culture midpoint approximately 3-7 days prior to transplantation, and on the day of transplantation.

Multiple sterility tests are performed. The culture medium is pooled on the day after harvest, at approximately 1 week prior to transplantation, approximately 3 days prior to transplantation and on the day of transplantation. The media are cultured for bacteria, fungus, and mycoplasma per the United States Pharmacopeia (USP). An endotoxin assay of pooled supernatant, using the limulus amoebocyte lystate as-

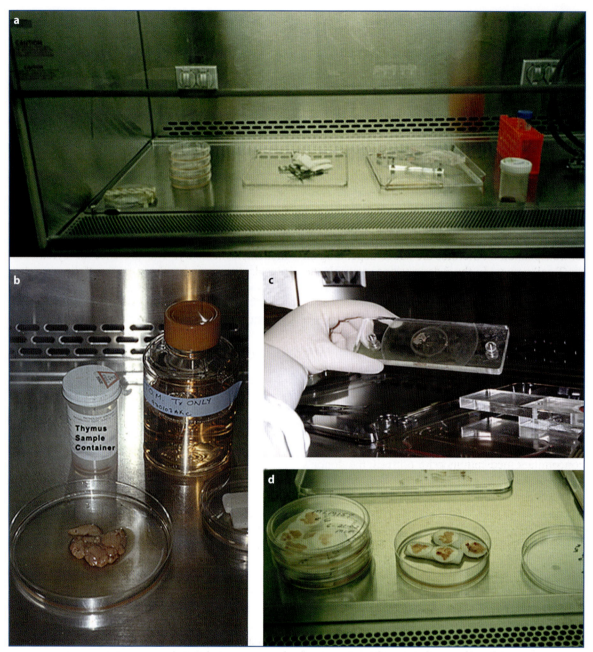

Fig. 30.1a-d Thymus processing. **a** Slicing equipment in the biosafety cabinet. Petri culture dishes are on the *left*, the thymus is on the *right* in the container. **b** The appearance of the thymus that is obtained from the operating room. **c** A slice of thymus. **d** Slices of thymus tissue that will be held in the tissue culture incubator until transplantation

say, is performed within 24 h of transplantation, and a Gram stain of pooled supernatant is assessed immediately prior to transplantation.

The dose of the thymus is ascertained the day prior to transplantation by physical measurement of all the pieces in each culture dish, estimating the length, width, and thickness of each piece. The dose range is between 4 and 18 g per meter squared of recipient body surface area.

Preparation of the Recipient for Transplantation

The initial immune screening of infants is used to determine if immunosuppression is required (reviewed in [26]). Infants with typical complete DiGeorge anomaly with low proliferative responses to PHA are not treated with immunosuppression before or after transplantation.

The use of PHA to determine the need for immunosuppression is problematic because PHA responses are not standardized. Three concentrations of PHA are used, and triplicate cultures of peripheral blood mononuclear cells are incubated for 3 days (or 3 and 4 days if sufficient cells are available). The highest proliferative result is used for the determination. Our laboratory uses a response of over 5,000 counts per minute (cpm) or greater than a 20-fold response over background as the threshold for requiring immunosuppression. Studies are underway to standardize the PHA assay so that responses are comparable.

All infants with atypical complete DiGeorge anomaly are treated with cyclosporine before and after transplantation. Steroids are added depending on the T-cell counts. In the 5 days prior to transplantation the atypical infants are treated with 3 doses of 2 mg/kg rabbit anti-thymocyte globulin concomitant with steroids, diphenhydramine, and acetaminophen.

Occasionally, subjects with typical complete DiGeorge anomaly have proliferative responses to PHA over 5,000 cpm and more than 20-fold over background. These subjects have very few naïve T-cells ($<50/mm^3$ or less than 5% of total T-cells). They do not have rash or lymphadenopathy. Because of the elevated proliferative response to PHA, they are also treated with rabbit anti-thymocyte globulin and the concomitant medications prior to transplantation. If the proliferative response reaches 75,000 cpm, they are treated with cyclosporine before and after transplantation as well.

Cyclosporine is carefully monitored to maintain trough levels between 180 and 220 ng/ml. Weaning of the cyclosporine (over 8-10 weeks) begins once naïve T-cells reach 5% of the total T-cells. A current focus of research is the management of atypical subjects who have detectable maternal T-cells in the circulation. Early weaning of the cyclosporine can lead to reappearance of the maternal T-cells in the blood. These maternal T-cells can threaten the integrity of the thymus allograft.

Surgical Procedure of Thymus Transplantation and Biopsy

Thymus transplantation is performed as an open procedure under general anesthesia in the operating room. As previously described [51], the thymus tissue is brought to the operating room in the dishes that have been used for culture. The tissue on the Millipore filters is transferred into sterile petri dishes on the operating table. The thymus tissue is placed into incisions in the quadriceps muscles bilaterally. Bleeding is minimized. Each piece is placed into its own pocket in the muscle and a suture is placed over the pocket to prevent the tissue from being extruding out of the muscle.

A biopsy of the transplanted tissue is performed 2-3 months after transplantation as an open procedure in the operating room. The initial incision is opened and the surface of the quadriceps muscle is accessed. Approximately four 5×5 mm pieces of tissue are obtained directly below 4 of the sutures that were used to close the muscle and that marked the location of the transplanted tissue. For each sample, part is frozen and part is placed in formalin and embedded in paraffin. Both parts are examined by immunohistochemistry. The presence of cytokeratin reveals the graft has been successfully sampled. Lymphocytes reactive with antibodies to CD3, CD1a, and Ki-67 (nuclear proliferation marker) are cortical thymocytes. The presence of these cells in the context of cytokeratin has been associated with development of naïve T-cells in the blood at 4-6 months after transplantation in all 23 biopsies with this finding to date. Figure 30.2 shows an allograft biopsy with cortical thymocytes and lacy thymic epithelium.

Clinical Outcomes

Subjects tolerate the surgical procedures with only occasional problems of dehiscence and inflammation around sutures. Figure 30.3 shows the Kaplan Meier survival estimate. Survival after transplantation is 73% with most deaths occurring in the first year after transplantation. These deaths are usually related to infection, cardiac, or pulmonary issues. One transplant recipient died of a sudden cardiopulmonary arrest 4 years after transplantation. The subject had undergone a second stage repair of her heart defect that had many complications 2 months prior to the event. It was assumed that the cause of death was a cardiac arrhythmia.

Prophylaxis for *Pneumocystis jarovecii* is stopped after the development of antigen-specific T-cell responses after 1 year. Discontinuing the prophylaxis has been possible in all subjects except for one who has ectodermal dysplasia and does not have T-cell proliferative responses to antigens. No subjects have developed pneumocystis infections after prophylaxis has been stopped.

Morbidity from infection is greatly reduced by 1 year after thymus transplantation. Viral infections that previously would have probably resulted in prolonged hospitalizations and that have resulted in the

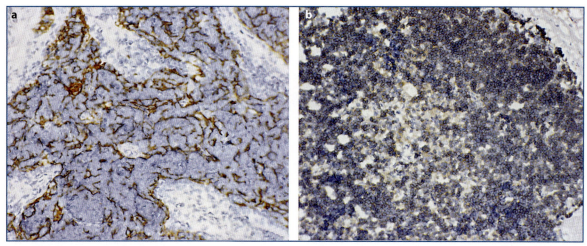

Fig. 30.2a,b Biopsy of thymus allograft. The biopsy from an atypical patient on day 66 after transplantation. **a** Cytokeratin. **b** CD3

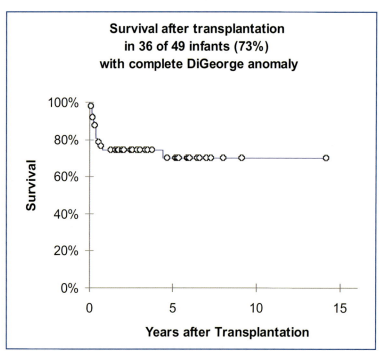

Fig. 30.3 Kaplan Meier Survival Function

death of patients (e.g., parainfluenza virus, RSV) have been associated with mild symptoms similar to those of other children, such as cough and fever. By 1 year, infections are usually followed in an outpatient setting without therapy. Problematic infections seen after 1 year are usually those caused by anatomic or neurologic problems, such as bronchomalacia leading to respiratory infections, abnormal ear and sinus anatomy (such as choanal atresia) resulting in otitis and sinusitis infections, and aspiration leading to recurrent aspiration pneumonias. The one exception in the author's series is one subject who had complete DiGeorge anomaly associated with ectodermal dysplasia. This subject developed naïve T-cells and a polyclonal repertoire but has not been able to mount antigen-specific responses. This subject has had significant viral infections requiring prolonged hospitalizations.

Autoimmune disease is a frequent complication after thymus transplantation found in 42% of subjects over 1 year post transplantation. Of the 31 infants who are more than 1 year after transplantation,

8 (26%) have developed autoimmune thyroid disease and are on replacement therapy. One of these infants developed alopecia totalis, which has not been responsive to therapy. A second of these infants with thyroid disease had previously developed nephrotic syndrome which responded to a 2-month course of steroids. (A renal biopsy was not performed.) Three additional subjects had transient episodes of thrombocytopenia. Two subjects developed autoimmune hemolytic anemia associated with viral infections. One of the subjects with anemia subsequently developed autoimmune hepatitis. These complications have responded to treatment. The one subject who developed autoimmune hemolytic anemia associated with HHV6 infection followed by autoimmune hepatitis continues on immunosuppression. These adverse events should be considered in the context of the high background of autoimmune disease in DiGeorge anomaly and in other primary immunodeficiencies such as severe combined immunodeficiency (SCID). Six subjects enrolled in transplantation protocols in the Duke series developed thyroid disease prior to transplantation. Thyroid disease has been described in partial DiGeorge anomaly [52-55] and in SCID after bone marrow transplantation [56]. Autoimmune cytopenias are a common and often severe complication of partial DiGeorge anomaly [57-59]. It is not clear at this time whether the autoimmune disease seen after transplantation is secondary to defective thymopoiesis or to the underlying genetic background of the recipient. Interestingly, neonatal thymectomy in an animal has been shown to increase the rate of spontaneous thyroiditis [60], suggesting that the mass of the thymus may be important for preventing thyroid disease.

The most severe adverse event occurred in the subject who received the largest dose of thymus tissue (23 g/m² body surface area). This subject presented with atypical complete DiGeorge anomaly. Most of the circulating T-cells were double negative (CD3⁺CD4⁻CD8⁻). Large expansions of TCRBV3⁺ T-cells were observed. Five months after transplantation, CD4⁺ T-cells became the predominant population and the TCRBV repertoire normalized, suggesting that T-cells were emerging from the thymus. No naïve T-cells were detected. At the same time the subject developed severe unrelenting enteritis and colitis. This condition required high doses of immunosuppression to reverse. The subject died from a fungal infection, likely related to the steroid therapy. Because of this adverse event the maximum dose of tissue was lowered to 18 g/m² body surface area.

Immune Outcomes

All 31 subjects who are now more than 1 year after transplantation have developed naïve T-cells with the exception of DIG208 who remains on immunosuppression for autoimmune hepatitis (Fig. 30.4). Outcomes of CD3, CD4, and CD8 counts and PHA responses have recently been reported [26] and show improvements in all subjects. The CD4:CD8 ratio is normal in all subjects after transplantation. The CD4 and CD8 numbers are at approximately the 10th percentile for age. Naïve CD4 and CD8 numbers also increase to the 10th percentile for age (Fig. 30.4).

The T-cell receptor beta variable chain family repertoire normalizes after transplantation and has been reported for both typical patients [61] and atypical patients [40]. An example of normalization of repertoire in an atypical patient is shown in Fig. 30.5.

T-cell function, as assessed by proliferative responses to antigens and alloantigens, normalizes within the first 2 years of transplantation. Antigen-specific T-cell proliferative responses to tetanus toxoid have developed in all subjects after 1 year with the exception of DIG208 (who is still on immune suppression) and DIG017 (who has ectodermal dysplasia). Mixed lymphocyte reactions show normal responses to alloantigens. Of interest, the recipients are tolerant toward their thymus donor in mixed lymphocyte reactions [62].

B-cell function is tested 2 years after transplantation when replacement immunoglobulin is stopped. Table 30.1 shows serum immunoglobulin levels. For IgG, these values in the table are the most recent obtained after stopping immunoglobulin replacement. The IgA, IgM, and IgE values included in this table are the most recent levels obtained 1 year after transplantation. Serum IgG levels are low for age in only 1 of 18 subjects tested. Of note, the subject with the

Table 30.1 Serum Immunoglobulins in patients over 1 year after transplantation

Isotype	#	High	Normal	Low
IgG[1]	19	1/19 (5%)	18/19 (95%)	0/19 (0%)
IgA	31	4/31 (13%)	25/31 (81%)	2/31 (6%)
IgM	31	1/31 (3%)	25/31 (81%)	5/31 (16%)
IgE	30	6/30 (20%)	23/30 (77%)	1/30 (3%)

[1] Serum IgG values are for subjects more than 2 years after transplantation who are off immunoglobulin replacement therapy (n=22) for whom levels are available.

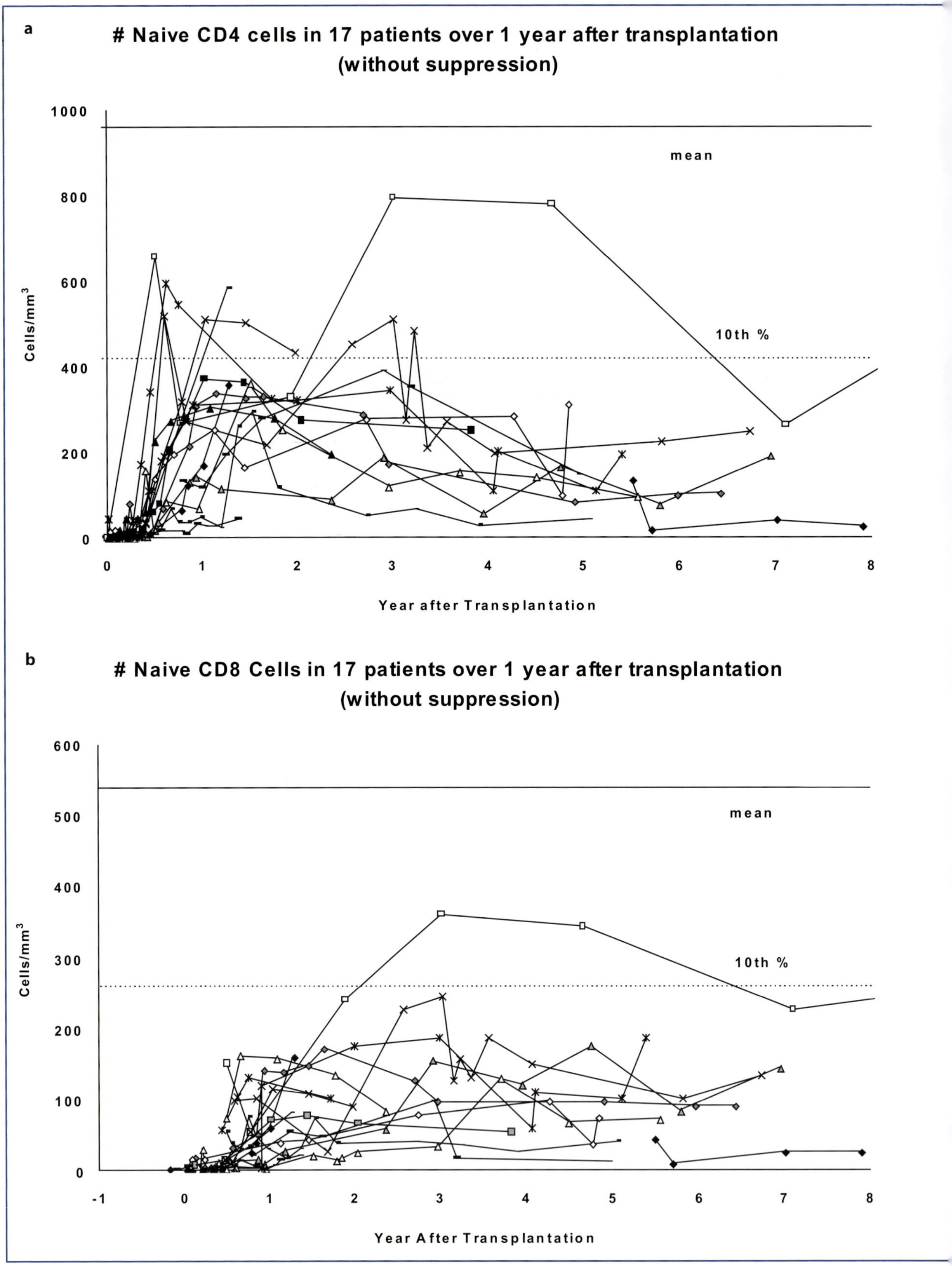

a # Naive CD4 cells in 17 patients over 1 year after transplantation (without suppression)

b # Naive CD8 Cells in 17 patients over 1 year after transplantation (without suppression)

Fig. 30.4a-d Development of naïve T cells after thymus transplantation. The 10th percentile and mean for children aged 2-6 years are shown [65]. Each subject is an separate line

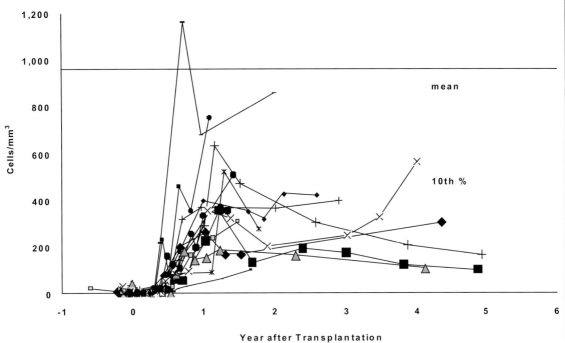

c Naive CD4 T cells in 14 subjects over 1 year after transplantation (with suppression)

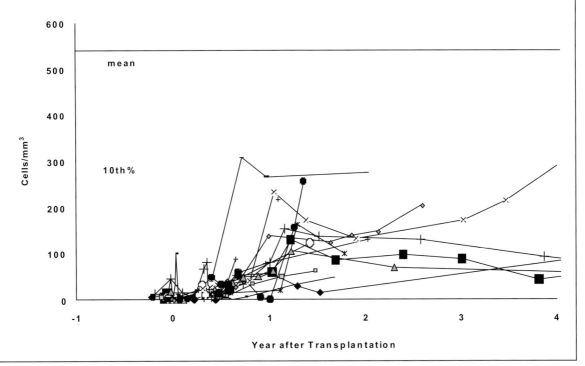

d Naive CD8 T cell counts in 14 subjects over 1 year after transplantation (with suppression)

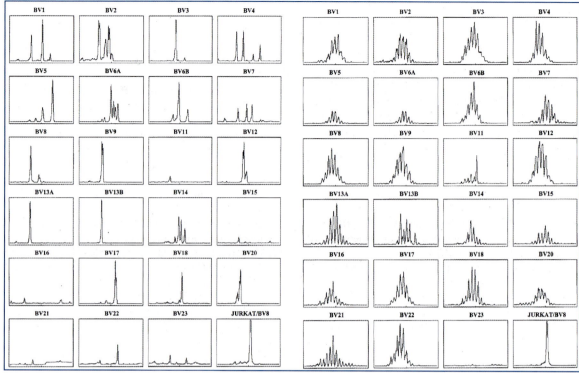

Fig. 30.5 Spectratype analysis of TCRBV diversity before and after transplantation in a subject with atypical complete DiGeorge anomaly. The panel on the *left* is day 19 with respect to transplantation. The panel on the *right* is day 301 after transplantation. Each profile represents a different TCRBV family. The *bottom right* profile in each panel is derived from Jurkat cells that express TCRBV8

Table 30.2 Specific antibody formation after thymus transplantation

Tetanus antibodies tested after 2 years (not done in 6)[1]	
Normal	17
Low	1
Pneumovax (CHO) antibodies after 2 years (not tested in 8)[1]	
Responses to 3 or more serotypes	14
Responses to 1-2 serotypes	2
No significant responses	0
Isohemagglutinins after 1 year (not done in 10)[2]	
Normal	7
Low	9
Negative	5

[1] 24 subjects are over 2 years after transplantation. Twenty-two are off immunoglobulin therapy, 2 are on immunoglobulin therapy (one because of chronic aspiration). These antibody titers were obtained after immunoglobulin replacement was stopped.
[2] All values listed were obtained at least 1 year from transplantation in the 31 subjects over 1 year after transplantation

low IgG level makes antigen-specific antibodies [26]. IgA is elevated in 4 subjects. Two have CHARGE, one of whom has recurrent sinusitis secondary to choanal atresia. Another with elevated IgA has recurrent aspiration pneumonias. Only 2 subjects have low IgA despite the finding being common in partial DiGeorge anomaly [63]. IgE levels are elevated in 20%. Several subjects had low IgM levels, which was an unexpected finding although recently 3 subjects with 22q11 deletion were reported as having selective IgM deficiency [64]. Antibody titers are shown in Table 30.2. Tetanus toxoid and pneumococcal anti-carbohydrate antibodies to unconjugated vaccines are shown. These titers are obtained after immunoglobulin replacement is stopped. Most subjects generate normal antibody responses. The serum isohemagglutinins remain low or absent in a majority of subjects. This observation may correlate with the low IgM values in some subjects. Antibody formation is a current area of research.

Summary

Thymus transplantation is a promising therapy for the athymia of complete DiGeorge anomaly. The survival rate after transplantation is 73%, with follow-up as long as 14 years. Only one subject has died more than 1 year post transplantation. Excellent T- and B-cell function and a diverse T-cell repertoire develop in most subjects. Over 90% are able to stop *Pneumocystis* prophylaxis and immunoglobulin replacement therapy. Immune reconstitution occurs when recipient T-cells develop in the donor thymus tissue. These recipient T-cells are tolerant toward the donor thymus. Autoimmune disease, especially thyroid disease and cytopenias, has been seen in a subgroup of subjects. The subjects continue to be followed for immune competence, thymic function, and adverse events.

References

1. Cleveland WW, Fogel BJ, Brown WT, Kay HE (1968) Foetal thymic transplant in a case of DiGeorge's syndrome. Lancet 2:1211-1214
2. August CS, Rosen FS, Filler RM et al (1968) Implantation of a foetal thymus, restoring immunological competence in a patient with thymic aplasia (DiGeorge's syndrome). Lancet 2:1210-1211
3. Wara DW, Golbus MS, Ammann AJ (1974) Fetal thymus glands obtained from prostaglandin-induced abortions. Cellular immune function in vitro and evidence of in vivo thymocyte activity following transplantation. Transplantation 18:387-390
4. Shearer WT, Wedner HJ, Strominger DB et al (1978) Successful transplantation of the thymus in Nezelof's syndrome. Pediatrics 61:619-624
5. Pahwa S, Pahwa R, Incefy G et al (1979) Failure of immunologic reconstitution in a patient with the DiGeorge syndrome after fetal thymus transplantation. Clin Immunol Immunopathol 14:96-106
6. Hong R (1986) Reconstitution of T-cell deficiency by thymic hormone or thymus transplantation therapy. Clin Immunol Immunopathol 40:136-141
7. Hong R (1983) Thymus transplantation. Birth Defects Original Article Series 19:259-265
8. Hong R, Schulte-Wissermann H, Jarrett-Toth E et al (1979) Transplantation of cultured thymic fragments. II. Results in nude mice. J Exp Med 149:398-415
9. Barry TS, Jones DM, Richter CB, Haynes BF (1991) Successful engraftment of human postnatal thymus in severe combined immune deficient (SCID) mice: Differential engraftment of thymic components with irradiation versus anti-asialo GM-1 immunosuppressive regimens. J Exp Med 173:167-180
10. Lobach DF, Scearce RM, Haynes BF (1985) The human thymic microenvironment. Phenotypic characterization of Hassall's bodies with the use of monoclonal antibodies. J Immunol 134:250-257
11. McFarland EJ, Scearce RM, Haynes BF (1984) The human thymic microenvironment: Cortical thymic epithelium is an antigenically distinct region of the thymic microenvironment. J Immunol 133:1241-1249
12. Haynes BF, Scearce RM, Lobach DF, Hensley LL (1984) Phenotypic characterization and ontogeny of mesodermal-derived and endocrine epithelial components of the human thymic microenvironment. J Exp Med 159:1149-1168
13. Haynes BF, Denning SM, Singer KH, Kurtzberg J (1989) Ontogeny of T-cell precursors: A model for the initial stages of human T-cell development. Immunol Today 10:87-91
14. van Ewijk W (1991) T-cell differentiation is influenced by thymic microenvironments. Annu Rev Immunol 9:591-615
15. Markert ML, Watson TJ, Kaplan I et al (1997) The human thymic microenvironment during organ culture. Clin Immunol Immunopathol 82:26-36
16. Picker LJ, Treer JR, Ferguson-Darnell B et al (1993) Control of lymphocyte recirculation in man. I. Differential regulation of the peripheral lymph node homing receptor L-selectin on T cells during the virgin to memory cell transition. J Immunol 150:1105-1121
17. Markert ML, Hummell DS, Rosenblatt HM et al (1998) Complete DiGeorge syndrome: Persistence of profound immunodeficiency. J Pediatr 132:15-21
18. Bastian J, Law S, Vogler L et al (1989) Prediction of persistent immunodeficiency in the DiGeorge anomaly. J Pediatr 115:391-396
19. Muller W, Peter HH, Wilken M et al (1988) The DiGeorge syndrome. I. Clinical evaluation and course of partial and complete forms of the syndrome. Eur J Pediatr 147:496-502
20. Thomas RA, Landing BH, Wells TR (1987) Embryologic and other developmental considerations of thirty-eight possible variants of the DiGeorge anomaly. Am J Med Genet (Suppl) 3:43-66
21. Hong R (1991) The DiGeorge anomaly. Immunodefic Rev 3:1-14
22. Conley ME, Beckwith JB, Mancer JF, Tenckhoff L (1979) The spectrum of the DiGeorge syndrome. J Pediatr 94:883-890
23. Barrett DJ, Ammann AJ, Wara DW et al (1981) Clinical and immunologic spectrum of the DiGeorge syndrome. J Clin Lab Immunol 6:1-6
24. Ryan AK, Goodship JA, Wilson DI et al (1997) Spectrum of clinical features associated with interstitial chromosome 22q11 deletions: A European collaborative study. J Med Genet 34:798-804
25. Robin NH, Shprintzen RJ (2005) Defining the clinical spectrum of deletion 22q11.2. J Pediatr 147:90-96
26. Markert ML, Devlin BH, Alexieff MJ et al (2007) Review of 54 patients with complete DiGeorge anomaly enrolled in protocols for thymus transplantation: Outcome of 44 consecutive transplants. Blood 109:4539-4547
27. Wilson DI, Goodship JA, Burn J et al (1992) Deletions within chromosome 22q11 in familial congenital heart disease. Lancet 340:573-575
28. Driscoll DA, Budarf ML, Emanuel BS (1992) A genetic etiology for DiGeorge syndrome: Consistent deletions and microdeletions of 22q11. Am J Hum Genet 50:924-933
29. Pagon RA, Graham JM Jr, Zonana J, Yong SL (1981) Coloboma, congenital heart disease, and choanal atre-

sia with multiple anomalies: CHARGE association. J Pediatr 99:223-227
30. Blake KD, Davenport SL, Hall BD et al (1998) CHARGE association: An update and review for the primary pediatrician. Clin Pediatr (Phila) 37:159-173
31. Vissers LE, van Ravenswaaij CM, Admiraal R et al (2004) Mutations in a new member of the chromodomain gene family cause CHARGE syndrome. Nat Genet 36:955-957
32. Wang R, Martinez-Frias ML, Graham JM Jr (2002) Infants of diabetic mothers are at increased risk for the oculo-auriculo-vertebral sequence: A case-based and case-control approach. J Pediatr 141:611-617
33. Gosseye S, Golaire MC, Verellen G et al (1982) Association of bilateral renal agenesis and DiGeorge syndrome in an infant of a diabetic mother. Helv Paediatr Acta 37:471-474
34. Markert ML, Alexieff MJ, Li J et al (2004) Complete DiGeorge syndrome: Development of rash, lymphadenopathy, and oligoclonal T cells in 5 cases. J Allergy Clin Immunol 113:734-741
35. Archer E, Chuang TY, Hong R (1990) Severe eczema in a patient with DiGeorge's syndrome. Cutis 45:455-459
36. Pirovano S, Mazzolari E, Pasic S et al (2003) Impaired thymic output and restricted T-cell repertoire in two infants with immunodeficiency and early-onset generalized dermatitis. Immun Lett 86:93-97
37. Omenn GS (1965) Familial Reticuloendotheliosis with Eosinophilia. New Engl J Med 273:427-432
38. Villa A, Sobacchi C, Notarangelo LD et al (2001) V(D)J recombination defects in lymphocytes due to RAG mutations: Severe immunodeficiency with a spectrum of clinical presentations. Blood 97:81-88
39. Rieux-Laucat F, Bahadoran P, Brousse N et al (1998) Highly restricted human T cell repertoire in peripheral blood and tissue-infiltrating lymphocytes in Omenn's syndrome. J Clin Invest 102:312-321
40. Markert ML, Alexieff MJ, Li J et al (2004) Postnatal thymus transplantation with immunosuppression as treatment for DiGeorge syndrome. Blood 104:2574-2581
41. Douek DC, McFarland RD, Keiser PH et al (1998) Changes in thymic function with age and during the treatment of HIV infection. Nature 396:690-695
42. Ocejo-Vinyals JG, Lozano MJ, Sanchez-Velasco P et al (2000) An unusual concurrence of graft versus host disease caused by engraftment of maternal lymphocytes with DiGeorge anomaly. Arch Dis Child 83:165-169
43. Gobbi A, Stoddart CA, Malnati MS et al (1999) Human herpesvirus 6 (HHV-6) causes severe thymocyte depletion in SCID-hu Thy/Liv mice. J Exp Med 189:1953-1960
44. Dictor M, Fasth A, Olling S (1984) Abnormal B-cell proliferation associated with combined immunodeficiency, cytomegalovirus, and cultured thymus grafts. Am J Clin Pathol 82:487-490
45. Borzy MS, Hong R, Horowitz SD et al (1979) Fatal lymphoma after transplantation of cultured thymus in children with combined immunodeficiency disease. New Engl J Med 301:565-568
46. Hanto DW, Frizzera G, Gajl-Peczalska KJ, Simmons RL (1985) Epstein-Barr virus, immunodeficiency, and B cell lymphoproliferation. Transplantation 39:461-472
47. Reece ER, Gartner JG, Seemayer TA et al (1981) Epstein-Barr virus in a malignant lymphoproliferative disorder of B-cells occurring after thymic epithelial transplantation for combined immunodeficiency. Cancer Res 41:4243-4247
48. 2006. Title 21-Food and Drugs; Chapter I-Food and Drug Administration, Department of Health and Human; Subchapter L-Regulations Under Certain Other Acts Administered by the Food and Drug Administration, Part 1270 Human Tissue intended for Transplantation. Code of Federal Regulations
49. Hong R, Moore AL (1996) Organ culture for thymus transplantation. Transplantation 61:444-448
50. 2006. Title 21-Food and Drugs; Chapter I-Food and Drug Administration, Department of Health and Human; Subchapter L-Regulations Under Certain Other Acts Administered by the Food and Drug Administration, Part 1271 Human Tissue Intended for Transplantation. Code of Federal Regulations
51. Rice HE, Skinner MA, Mahaffey SM et al (2004) Thymic transplantation for complete DiGeorge syndrome: Medical and surgical considerations. J Pediatr Surg 39:1607-1615
52. Ham Pong AJ, Cavallo A, Holman GH, Goldman AS (1985) DiGeorge syndrome: Long-term survival complicated by Graves disease. J Pediatr 106:619-620
53. Brown JJ, Datta V, Browning MJ, Swift PG (2004) Graves' disease in DiGeorge syndrome: Patient report with a review of endocrine autoimmunity associated with 22q11.2 deletion. J Pediatr Endocrinol Metab 17:1575-1579
54. Choi JH, Shin YL, Kim GH et al (2005) Endocrine manifestations of chromosome 22q11.2 microdeletion syndrome. Horm Res 63:294-299
55. Scuccimarri R, Rodd C (1998) Thyroid abnormalities as a feature of DiGeorge syndrome: A patient report and review of the literature. J Pediatr Endocrinol Metab 11:273-276
56. Mazzolari E, Forino C, Guerci S et al (2007) Long-term immune reconstitution and clinical outcome after stem cell transplantation for severe T-cell immunodeficiency. J Allergy Clin Immunol 120:892-899
57. Levy A, Michel G, Lemerrer M, Philip N (1997) Idiopathic thrombocytopenic purpura in two mothers of children with DiGeorge sequence: A new component manifestation of deletion 22q11? Am J Med Genet 69:356-359
58. DePiero AD, Lourie EM, Berman BW et al (1997) Recurrent immune cytopenias in two patients with DiGeorge/velocardiofacial syndrome. J Pediatr 131:484-486
59. Duke SG, McGuirt WF Jr, Jewett T, Fasano MB (2000) Velocardiofacial syndrome: Incidence of immune cytopenias. Arch Otolaryngol Head Neck Surg 126:1141-1145
60. Welch P, Rose NR, Kite JH Jr (1973) Neonatal thymectomy increases spontaneous autoimmune thyroiditis. J Immunol 110:575-577

61. Markert ML, Sarzotti M, Ozaki DA et al (2003) Thymic transplantation in complete DiGeorge syndrome: Immunologic safety evaluations in twelve patients. Blood 102:1121-1130
62. Chinn IK DB, Li YJ, Markert ML (2008) Long-term tolerance to allogeneic thymus transplants in complete DiGeorge anomaly. Clinical Immunol 126:277-281
63. Smith CA, Driscoll DA, Emanuel BS et al (1998) Increased prevalence of immunoglobulin A deficiency in patients with the chromosome 22q11.2 deletion syndrome (DiGeorge syndrome/velocardiofacial syndrome). Clin Diagn Lab 5:415-417
64. Kung SJ, Gripp KW, Stephan MJ et al (2007) Selective IgM deficiency and 22q11.2 deletion syndrome. Ann Allergy Asthma Immunol 99:87-92
65. Shearer W, Rosenblatt HM, Gelman RS et al (2003) Lymphocyte subsets in healthy children from birth through 18 years of age: The Pediatric AIDS Clinical Trials Group P1009 study. J Allergy Clin Immunol 112:973-980

Subject Index

A

Acetylcholine 46, 77, 86, 90, 95, 97, 98, 108, 138, 139, 142, 143, 149, 153, 187, 191, 247
Acetylcholine receptor 46, 77, 95, 97, 98, 108, 149, 153, 187, 191, 247
ACh 89-91, 95, 142, 193, 248, 249
AChE 95, 247-249, 252, 253
AChR 46, 89-93, 95, 149, 187, 247, 248
Adipose body 13, 17
Anesthetic agents 141, 143, 145
Anterior chest wall lifting method 190, 191
Anterior mediastinum 14, 35, 61, 66, 99, 100, 102, 104, 106, 107, 111, 116, 119, 121, 124-130, 132, 133, 159, 162-164, 178, 183, 184, 188, 189, 198, 201, 203-205, 210, 217, 222, 224, 235
Anterior mini-mediastinotomy 125, 128-130
Anticholinesterase agents 138-144, 146
Athymia 256, 264
Atypical complete DiGeorge anomaly 256, 259, 261, 264
August Charles S 10
Autoimmune 11, 16, 21, 26, 27, 33, 39, 41, 43-47, 52, 53, 70, 73, 77, 78, 80, 84, 89, 91-93, 97, 100, 108, 138, 149, 154, 157-159, 161, 186, 198, 206, 211, 247-249, 251-254, 257, 260, 261, 265, 266
    disorders 41, 52, 91, 93, 97, 251, 252, 254
Autoimmunity 19, 27, 52, 53, 70, 83, 84, 92, 149, 266
Autoreactivity 19
Azathioprine 47, 52, 92, 139, 170, 184, 251-253

B

Beard John 9
Berengario da Carpi 2, 3, 11
Biphasic thymoma 75
Blalock Alfred 10
Brachiocephalic vein 14, 175, 176, 178, 188, 189, 194, 197, 204, 206
Bulbar palsy 89

C

Central tolerance 19, 21, 27, 70
Cervical approach 206

CHARGE syndrome 32, 70, 266
Chemoradiation 233
Chemotherapy 24, 25, 29, 35, 39, 41-43, 49, 50, 51, 79, 80, 87, 100-102, 107, 112-114, 118-121, 162, 164, 166, 214, 217-220, 222-229, 232, 233, 235-237, 241, 245
    and thymus enlargement 41
Chylothorax 136, 176, 178, 205
Cochrane review 249, 250
Cooper Astley Paston 6
Corticosteroids 35, 43, 91, 139, 167, 184, 219, 224, 225, 241, 244, 245, 249, 252, 254
Cosmetic results 177, 194, 207, 210
CT images 111, 116, 119, 122
Cyclophosphamide 139, 166, 224-228, 233, 251, 252
Cyclosporine 48, 139, 251, 252, 259
Cytoreticulum 13

D

Da Vinci robotic system 207, 209, 210
Debulking approach 217, 218, 223
Decremental response 96
DeFilippi classification 196, 197
22q11 deletion 70, 72, 73, 84, 264
Depolarization 90, 91
Differential diagnosis 40, 49, 50, 58, 81, 94, 97, 101, 105, 106, 119, 121, 129, 224
DiGeorge Syndrome 31, 36, 37, 70-73, 83-85, 265-267
Drug induced MG 248

E

Ectopic thymus 31, 35, 36, 77, 79, 196, 197
Edrophonium (tensilon) test 95
EMG 96, 153
Epitheliocytes 13-15
Eustachio Bartolomeo 4
Extraocular muscle 90, 93, 95

F

Fluctuation 93
Fused images 119

G
Galen of Pergamon 2
Germ Cell Tumors 40-42, 50, 61, 63, 66, 75, 79
Germinal center 46, 52
Glisson Francis 5

H
Hassall Arthur Hill 7
Hassall's corpuscles 13-15, 18, 27, 33, 55, 56, 57
Hemangioma 57, 64
22q11 hemizygosity 256
Hepatoid carcinomas 75
Hewson William 6
HIV infection 47, 48, 53, 82, 83, 87, 266
Human immunoglobulin 139
Hyperplasia
    and growth hormone 43
    follicular 45, 46, 47
    in autoimmune diseases 44
    in Cushing's syndrome 43, 44
    in Graves' disease 47, 52, 53
    massive thymic 44, 45
    post-chemotherapy 41, 42
    true thymic 39, 40, 41
Hypocalcemia 32-34, 70, 72
Hypogammaglobulinemia 44, 77, 78, 103, 106, 131, 161, 246

I
Ice pack test 95
Immunodeficiencies 37, 255, 261
Immunoendocrinopathy 77
Immunogenic mechanisms 91
Immunosuppression 41, 92, 150, 170, 249, 251-253, 256, 258, 259, 261, 266
Infectious mononucleosis 48, 53
Innominate vein 133-136, 151, 169, 182, 183, 209, 215, 234
Intravenous immunoglobulin (IVIg) 91, 146, 150, 206, 247, 249, 250-254

J
Jitter 96

K
Karnofsky performance status 78

L
Lambert-Eaton syndrome 94, 95
LEMS 95-97
Lymphoid organs 13, 14, 16, 23, 27, 49, 83, 246
Lymphomas 40, 41, 64, 67, 73, 74, 79, 80, 87, 102, 106, 121, 122, 124, 130, 246

M
MRI 36, 100, 102, 103, 105, 106
Masaoka staging 75, 76
Mediastinal mass 37, 40-44, 47-51, 63, 74, 77-79, 81, 101, 105-108, 125, 161, 162, 177, 244, 248
Mediastinum 2, 3, 12, 14, 31, 35, 36, 40, 41, 43, 44, 49, 55-58, 61, 62, 64-67, 78-80, 86, 87, 96, 99-102, 104-107, 111, 115, 116, 119-121, 123-136, 152, 157-159, 161-164, 167-169, 173, 176, 178, 183, 184, 187-189, 198, 201, 203-205, 209, 210, 217, 222-224, 234, 235, 239, 251
Mesenchymal neoplasms 64
MGFA clinical classification 93, 94
MHC 19
Micronodular thymoma 75
Minimally invasive 10, 121, 123, 125, 127-131, 134, 147, 154, 171, 173, 176-178, 196-198, 206, 207, 210, 231
    surgery 125
    techniques 125, 129, 130, 210
Müller-Hermelink classification 74, 76
Multilocular thymic cyst 48, 52, 53, 55, 56, 64, 108
Multimodality treatment 79, 159, 166, 218, 225-228, 236, 237, 239
Muscarinic effects 139, 249
MuSK 90, 92, 93, 149, 153, 154, 187, 247
MuSK antibodies 92, 93, 96, 154
Myasthenia gravis (MG) 9-12, 35, 39, 44-46, 48, 49, 52, 57, 69, 76-79, 81-83, 86, 89, 91-97, 100, 107, 108, 134, 136-147, 149, 153-155, 157, 158, 161, 187, 247
Myasthenic crisis 93, 153, 167, 196, 206, 250
Myasthenic patient 9, 89, 137, 138, 143, 144, 146, 147
Mycophenolate mofetil 139, 251, 253, 254

N
Naïve T-cells 262
Natural killer T-cell 16, 22, 23
Negative selection 19, 20-22, 26, 27
Neoadjuvant therapy 233
Neuroendocrine carcinomas 60, 65, 75, 217
Neurological results 157, 159
Neuromuscular junction (NMJ) 46, 77, 89-92, 94-96, 140, 141, 149, 247, 248, 254
Nezelof syndrome 31, 34-36

O
Ocular MG 92, 96, 97, 150, 247-249, 253
Osserman classification 137

P
Paltauf Arnold 8
Pancoast Henry K 9

Paraganglioma 57, 58, 64, 81
Parathymic syndromes 77, 78, 124
Parathyroid 13, 31, 32, 34, 36, 57, 58, 64, 69-72, 81, 84, 182, 205, 255
Paré Ambroise 11
Pericardium 14, 56, 75, 78, 80, 105, 124, 134, 151, 161, 163, 165, 169, 183, 184, 189-191, 204, 209, 214, 215, 217-223, 229
PET/CT device 111
Pharmacological interactions 140
Pharyngeal pouches 13, 31, 36, 69, 255
Phrenic nerve 69, 129, 136, 157, 164, 175, 183, 184, 189, 191, 194, 195, 201, 203-205, 209, 210, 222
Plasmapheresis 91, 138, 139, 142, 146, 165, 167, 170, 184, 193, 196, 206
Plater Felix 5
Pleura 56, 65, 66, 75, 78-80, 104, 105, 124, 136, 151, 152, 158, 161-164, 169, 183, 184, 189, 194, 204, 209, 217-221, 223, 229, 232, 234, 236, 237
Pleural invasion 234, 237
Polymyositis 47, 77, 94, 96
Positive selection 16, 19-21, 27
Positron Emission Tomography 86, 111, 120
Postoperative Radiation Therapy 225, 227, 230, 232, 238, 239
Prednisone 86, 94, 154, 170, 184, 224-228, 242-247, 249, 251, 253
Pyridostigmine 139

R

Radical surgery 165
Radiologic
    diagnosis 99, 101, 103, 105, 107, 109
        diseased thymus 100
        normal thymus 99
Radiotherapy 43, 79, 80, 100, 121, 162, 164-166, 205, 214, 217, 219, 220, 222, 223, 225, 226, 229-235, 237-239, 248
    techniques 234
Red cell aplasia 47, 53, 77, 86, 108, 219, 245
Regulatory T-cell 27
Rehn Ludwig 9
Reinterventions for thymoma recurrences 219, 221, 223
Repetitive nerve stimulation 89, 95, 96
Rethymectomy 184
Robot 208
Robotic techniques 207, 209, 211
Rufus of Ephesus 1
Ryanodine 92, 93, 97, 247, 249, 252

S

Sauerbruch Ernst Ferdinand 10
Sclerosing mediastinitis 56, 64

Seronegative MG (SNMG) 47, 92, 98, 149
Seropositive MG (SPMG) 92
SFEMG 95, 96, 248
Shprintzen's syndrome 73
Simon John 7
Simpson test 95
SNAREs 91
Somatostatin 78, 219, 227, 228, 241-246
    receptor 78, 227, 242, 243, 246
        scintigraphy 78, 242
Staging 42, 59, 65, 66, 75, 76, 86, 104, 105, 108, 111, 119-122, 130, 131, 137, 161, 165, 217-219, 230, 238
Status thymolimphaticus 8
Sternotomy 10, 41, 79, 129, 133, 134, 136, 150, 152, 154, 157-159, 162, 166, 168-170, 173, 176, 178, 185-188, 190, 193, 196, 201, 203-206, 210, 211, 215, 219, 220, 222
Steroids 25, 30, 35, 78, 167, 170, 184, 186, 187, 190, 191, 214, 225, 241-245, 249, 251-253, 259, 261
Subxiphoid 128, 173-179, 181-186, 201
Superior vena cava syndrome 69, 77, 81, 125, 126, 132, 213, 215, 216
Surgical
    approach 125, 150, 152, 153, 157, 162, 164, 176, 187, 207
        bilateral with anterior chest wall lifting VATS 187
        cervicotomy 149
        manubriotomy 10
        median sternotomy 157
        subxiphoid 173
        transthoracic 161
    indications 161
SUV value for mediastinal malignancy 114, 119

T

T-cell receptor 20, 26, 74, 256, 261
    beta variable chain repertoire 20
    rearrangement excision circles 20
T-lymphocytes 13, 15-17, 19, 22, 23, 40, 43, 45, 46, 48, 74, 79
Tacrolimus 139, 227, 228, 251, 252
TE 198, 206, 247, 248, 250, 251, 253
Thoracic 6, 10, 16, 75, 99, 100, 102, 103, 105, 122, 132, 136, 143-147, 151, 153, 159, 160, 166, 168, 171, 173, 175-178, 181-185, 188, 189, 195-198, 201, 203, 204, 209-211, 214, 216, 218, 220-223, 226, 228, 234, 235, 238, 239, 243, 248
    duct 6, 136, 175, 178
Thoracoscopic 10, 12, 43, 79, 133, 147, 160, 169, 173-179, 184, 186, 187, 189-191, 193-199, 201-203, 205-207, 210, 211, 233

Subject Index

thymectomy 147, 173, 177-179, 186, 191, 193-199, 203, 205-207, 210, 211
Thoracoscopy 10, 12, 131, 132, 147, 173, 175-177, 179, 198, 207
Thoracotomy 43, 44, 108, 133, 162, 163, 166, 188, 204, 205, 214, 219-223, 232
Thymectomy 9, 10, 12, 24, 40, 44, 46, 47, 49, 52, 53, 64, 78-80, 83, 89, 91, 92, 107, 133-139, 143-147, 149, 150, 152-155, 157-160, 162, 163, 165-171, 173, 174, 176-178
- basic 207
- complete 150
- extended 133, 207
- maximal 207
- radical 165
- standard 174, 207
- thoracoscopic
  - left-sided 193
  - right-sided 201

Thymic
- asthma 8
- cortex 20, 26, 48, 74, 82
- death 8
- epithelial tumors 65, 74, 75, 81, 85, 108, 109, 119, 120, 131, 166, 223, 224, 237, 241, 246
- epitheliocytes 13, 14
- epithelium 12, 13, 18, 34, 53, 60, 65, 217, 235, 245, 259, 265
- hormones 15, 17, 19, 23, 25, 28, 29, 34, 241
- humoral factor (THF) 17, 23, 25
- hyperplasia 35-37, 39-41, 44, 45, 47, 49-53, 78, 89, 92, 96, 100, 101, 106, 107, 114, 119, 120, 173, 175, 227, 243
- macrophages 16
- medulla 13, 21, 39, 45, 46, 74, 243
- neoplasms
  - chemotherapy 225
  - clinical features 74
  - complementary treatments 241
    - octreotide 242
    - steroids 241
  - PET features 111
  - radiotherapy 229
  - WHO classification 74
- rebound 49, 50, 80, 87, 107

Thymitis 39, 45, 49, 82, 93
Thymocytes 13-16, 19-23, 25-28, 31, 33, 47, 51, 241-243, 257, 259
Thymoma 7, 9, 10, 40, 46-48, 52, 53, 58-60, 62, 65, 69, 74-81, 83, 85-87, 89, 92, 93, 96-97, 99-106, 108, 111, 114, 117, 119-122, 124, 129, 131, 132, 144, 149, 150, 154, 157, 161-166
- recurrences 217-219, 221, 223
Thymopentin 17, 24

Thymopoietin 11, 17, 23, 24, 28, 29
Thymosins 17, 23, 24, 28, 29
Thymulin 17, 23-25, 29
Thymus
- anatomy and embriology 13
- benign tumors 55
  - cystic lesions 55
  - hemangioma 57
  - multilocular cyst 55
  - paraganglioma 57
  - sclerosing mediastinitis 56
  - thymolipoma 56
- congenital malformations 31
- endocrine functions 17, 23
- follicular hyperplasia 45, 46, 47
- immunology 17
- infectious diseases 47, 82
- malignant tumors
  - carcinoid 60, 61
  - carcinoma 60, 79
  - choriocarcinoma 63
  - embryonal carcinoma 63
  - ganglioneuroblastoma 61
  - lymphoma 64, 79
  - neuroblastoma 61
  - seminoma 62
  - thymoma 59, 74
  - yolk sac tumor 63
- neuroendocrine control 17, 25
- pathology 69, 71, 73, 75, 77, 79, 81-83, 85, 87
  - anesthesiological problems 137
  - conventional surgical techniques 149, 157, 161
  - diagnostic techniques 121
    - endoscopic
      - EBUS 123
      - EUS 123
      - TBNA 122
    - interventional radiology
      - CNB 121, 124
      - FNAB 121, 124
    - surgical
      - anterior mini-mediastinotomy 128
      - VA minithoracotomy 129
      - pericardioscopy (PSC) 128
      - videomediastinoscopy (VAM) 126
      - videothoracoscopy (VATS) 125
      - conventional open techniques 129
    - PET features 111
    - radiologic diagnosis 99
- physiology 19
- surgical anatomy 133
- transplantation 255
- true hyperplasia 39, 40, 41

tubercolosis 49, 83
Titin 92, 93, 97, 153, 247, 249
Traditional "open" surgery 129, 130
Typical complete DiGeorge anomaly 258, 259

U
Unresectable disease 226, 235, 237

V
Vagus nerve 183

VATS 125-127, 129, 130, 133, 134, 157, 159, 176, 178, 185-190, 198, 201-203, 205-207, 210, 214
Velocardiofacial syndrome 32, 70, 73, 83-85, 266, 267
Vesalio Andrea 3
Vesicles 90, 91
VGCCs 91
Videoassisted thoracoscopic surgery 79, 187

W
Wirchow Rudolf 8

Printed in July 2008